"Aside from its wealth of factual details and scien[tific...] helps highlight the broader need for awareness and action against toxic substances threatening our families. In a world where such poisons are increasingly prevalent, it is akin to a survivor's manual. It should assist public policy–makers and parents alike."

—Connecticut attorney general Richard Blumenthal

"A lucid and honest volume that offers parents practical, balanced advice on how to protect their children against environmental hazards."

—Philip J. Landrigan, M.D., M.Sc., F.A.A.P.; professor and chairman, Department of Community and Preventive Medicine; professor of pediatrics, Mount Sinai School of Medicine

"Mercury in seafood, dioxins, and PCBs in our diet; industrial chemicals in our water and air; 'toxic' molds growing in our homes—the list goes on and on. Are these chemical hazards *really* a threat to our health? Just how much should we worry about them? Are there ways to reduce our risks? Unfortunately, the real truth is often difficult to discern. Ginsberg and Toal now offer a user-friendly citizen's guide to the everyday world of toxic chemicals. Throughout the book, the authors successfully consolidate the sometimes mammoth amounts of scientific information on specific chemical hazards into understandable and useful information—information that will both help protect consumers from potentially hazardous situations and alleviate unfounded fears of chemical risks that are often overhyped in the media. Ginsberg and Toal provide a reasoned, but appropriately cautious, approach to evaluating the health risks from chemicals in our environment."

—David L. Eaton, Ph.D., D.A.B.T., F.A.T.S.; associate vice provost for research, University of Washington; former president, Society of Toxicology

Visit the authors' website at
www.whatstoxic.com

WHAT'S TOXIC, WHAT'S NOT

Dr. Gary Ginsberg & Brian Toal, M.S.P.H.

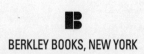

BERKLEY BOOKS, NEW YORK

THE BERKLEY PUBLISHING GROUP
Published by the Penguin Group
Penguin Group (USA) Inc.
375 Hudson Street, New York, New York 10014, USA
Penguin Group (Canada), 90 Eglinton Avenue East, Suite 700, Toronto, Ontario M4P 2Y3, Canada
(a division of Pearson Penguin Canada Inc.)
Penguin Books Ltd., 80 Strand, London WC2R 0RL, England
Penguin Group Ireland, 25 St. Stephen's Green, Dublin 2, Ireland
(a division of Penguin Books Ltd.)
Penguin Group (Australia), 250 Camberwell Road, Camberwell, Victoria 3124, Australia
(a division of Pearson Australia Group Pty. Ltd.)
Penguin Books India Pvt. Ltd., 11 Community Centre, Panchsheel Park, New Delhi—110 017, India
Penguin Group (NZ), Cnr. Airborne and Rosedale Roads, Albany, Auckland 1310, New Zealand
(a division of Pearson New Zealand Ltd.)
Penguin Books (South Africa) (Pty.) Ltd., 24 Sturdee Avenue, Rosebank, Johannesburg 2196,
South Africa

Penguin Books Ltd., Registered Offices: 80 Strand, London WC2R 0RL, England

This book is an original publication of The Berkley Publishing Group.

Publisher's Note: While the author has made every effort to provide accurate telephone numbers
and Internet addresses at the time of publication, neither the publisher nor the author assumes any
responsibility for errors, or for changes that occur after publication. Further, publisher does not
have any control over and does not assume any responsibility for author or third-party websites
or their content.

PRINTING HISTORY
Berkley trade paperback edition / December 2006

Library of Congress Cataloging-in-Publication Data

Ginsberg, Gary.
    What's toxic, what's not / Gary Ginsberg & Brian Toal.
        p.   cm.
    Includes bibliographical references.
    ISBN: 0-425-21194-0
    1. Health risk assessment.   2. Environmental toxicology.   3. Consumer education.   I. Toal,
Brian.   II. Title.

RA566.27.G57 2006
615.9'02—dc22

                                                                                              2006043008

PRINTED IN THE UNITED STATES OF AMERICA

10   9   8   7   6   5   4   3

Contents

Introduction

Hello, my house has an unusual odor coming from the basement.... Hello, we just broke a thermometer in the bedroom and there are little silver beads everywhere.... Hello, the roof leaks at my daughter's school, and she comes home feeling sick every day.... Hello, my son plays down by the river near an old abandoned factory.... Hello, my neighbor just told me that she's not eating fish for the rest of her pregnancy.... Hello, there have been three cases of cancer on my street in the last six months....

These kinds of calls are coming into toxics hotlines across the country. As much as we would like to believe that our homes, schools, and workplaces are free from toxic substances, the reality is our society has grown up with a heavy reliance on industrial chemicals. Such substances have ushered in cultural breakthroughs, such as the green revolution and the plastics era, but they have also led to widespread chemical exposure—sometimes in the places where we least expect it.

Toxic chemicals are a legitimate source of worry: certain contaminants are associated with serious health effects, ranging from cancer to birth defects to asthma. While it's easy to document these effects at high doses (for example, workers subjected to a chemical on a daily basis for many years), the key question is whether toxics can be harmful at lower doses more typical of exposure to the general public. It's common sense that high doses of toxic substances can cause illness, and can even be fatal, but what kind of effects do these chemicals have at low doses—the doses we encounter every day, perhaps without even knowing it? And how can we recognize and prevent such exposures? These are the questions we're going to answer in this book.

When people hear about chemicals in their environment, the natural tendency is to assume the chemicals are causing disease. It's important that we not overlook the role of our increasingly sedentary and stressful lifestyle

WHAT IS TOXICOLOGY AND EPIDEMIOLOGY?

The fields of toxicology and epidemiology are both concerned with understanding the link between chemical exposure and disease; they form the basis for public regulations on toxics. But what exactly are these two sciences?

Toxicology Toxicology is the study of the toxic (harmful) effects of chemicals, including cancer, birth defects, and damage to internal organs or various life support systems (nervous, endocrine, or immune). Testing is usually done on rats and mice because there is a lot we can learn about chemical hazards by testing on these animals.

One key concept in toxicology is that too much of even the most innocuous chemicals, such as water or sugar, can kill you. Here's where the concept of potency comes in: the more potent the chemical, the more likely it can be risky even at low levels of exposure. You may be familiar with this concept from alcoholic drinks. Rum is much more potent than beer or wine—it takes less rum to produce a drunken state. Toxicologists calculate the potency of chemicals to harm the body. That's how we know that certain chemicals (dioxin, PCBs, cyanide) are more potent than others (acetic acid in vinegar, acetone in nail polish remover, heptane in rubber cement).

Epidemiology The key to understanding epidemiology is the "dem" in the middle of the word. The Greek root "dem" means "people," and epidemiology is the study of how disease occurs in the human population. Epidemiology studies collect information on people and their environment in order to establish links between disease and personal risk factors. It's a natural companion to toxicology because, when one finds a chemical is toxic in animals, it's important to see if people exposed to that chemical in the real world are getting sick. Officials can then intercede and stop any further exposure. Among the great successes of epidemiology are the public health campaigns to remove cigarette smoke, arsenic, lead, and asbestos from the human environment.

in the rise of various diseases. These risk factors can be compounded by our exposure to toxic chemicals, some of which *are* potent enough to cause health risks, even at low doses.

Being an educated "consumer" of air, drinking water, sunshine, food, and everything else is a difficult task, given the variety of claims about health risks from different experts. You can find books that warn of just about every household product, providing creative recipes for toxic-free living. For most people, living "toxic-free" would be more than what is necessary for a healthy lifestyle—not every kind of chemical exposure is unnatural and unhealthy. But, ignoring toxic risks altogether would be foolish and even dangerous. Striking a sensible balance requires understanding the degree of risk on a case-by-case basis.

That's where we come in. This book sorts out the chemical risks that are serious from those that are not. Our goal is to provide a healthy-living handbook on toxics that provides practical step-by-step advice for avoiding the most significant risks, and helps people experience less exposure, less risk, and less worry.

Where Do Toxic Chemicals Come From?

The most important information we can provide is where your exposures come from and how you can prevent them. A lot of people think that toxic chemicals come from giant chemical companies belching out air and water pollution that finds its way to our doorstep. Certainly that can happen, but as outlined below, sometimes our greatest risks have nothing to do with factory pollution. (For more information on particular toxics, refer to the individual chapters.)

HIDDEN CHEMICALS

Some products have chemicals hidden in them. The purposeful addition of things like lead to paint (now banned), solvents to paints and glues, and pesticides to wood has put toxics into the hands of unsuspecting homeowners, and into their children's as well. For example, most people don't realize that pressure-treated wood that was sold from the 1950s until December 2004 contained high levels of pesticides that were a hazard to carpenters and are still a risk for children (see Chapter 12).

SKULL-AND-CROSSBONE PRODUCTS

Look around under your sink or in your garage—it won't take long to find products that are loaded with toxic chemicals. Granted, most people who buy ant killer know there is a pesticide in it and don't use it like air freshener. But putting hazardous materials into the homeowner market will lead to mistakes and toxic exposures. You can't assume people will always do the right thing. Take the case of the woman who had a recurrent problem with bed fleas. Normal laundering didn't work, so she treated the bed, pillows, and sheets with a bottle of pesticide. If that's not bad enough, the bottle was from the 1980s and contained chlordane, a pesticide banned in 1988 because of its persistence and toxicity. This mistake led to acute illness in her family, and once the problem was diagnosed, it cost thousands of dollars to remove it from their home. Toxic chemicals in the home are accidents waiting to happen. It takes a great deal of education and vigilance to use these products safely (see Chapter 7). Keeping them away from children is essential, as children have been fatally poisoned from accidental ingestion of things like antifreeze, home pesticides, and bleach.

FOOD

Almost all food contains trace levels of heavy metals, pesticides, or persistent chemicals like PCBs or dioxins. These chemicals are not added to food on purpose, but rather are present as unavoidable contaminants. In most cases, such low-level background exposure can't be singled out as a definitive health risk. However, in certain cases, such as mercury levels in fish, the toxic risk is clearer, and warnings are needed (Chapter 5). Food also contains chemicals added on purpose, like colorings, preservatives, and artificial sweeteners. Food additives must pass strict safety standards, but they can still be controversial. For example, certain food additives were banned only after millions of people had already been exposed to them (Chapter 5).

NATURALLY OCCURRING SUBSTANCES

There are many naturally occurring toxic chemicals that have been with us for millennia. Highest on the list is radon, a radioactive gas that seeps into basements and can increase your odds of getting lung cancer (Chapter 2). Modern-day construction creates homes that are airtight, which makes radon a bigger risk than ever before. Also in this category are naturally occurring contaminants in groundwater such as arsenic, uranium, and manganese (Chapter 6). Some folks are unlucky enough to have high levels of these natural but risky chemicals in their well water. Finally, mold belongs in the "naturally occurring" category because it has been growing in damp, dark corners since the time of the caveman (Chapter 3).

AIR POLLUTION

Some people think the solution to air pollution is dilution (namely, a lot of air to spread out the toxins.) But that's not the case if the pollution leaving a nearby smokestack is heading right toward your house. Even with modern controls, thousands of pounds of toxins are released every year from individual factories across the country, causing both polluted skies and health effects. Industry is not necessarily the main culprit: car exhaust is a large problem and potentially getting worse due to the ever-increasing number of miles we drive (Chapter 11).

POLLUTION FROM BELOW

The areas surrounding many factories have become contaminated due to relaxed waste disposal practices in the past. In some cases, the pollution lasted many years and traveled off-site via groundwater to affect nearby homes and businesses. Town landfills can also be a source of groundwater pollution that spreads out into neighborhoods. These pathways can contaminate both drinking water wells and indoor air. Chapters 6 and 15 describe the potential hazards from these sources.

The bad news: you probably have at least one of these exposures. The good news: there are some cases where you don't need to do anything about them, because the risks are too low to be a health concern. Remember, some toxics are more potent than others, and some exposures are too minor to be a real concern. How can we tell which is which? We use a tool called risk assessment to bring into focus what a particular exposure can mean to your health.

Risk Assessment?

Scientists in the field of risk assessment recognize that chemicals in the air, water, soil, or food will inevitably end up inside your body. The first major question is, how much will be taken in? The answer comes from data kept on your behaviors: the amount of air you inhale, water and food you ingest, and soil you contact when participating in your daily activities. This information enables us to calculate the dose of a contaminant, to you and your family, regardless of where it is in your environment and how you come into contact with it. The second major question is, how toxic is the chemical? We rely on the toxicology and epidemiology studies described earlier to determine a chemical's toxicity. Risk assessment combines these two factors—exposure and potency—to estimate the likelihood or risk for someone's health to be affected. The greater the exposure and potency of the chemical, the greater the risk. In the end, it is this risk that determines what's toxic and what's not to you and your family.

Risk Comparisons

Risk comparisons are all around us. To use a mundane example, you may hear from your doctor: "The risk of driving to my office is greater than the risk of your child having a problem from you eating tuna during pregnancy." In other words, don't worry about exposing your developing baby to mercury in tuna fish, since you already take larger risks every day. That's an unfair risk comparison: you might willingly take a calculated risk that is an essential part of daily living (driving to the doctor), but would choose to avoid any type of chemical risk that might harm your baby. Risk comparisons are fraught with value judgments, uncertainty, and bias. They are often apples-to-oranges comparisons framed in a way that makes the layperson feel foolish he or she ever worried about the issue.

That said, not all risk comparisons are misleading. The best kind compare exposures from the same chemical. For example, people can be up in arms over neighborhood pesticide spraying (which has become more common in recent years due to West Nile virus). But the reality is, the pesticide being sprayed from the trucks is a pyrethroid, the same ingredient in flea

MAKING RISK ASSESSMENTS

Risk assessment is far from cut-and-dry—in fact, it is filled with uncertainty. It's a little like being a weatherman, but with a big disadvantage. Both types of scientists make predictions of risk, but weathermen get to see very quickly whether they were right, which allows them to refine their predictions and achieve a higher batting average. By contrast, it's rare for a risk assessor to see whether his prediction of disease is correct. That's because a disease like cancer takes years to develop and involves many factors, only one of which is exposure to a particular chemical.

So, how does risk assessment work? Usually, in the face of uncertainty, the risk assessor makes educated guesses of potency and exposure that are somewhat on the high side, so as to be sure not to underestimate a risk or allow standards that are too lenient. However, the risk estimates are still realistic and generally don't produce unreasonably strict standards.

shampoos, tick collars, and many other products you can buy from the hardware, drug, or pet store. The general public's dose from home use of these products is much greater than what they might be exposed to from the tanker truck cruising down the street. That kind of apples-to-apples comparison can put an exposure into perspective, using other exposures that the public readily accepts. One of our tasks in this book is to dispel faulty risk comparisons and help you determine which of your exposures truly are toxic risks.

Calculating Your Risk Index

This book uses the most up-to-date information in toxicology, epidemiology, and risk assessment to rank types of chemical exposure by how much risk they present to the general public. We will comprehensively discuss your potential exposures at home, work, school, and in the neighborhood, including what to watch out for when buying a new house, consumer goods, or food. As such, we've divided our chapters into four major sections: Major Toxics at Work and Home; Toxics in What We Eat, Drink, and Buy at the Store; Toxics in the Air We Breathe; and Toxics in Your Yard and Neighborhood. The information contained in these sections is consolidated into a Home-Buyer's and Consumer's Guide to Toxics at the end of the book. Within the chapters, you'll find facts and information about toxic substances, as well as commonly asked questions and answers, widely misperceived myths and realities, and real-life stories of toxic exposure from our Toxic Files. Each chapter closes with a special risk index chart, which shows not only how risky something is, but also why. The following factors appear in the charts:

- Exposure: First and foremost is your likelihood of coming in contact with the chemical. If there's no exposure, there's no risk, no matter how toxic the chemical might be. We have evaluated how likely and how often people will contact a chemical; we have also taken into account the magnitude of the exposure. A high exposure ranking is reserved for chemicals known to cause health effects at levels which are commonly encountered by the general public.

- Toxicity: The next factor is the potency of the chemical to produce a toxic effect. As described previously, potent chemicals are those that can produce serious harm (birth defects, asthma, cancer, even death) even at low levels of exposure.

- Risk Ranking: Each chart features an overall risk-ranking score, which is a composite of the exposure and toxicity scores. A ranking of 0–4 signifies a low risk (no action needed), 5–7 a moderate risk (avoid if possible), and 8–10 a high risk (definitely avoid). In this ranking we take into account how much we know about a chemical's risk—a high level of uncertainty about how toxic a chemical is will increase the risk ranking, because we cannot be sure how dangerous it is.

Also at the end of each chapter is a toxic checklist, your quick reference guide for identifying the toxic substance and taking steps to limit exposure.

On the following pages, we have ranked our top-ten toxic risks and myths to highlight the information you will find in the rest of the book. These top risks and myths do not appear in any particular order. Depending upon your individual circumstance, any one of these may be most important to you. (Consult the individual chapters for more detailed information on how to prevent exposure to specific toxics.) We also provide a listing of the top toxic uncertainties, toxic issues that are controversial and may become leading risks in the future. We invite you to read on to find out what is behind these rankings, and about other chemicals that you may be knowingly or unknowingly exposed to. Our main goal is to make you an educated consumer of risk information. After reading this book, we're confident that you'll be better able to tell the difference between "what's toxic and what's not."

TOP 10 TOXIC RISKS

Particulate air pollution .... Chapter 11

Ozone air pollution .... Chapter 11

Radon in homes .... Chapter 2

Lead paint .... Chapter 1

Carbon monoxide .... Chapter 8

Dioxin in food .... Chapter 5

Mercury in fish .... Chapter 5

Arsenic at home[1] .... Chapters 6, 12

Heating with wood [2] .... Chapter 11

Volatile chemicals[3] ...... Chapters 7, 15

[1] Arsenic in decks and drinking water

[2] Wood stoves and backyard wood furnaces

[3] Volatile chemicals in consumer products and from groundwater pollution

TOP 10 TOXIC MYTHS

Mold found in homes is toxic.. Chapter 3

Most cancer is caused by environmental chemicals .... Chapter 16

Air purifiers clear the indoor air .... Chapter 8

Formaldehyde insulation (UFFI) is an indoor air hazard .... Chapter 14

Most air pollution comes from industrial smokestacks .... Chapter 11

Bottled water is purer than city tap water........................... Chapter 6

Pesticide residues in food are a major toxic risk .... Chapter 5

Testing indoor air for mold and other compounds is useful .... Chapters 3, 8

Consumer products are well tested for toxic risks .... Chapter 7

Asbestos is a significant indoor air risk factor........................ Chapter 4

TOP TOXIC UNCERTAINTIES

Risk from fluoride in drinking water .... Chapter 6

Risk from power lines and EMF .... Chapter 13

Risk from phthalates in cosmetics .... Chapter 7

Risk from emerging chemicals (flame retardants, Teflon) .... Chapter 5

Causes and prevention of Multiple Chemical Sensitivity .... Chapter 8

SECTION 1

Major Toxics at Home and at Work

CHAPTER 1

Lead

Lead is a metal with many toxic effects. Among the most troubling is that it makes us less smart. Lead has been insidiously affecting our learning abilities and IQs since the time when its economic and industrial uses were first exploited centuries ago. By the twentieth century, we obviously had still not learned lead's toxic lessons, as we brought it into our homes and yards via paint, plumbing, and gasoline. While lead helped make those products better, it also made our living environment more toxic, especially to young children. We've corrected most of those mistakes, but there are still plenty of opportunities for lead exposure around the home.

Lead is a bluish-gray metal that is naturally present in the earth's crust, at low levels in bedrock and soil. It does no harm to people when left there. However, we have been mining lead for thousands of years, putting the heavy metal into consumer products and spreading it throughout the environment. Extremely versatile, lead has been used in products ranging from batteries to bullets, pencils to pipes. Early industry favored lead because it was easier to forge: it melts at a low temperature and is malleable, yet at the same time it is strong and doesn't rust. Lead was often used in early plumbing and drinking goblets, both of which caused Romans to get a dose of the metal every time they quenched their thirst. In fact, lead poisoning is believed to underlie the aberrant behavior of Rome's ruling elite and the eventual fall of the Roman Empire (Lewis, 1985).

Unfortunately, modern civilization has repeated antiquity's mistakes. By 1980, the United States was using ten times more lead per person than

Caesar's Rome. This toxin that surreptitiously causes hyperactivity, learning disabilities, and criminal behavior was brought into nearly every U.S. home in the form of a paint additive. At the same time, it infiltrated our air through its use as an octane booster in gasoline. When leaded gasoline is burned, lead enters the atmosphere only to be inhaled into the lungs of those living closest to traffic. To make matters worse, the group receiving the greatest exposure, young children, was also the most vulnerable. Lead can damage the brain at relatively low doses, especially in a developing fetus or young child. Lead poisoning leads to decreased attention span, slower learning, and behavioral changes. And those are its mild effects.

There is a silver lining: we're not going to end up like ancient Rome. In fact, lead has turned into one of the greatest toxics success stories in history. Epidemiologists, toxicologists, and experimental psychologists became public health heroes by uncovering the chronic dangers of lead. This resulted in lead being banned from paint in 1978 and from gasoline by 1995. Since then, the amount of lead in our air, water, food supply, and, most importantly, in the bodies of children and adults across the U.S. has dropped dramatically.

But there's still work to be done.

> **MYTH:** Banning leaded products has ended the threat from this toxic metal.
>
> **REALITY:** Unfortunately, lead contamination of yards, homes, and playing fields continues today.

The lead legacy lives on in the layers of paint that still coat the walls in millions of homes built before 1978. It lives on in the lead-contaminated soil present in urban neighborhoods and surrounding older homes. Lead's legacy lives on in the approximately 400,000 children who are overexposed to lead each year (Meyer, et al., 2003). The problem is, lead doesn't break down or migrate: it will stay where it was deposited for generations. Which means that, if you and your children are unlucky enough to live in its midst, you're at a high risk of experiencing some degree of lead poisoning, ranging from mild to severe.

Q *We live in a beautiful old Victorian house, but it's been a project. Fortunately, my husband is very handy and has saved us money by fixing it up. His latest project is to create a baby room out of a small sitting area, as we*

are expecting our first child in five months. How can we make sure the new
room is environmentally friendly for our baby?

A It's certainly a good idea to complete the construction project, including finishing work such as painting, before you bring the new baby into your
house. Buying low-emission furniture, carpeting, and drapes and giving
these time to air out before the baby is moved into the room are important
steps (see Chapter 8). However, the first and most important step is to protect yourself and the baby growing inside you from the toxic effects of lead.

Most people are not aware of how dangerous remodeling projects in
older homes can be. Your home probably has lead paint on the walls and
woodwork because it was built before 1978. Even lead paint buried beneath
several newer coats of paint can find its way to the floor and into your body
through normal peeling and chipping. Home remodeling greatly increases
this problem: large amounts of lead can be released from walls and woodwork in the dust created by gutting rooms. Even if you are not doing the work
yourself, you can unknowingly come in contact with lead dust via inhalation,
or simply getting it on your clothes and hands. From there, you can end up
swallowing it if it gets into your food, or from normal hand-to-mouth activity.

Any lead that you, as the pregnant mom, absorb can be passed along
to the fetus. Lead readily crosses the placenta, and the fetal period is the
most sensitive time for lead toxicity to the brain. To safeguard your baby as
you prepare its room, follow lead-safe remodeling practices that keep the
lead dust under control. You need to make your husband aware of these
practices. If you use a contractor for part of the work, make sure that they
follow lead-safe construction practices.

As this Q and A makes clear, remodeling projects in old houses can be
a lead hazard. And we're not just talking about the demolition of walls—
many homes have attractive woodwork underneath layers of paint. It has
been common practice for homeowners to strip away paint by scraping,
sanding, using chemical strippers, or heat guns. This kind of disturbance
can release large amounts of lead dust into your home. You should keep in
mind this warning from the federal Consumer Product Safety Commission
(CPSC): "There is no completely safe method for do-it-yourself removal of
lead paint. Only experts should remove lead paint" (Farley, 1998).

Even without such aggressive disturbance of paint, lead can be released from walls from normal wear and tear. As paint ages, it becomes

brittle, and flakes and chips. Once it hits the floor, it becomes ground into dust which is readily taken up on little hands crawling on floors. The frequent hand-to-mouth activity of toddlers makes it impossible to wash their hands often enough. They *will* ingest dust and dirt from your floors—your responsibility is to keep this dust as lead-free as possible. Cleaning floors often is important, but the best way to prevent lead exposure is to keep it from flaking off the walls in the first place.

There are two ways to prevent lead flaking. The first is a complete, professional lead removal (or "de-leading") of the house, which entails a removal of the lead paint from all surfaces. This can be a huge job and, as pointed out above, if not properly done can cause large quantities of lead to be spread around your house. In recent years, the prevailing wisdom has turned toward a more practical solution: sealing the lead hazard in place. A variety of lead encapsulants that go onto walls and molding like a heavy, thick paint have been developed. These sealants don't become brittle and flake the way normal paint does, and stand up to physical blows and heavy scrubbing. The problems with this approach are: 1) encapsulants are not effective on surfaces subject to a lot of friction, such as floors, stairs, and window frames; 2) house remodeling can still liberate the underlying lead paint, creating a dust hazard; and 3) the encapsulant will not necessarily stand up to another key exposure pathway: children chewing on wood molding. If you are planning on remodeling, or have small children, careful removal of the lead paint may be your best option. This goes for high-friction areas of your home as well.

TOXIC FILE · ONE MOTHER'S STORY

As a Realtor, I was of course aware of the requirement that any wood molding at a toddler's height be tested for lead. And we had been told that toddlers might chew on any surfaces sticking out from walls that they can get their mouth around. However, I was shocked to see it happening in my own home. My two-year-old daughter was face-to-face with some floor molding, mouth pressed against the woodwork. Sure enough, when I pulled her away, there were teeth marks on the paint; fortunately, she hadn't yet chipped off a piece. We had already made sure that the low-lying painted surfaces in our home did not contain lead, so we didn't run out and get her blood tested. However, we were horrified by her behavior and quickly taught our daughter to leave the woodwork alone.

This Toxic File describes a form of pica (Latin for magpie, due to the bird's omnivorous diet); it refers to the insertion of foreign (non-food) objects in the mouth. Of course, some mouthing behavior is normal, and keeping clean toys in your child's environment is important. However, he or she may still choose to stick handfuls of dirt in his mouth or ingest paint chips. It's a myth that only kids from poorer or less educated families chew on woodwork and eat paint chips—this is truly a universal issue. The more attention parents pay to their child's behavior, the more likely that pica-related lead ingestion can be recognized and prevented.

WINDOWSILLS ARE LEAD HAZARDS.

TOXIC FACT

Windowsills are an important lead hazard that can be harder to deal with. Lead paint on the inside surfaces of window tracks and the surrounding molding inevitably peels fastest due to vibration, rubbing, and exposure to outdoor weather. Think about where in your home you might be most likely to find paint chips—in window wells. It follows that windowsills are a primary source of lead exposure. Children like to spend time in front of windows, looking outside and even playing with items (like toy cars) that can fit within the window tracks. Here they have ample opportunity to pick up lead chips and dust on their hands and ingest it from routine hand-to-mouth contact. Perhaps even more dangerous, the paint chips that fall in window wells get ground into a dust that can blow into the house. In fact, one of the primary sources of lead on the floor is peeling window frames and sills. Therefore, it is especially important to address lead paint in these areas of your house. Refer to the lead-prevention steps described at the end of this chapter to help you accomplish this.

IS YOUR CHILD SAFE FROM LEAD AWAY FROM HOME?

TOXIC FILE

The Jones family received some disturbing news a month ago after two-year-old Billy had his annual visit to the doctor's office. Part of the check-up was drawing a finger-prick blood sample that was sent off to the lab. Mary Jones was surprised when she got a call from the doctor regarding Billy's blood test. "We need to have Billy back in for a follow-up blood test," he said. "The lead result was above what we like to see: twenty-two, and normal is below ten. But the way that particular test was done is crude. It may have been what we call a false positive—contaminated by lead on your son's skin but not in his blood. Let's double-check with a more reliable test, a venipuncture. We can take the sample right here in our office. Can you bring him in tomorrow?"

Mary said yes and then immediately called her husband. They discussed what little they knew about lead—their home was built ten years ago, so it shouldn't have lead paint. The plumbing was also modern, though they'd never tested their water. But their biggest concern was the safety of their child: had Billy been permanently hurt? Was he at risk for contracting a disease like cancer?

The retest came back four anxious days later. Mary learned that her son's result was similar—nineteen, roughly two times above the safe limit. But the doctor met her anguished expression with calm reassurance.

"I know you're worried about Billy, but he'll probably be fine. By today's standards, he's got more lead in his blood than should be there. But twenty years ago this result was normal, and that generation of kids turned out OK. It takes two times more lead than Billy's blood test shows—around forty—to be dangerous. He is in the precautionary zone, and his result means that he's getting lead somewhere in his environment. If we remove him from the source, his blood level should go down quickly and he'll be fine. So tell me about your house . . ."

Mary calmed down, and realized that she'd better give the doctor all the facts she could for Billy's sake. The more she described her house and its plumbing, furnishings, dishes, glassware, and consumer products, the more convinced the doctor became that the problem was not at home. "Mrs. Jones, does Billy go to day care?" Light bulbs went off in Mary's head as she described Billy's half-days with Mrs. Dawson, a lovely older woman who did a small amount of child care. The doctor sat up straighter as he asked, "Where does Mrs. Dawson live, and what kind of house is it?" Mary knew it was a colonial in the older section of town. "I'm going to ask you to not take Billy there until we check this out. I need to report Billy's blood test to the state and I'm going to let them know where he spends half the day. Do you know if Mrs. Dawson is a licensed day care provider?" Mary was embarrassed to admit that she had never asked.

It turns out that Mrs. Dawson wasn't licensed because she felt that her business was too small and informal to be worth going to the trouble. Within the week, the state sent in an inspector who found lead on all the woodwork and in the floor dust. She was fined and prohibited from taking on any more children until she obtained a license and the lead problem in her home was cleaned up.

This Toxic File reminds us that every environment where young children spend time, whether it be Grandma's house, school, or of course, day care, must be lead safe. There are state and federal requirements for schools and day care facilities for lead testing and removal—however, this is not the case for your neighbor's house. You need to be watchful for lead hazards away from home. Don't be shy about asking questions! If your child regularly goes over to a particular friend's house, especially an older home or one being remodeled, ask about lead paint. Regarding day care, only use state-licensed providers, but still ask them questions to make sure that their facilities have been inspected and had any lead paint removed or sealed in place.

Testing Your Child's Blood Lead Level

As we've learned, lead exposure is still common, and it's hard for a parent to control all the potential sources. Therefore, blood lead testing is strongly recommended at least twice, generally at one and two years of age. This testing is available at doctor's offices and medical clinics, and is typically either offered for free or is covered by medical insurance. The following chart shows you what the results mean.

BLOOD LEAD LEVEL	HEALTH EFFECTS	RECOMMENDED ACTION
Less than 10 ug/dl	None	None
10–19 ug/dl	Subtle effects on learning and behavior are possible	1. Look for and remove sources of lead 2. Retest blood in 3–6 months
20–44 ug/dl	Mild effects on learning and behavior are probable; symptoms such as stomachache, tiredness, and irritability are possible	1. Retest blood immediately 2. Look for sources of lead 3. Keep child away from any possible sources until they can be tested 4. Remove lead sources from child's environment 5. Test other children in household
Greater than 44 ug/dl	Symptoms described above are likely; moderate to severe effects on brain function and development. Exposure can be life-threatening above 80 ug/dl	1. Immediately obtain full medical check-up for child 2. Follow doctor's treatment orders, which may involve chelation therapy 3. If your home is the source, move child out until lead is removed

TOXIC FACT

GOOD NUTRITION IS IMPORTANT FOR PREVENTING LEAD POISONING.

Lead is taken up into blood by the same system that absorbs calcium. Diets rich in calcium (e.g., dairy), iron, and Vitamin D will allow less lead to be absorbed. The worst cases of childhood lead poisoning are in undernourished children.

> **MYTH: I'm on city water which comes from a reservoir, so it doesn't have lead in it.**
>
> **REALITY: Even if the water itself is uncontaminated, it can pick up lead as it travels through household plumbing.**

Water companies test the water they sell you; the burden of proof is on them to show that it's below the safety standard (15 ug/liter). However, it could be much higher than that at your tap if you have old pipes. Lead-containing pipes stopped being used in 1963, although lead solder was used in plumbing joints into the mid-1980s. If your plumbing was installed before 1987, you need to test for lead.

When water sits in pipes for long periods of time (even overnight), it has time to dissolve lead out of the plumbing and build up unhealthy

CHELATION THERAPY

The only antidote to lead poisoning is chelation therapy. One of a number of drugs—EDTA, penicillamine, dimercaprol, or succimer—is injected or taken orally by the patient. It binds to lead in blood and renders it harmless. The bound lead ends up excreted in urine. Chelation therapy can't undo any damage lead has already caused, but it can prevent more damage from occurring. It does, however, have its own side effects and usually requires hospitalization. Therefore, it is done only if lead levels are above 45 ug/dl.

Since most of the body's lead is stored in bone, it is common for blood levels to go back up after chelation therapy stops. This is because lead can leave bone to replace that which was taken out of the blood. Chelation therapy is most effective in patients who have had a short-term exposure to lead, so that there hasn't been a chance for much to be stored in bone.

concentrations in the water. However, running plenty of cold water through the faucet prior to your first drink in the morning can remove much of the danger. Fresh water that hasn't been sitting in the pipes is much lower in lead. An important point to remember is never to drink hot tap water or use it for cooking. Water that's been sitting in a hot water heater can leach more lead from plumbing and is not fresh. Only use it for washing.

Being on city water does have some advantage, though. One of the requirements placed on water companies is that their water be pH neutralized so that it won't dissolve your pipes. If your water is on the acidic side, it will more aggressively leach lead out of your pipes. If you are on a private well, there is no one at the controls to test and adjust your water—thus it may not be properly balanced, which increases your chances of having a lead problem in your drinking water. This is especially true if you have naturally "soft" (low mineral content) as opposed to "hard" (high magnesium and calcium) water. People living in older homes who have private wells need to test their water for lead when they move in. Assuming the test comes back fine, retesting is warranted every two to four years to make sure that changes in water quality haven't increased its ability to dissolve lead from your pipes. Follow the instructions in Chapter 6 regarding how to test your tap water.

Other Sources of Lead in the Home

Lead isn't just in paint and pipes. There are other important sources of lead in the home, including:

LEAD GLAZE ON POTTERY

Pottery bowls and mugs may beautify your kitchen, but some caution is warranted: the glaze finish can contain enough lead to be hazardous. Mass-produced pottery is not a lead hazard because it is prepared and fired in such a way to prevent the breakdown of the glaze finish. However, pottery made in small shops, especially from abroad, have glazes that can break down and leach lead into your food or drink. This has led to occasional cases of lead poisoning (Blumenthal, 1989). This problem has been documented most with pottery made in Mexico (Azcona-Cruz,

2000). In fact, the Washington Department of Health recently released an explicit warning regarding lead and Mexican pottery (Washington DOH, 2005). Lead might also be an issue with pottery from other countries and from small shops in the U.S. Unless you are sure the pottery is lead-safe, you should not use it to drink or eat. In general, note that acidic liquids such as tomato products, fruit juices, wine, and vinegar leach lead from pottery most easily.

LEAD CRYSTAL GLASSWARE

Putting lead into glassware makes it sparkle more brightly. But the lead doesn't necessarily stay put, and acidic liquids can slowly leach lead from the vessel and into your drink. This type of glassware is not safe for use on an everyday basis, especially if you are pregnant. In fact, pregnant women and young children should not drink from leaded glassware at all. Be wary of crystal glassware or any glassware that is particularly shiny or carved, as it may be leaded.

LEAD IN SOIL

A major fallout from leaded gasoline is the contamination of soil and street dust, greatest near busy roadways. Urban areas generally have higher lead levels than suburban or rural areas for this reason. Inner-city children playing on pavement or soil may still receive unhealthy amounts of lead exposure. Street dust levels have fallen with the removal of lead from gasoline, but can still be elevated above safe levels.

Another source of lead in soil is house paint. Lead was banned from exterior house paint in 1978, but plenty of lead paint remains on the shingles and window frames of homes across America. As this paint flakes off, the soil nearest to the foundation becomes lead-contaminated. Therefore, children's sand boxes and play areas should be kept away from the house or any other painted structures that were built before 1978 (e.g., sheds, fences).

It's a good idea to test your yard's soil for lead. The test will show whether exterior house paint or leaded gasoline has left you with potentially dangerous levels of the metal, and should also give you an idea of where in your yard is safest for children to play and for you to grow a garden. Lead uptake into plants is a distinct possibility. This can be minimized by keeping the soil neutral or slightly basic, and enriching it with phosphate-containing fertilizer. Your soil should contain less than 400 ppm of lead. You may be able to find parts of the yard with lower levels, so follow-up testing may be warranted if initial tests come back high.

MISCELLANEOUS SOURCES

There have been sporadic reports of household products that contain lead. The list includes certain brands of imported vinyl blinds, hair dyes, cosmetics from the Middle East, and some candy from Mexico. When the lead hazard is discovered, the product is usually taken off the market, but what has been sold may still exist in homes. For example, plastic mini-blinds from Mexico and Asia were found to contain high levels of lead in the mid-1990s, at which point most stores stopped carrying the product (CPSC, 1996). However, you may move into an apartment or house that still has them covering the windows. If so, they should be discarded. Aluminum and wood blinds are alternatives that do not contain lead, and newer plastic mini-blinds that have a "No Lead Added" sticker are safe.

Regarding lead acetate in hair dyes: studies have shown that the lead is not absorbed. The FDA has determined that this use of lead does not constitute a hazard.

WORKPLACE EXPOSURES: BRINGING LEAD HOME

Certain occupations may still involve lead exposure. Painters scrape a lot of paint, some of which may cling to their clothing and skin. Home repair and remodeling trades can lead to exposure because of the lead-containing dust they generate. Lead is still used in battery manufacture, and it is also reclaimed from batteries and then smelted. Workers in these lead industries can be exposed to particularly high amounts. Another workplace of concern is firing ranges due to the residue that can come off of lead bullets. A listing of over fifty occupations with lead exposure can be found at http://www.haz-map.com/lead.htm. To prevent workplace lead from contaminating your home, you should change clothes and thoroughly wash up before entering your house.

THE RISK INDEX FOR LEAD

By now, you've realized that lead is highly toxic and that you should do everything in your power to keep it away from your children. On our risk index chart below, lead gets a high toxicity ranking because of its well-recognized effects on many organs, most notably the brain. These effects can occur at low doses if exposure is chronic. Lead gets a moderate ranking for exposure. Ten years ago, this ranking would have been higher, and twenty years ago, it would have been off the chart. Fortunately, lead exposures have gone down considerably over the past two decades. However, there are still hundreds of thousands of children who are overexposed. Lead's overall risk is high because of its potent effects and because of all the lead paint that still exists in homes and other places where children spend time. Bottom line: lead hazards need to be controlled or eliminated if they exist in your home.

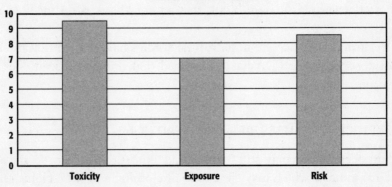

RISK INDEX FOR LEAD

LEAD CHECKLIST

LEAD IN YOUR HOME OR APARTMENT

❑ **Find out if your house has lead paint (only necessary if built before 1978).**

    ❑ Hire a certified lead inspector to evaluate your home.
A professional should use an XRF machine to scan all painted surfaces. Note that do-it-yourself test kits from hardware stores are not very reliable.

    ❑ Make sure any lead hazards are revealed when you buy your next house. (See Chapter 17 for more details on lead issues when buying a house.)

❑ **Keep any lead-painted surfaces in good repair** to avoid chipping and flaking of paint; be especially watchful of windowsills.

❑ **Consider using a lead encapsulant** to coat lead-painted surfaces. Use an encapsulant that has been certified as being effective by a governmental agency. The painted surface you are encapsulating must be intact (not peeling) and clean. Carefully follow lead-encapsulation procedures or hire a certified lead-abatement contractor to make sure the encapsulation job is done right.

❑ **Consider having lead paint removed from molding at floor level** where children can chew on the wood. Any paint removal should be done by a lead-abatement professional. You can call 1-800-424-LEAD to find out who is certified to conduct lead-safe paint removal in your area.

❑ **Clean floors and window wells regularly** to minimize the amount of lead dust available for children to ingest.

❑ **Be careful when painting or working on remodeling projects** in homes with lead paint; be sure to contain lead dust within the work zone and properly clean it up.

    ❑ Paint should not be removed by sanding or with a heat gun. All paint chips scraped off walls should be captured and home furnishings covered or moved out of the area.

    ❑ Contact the United States Environmental Protection Agency at 1-800-424-LEAD and obtain their fact sheet "Reducing Lead Hazards When Remodeling Your Home." Make sure your remodeling contractor follows the safety precautions described in this fact sheet.

❑ **Test your drinking water for lead** if the plumbing in your house is from before 1985. If lead is high, consider replacing the pipes. Check the pH of the water to see if it is too corrosive and needs to be adjusted. At a minimum, thoroughly flush the water before drinking it the first time it is used in the morning.

KEEPING YOUR CHILD LEAD-SAFE

❑ **Have your child's blood lead tested at ages one and two.** You cannot be sure that you've eliminated all sources of lead from your child's environment. The blood test will show whether your child is lead-exposed.

❑ **Clean children's hands and toys frequently.**

❑ **Prevent children from ingesting paint chips, dirt, and dust.**

❑ **Feed your child a healthy, varied diet** that has plenty of calcium, iron, and Vitamin D.

❑ **Select day-care providers that are licensed by the state.** Double-check to make sure the facilities have been tested for lead.

OTHER SOURCES OF LEAD

❑ **Test the soil in your yard for lead,** particularly near the house or other painted structures. If levels are above 400 ppm, make sure the area is well covered with grass or mulch. Keep vegetable gardens and children's play areas away from high lead areas.

❑ **Avoid drinking out of lead crystal glassware or eating/drinking out of ceramic pottery** imported from Mexico. It's especially important to not consume acidic foods in these containers.

❑ **Do not bring lead home from work.** If your job involves handling some form of lead, make sure to wash thoroughly and change into clean clothes before leaving work.

CHAPTER 2

Radon

Of all the environmental chemicals that have the potential to cause cancer, radon may be the greatest risk of all. This potent human carcinogen is a radioactive gas that exists at elevated levels in many homes across the country. While the radioactive dose from radon is far smaller than what is possible in, say, a nuclear catastrophe, radon still deserves a high degree of respect.

Radon was not thought to be a significant public health hazard until 1985, and at that point it was lucky to be detected at all! The story of its discovery involved a man named Stanley Watras, who worked at a nuclear power plant in eastern Pennsylvania. He came to the attention of his supervisor when he kept setting off radiation alarms on his way *into* work! It turns out that the power plant had radiation sensors at the exits to make sure workers didn't wear contaminated clothing home. When Mr. Watras set off the alarms on the way in, the company decided to check his home. There they found amazingly high levels of radon, nearly 1,000 times greater than the safe level. Geologists identified the area where Mr. Watras lived as the Redding Prong, a geologic formation that had high levels of uranium and therefore radon (see next section for explanation). The discovery at this one home led to an investigation throughout the Redding Prong areas of Pennsylvania and New Jersey. The high levels of radon found in these areas led to the birth of a nationwide radon testing campaign.

Radon is a naturally occurring element that is common in soil and bedrock. It forms through the breakdown of uranium, a radioactive element (the same uranium that is processed into nuclear bombs and used in power plants). Over time, uranium decays or breaks down into radon gas, which will move upward in the direction of anything that pulls air out of the soil. Your house can do just that, especially in the wintertime (see Chapter 15). As heated air rises through the house toward the attic, the basement temporarily has a little less air and thus a little less pressure than the rest of the house. Nature abhors a vacuum, and air rushes in to fill in this gap. The replacement air can come from outdoors, but in weather-tight homes, it's hard for outdoor air to get in via leaks around windows and doors. Instead, much of the replacement air comes from soil gas. This is where radon is lurking, waiting for the nearest house to take a deep breath of soil gas and inhale the contaminant into the home. The gas can enter via cracks, utility openings and sump pits in the basement floor. Through this process, homes can build up radon levels that are many times higher than those found outside. And while radon can move throughout the entire house, its levels are typically greatest in the basement.

When radon gets into your home, every breath you take sends a new dose of radioactivity to your lungs. Radon doesn't stay in its gaseous state very long, but decays further into tiny particles of polonium, another radioactive element. These smaller radioactive particles can become lodged in your lungs and emit rays of damaging ionizing radiation that can affect DNA, leading to mutations. After a latency period of twenty to thirty years, these mutations can give rise to lung cancer. The National Research Council estimates that between 20,000 and 30,000 lung cancer deaths are caused by radon annually in the United States (NRC 1999).

With such serious consequences, you would hope that there would be telltale signs of radon's presence. Unfortunately, this is not the case. Radon is a silent killer, providing absolutely no warnings. It is colorless and odorless, it causes no symptoms that residents might notice, and its harmful effects are delayed by many years, so you can't tell that it is doing any damage until it's too late. Some people who get lung cancer may never know that radon had a hand in the disease.

> **MYTH:** If inhaling radon is bad, drinking it in your tap water must be even worse.
>
> **REALITY:** Inhaling radon is actually more dangerous than drinking it. Radon ingested in drinking water has a good chance of being flushed out of the body. By contrast, inhaled radon forms tiny particles in the lung that can get trapped and create local damage for long periods of time.

Another source of exposure to radon is drinking water. Radon deep within the bedrock can dissolve in groundwater and be present at fairly high levels in your well.

The major problem with radon in tap water is that it can evaporate into the air of your home, adding to the radon that comes in from soil gas. A high radon test result in your air may be a sign that your drinking water is also contaminated. This can easily be checked with a radon water test. The USEPA guideline for radon in water is 4,000 picocuries per liter (pCi/liter), a level set to ensure that radon in water would not make much contribution to radon in your home's air. Of course, if your radon air level is low, there is little need to test the water.

If you are on a public water supply, you probably don't have a water radon problem. Water from reservoirs has very little radon, since the gas can escape into the outdoor air during storage. Public water from underground supplies may contain radon, but normal storage and treatment will reduce the levels significantly. If you are on a small public water system (less than 25 customers), there may be less opportunity for dilution and removal prior to the water reaching your tap. In that case, testing your water for radon is a good idea if your overall indoor air level is elevated.

RADON IN MY HOME?

TOXIC FILE

David had only vaguely heard of radon. When he and his young family moved into the neighborhood six years ago, he was told that the town was a low-radon area because it was located in a river valley. Such valleys fill up with sediment over the course of geologic time, burying the bedrock deep beneath layers of soil. The deeper the bedrock layer, the less chance that radon formed from bedrock can spread up toward homes. But this belief was shattered when David's neighbor put his house up for sale and a potential buyer asked for a radon test. Surprisingly, the neighbor's house had levels in the air over recommended guidelines (4 picocuries per liter, or pCi/l). This started David thinking that he should test his own home. He was afraid of what he might find, since his family had lived there all this time.

David found the USEPA website for radon (www.epa.gov/radon). This gave him the basic information on testing. He bought two simple test kits at a local hardware store and, following the directions, placed one in the basement and one on the first floor. After a three-day test period, he mailed the kits back to the laboratory, and a week later the answer arrived. The news was not good: his basement had 8.5 pCi/l and his first floor had 4.1 pCi/l. David wasn't really sure what the alarming results meant.

The USEPA website listed a phone number at his state health department for more detailed radon information. He was told that his family has a slightly elevated cancer risk, but that the findings were not that bad. The worst location was the basement, but they spent very little time down there. The radon level on the first floor was barely above the recommended goal of 4 pCi/l. They had only been in the house six years, and no family member smoked cigarettes. Those factors helped decrease the house's overall risk. However, the health department strongly recommended that he lower the radon level in his house to ensure the basement would be safe and that his family could avoid any further cancer risk in the rest of the house. They gave him a list of contractors who could fix radon problems. David selected one, and the contractor installed a radon-reduction system in his basement for $1,350. Testing after the system was installed showed that it worked well: radon levels were less than 1 pCi/l.

As this Toxic File illustrates, all homeowners should have their homes tested for radon. But even though radon testing and remediation is easy, few homeowners do it. The USEPA estimates that 18 million homes in the United States have been tested, with most of those tests occurring when the home was sold (Gregory and Jalbert, 2004). That may be fine for the new occupants, but what about the people who were living there for the past twenty years? As David's story points out, you should test your house, even if you don't intend to sell, for the sake of your own family's health. Of course, the best time to get this information is when you are first buying the house, but if for some reason you didn't do it then, you still need to find out the radon level.

Testing is necessary no matter where your house is located. Many states have mapped out radon levels, providing a rough sketch of where radon is most likely to be found. Hilly, rocky areas tend to be higher in radon while river valleys tend to be low. However, these are broad generalizations and there can be many exceptions. It is not unusual for the results in one area to seem random, with adjacent neighbors having very different levels. There are many possible explanations for this: for example, one basement may be closer to bedrock than another, or the amount of uranium in adjoining sections of bedrock may differ. The properties of the soil and house foundation all influence how easily radon will get into the home. Having a neighbor with high radon is a warning that there's some uranium-bearing bedrock in your area. However, having a neighbor with low radon is no guarantee of safety at your house. The only way to be sure is to test.

It's been estimated that five percent of homes in the United States have radon levels that are unsafe. That may seem like a low percentage (one in twenty homes), but given the seriousness of the health risk and how easy it is to test, there are no excuses not to. The do-it-yourself test kits, available at your average hardware store, are accurate, easy to use, and inexpensive. If the test is not for a house sale, there is no need for expensive consultants—simply buying a test kit and following the instructions will give you reliable results. Radon tests for real estate transactions usually require that a third party (e.g., a home inspector) set up the test and report the results.

The major exception to the radon-testing rule is if you live in an apartment or condominium that is higher than the second floor. Radon is a ground-level contaminant, and your risk of exposure goes down as you go up from the ground floor.

Q *I know a smoker who got lung cancer. After he passed away, his wife sold the house and it was discovered that the home was high in radon. Do you think he got cancer from cigarettes or from radon?*

A Very possibly from both. Radon can interact with cigarette smoke to create a highly dangerous combination, much more lethal than either of the factors by themselves. Many of the estimated 20,000 annual lung cancers caused by radon are in smokers who might not have been affected if not for the combined effects of radon and smoking.

The main reason for this potent interaction is that smoking puts lots of particles into the air, giving radon and its radioactive offspring (polonium) more surfaces to attach to. When inhaled on a particle, radon has a better chance of lodging in your lungs. Even secondhand smoke in a high-radon house can help transport radioactivity into the lungs. This increases everyone's cancer risk, even non-smokers.

The moral of the story is, if you stop smoking, or at least don't smoke in your house, you'll cut down on the amount of particles in the air, which will decrease the amount of radioactivity reaching your lungs. Of course, you should monitor your home's radon level regardless of whether anyone in the house smokes. (And, of course, the best way to decrease your lung cancer risk is to quit smoking altogether.)

TOXIC FACT

RADON IS THE GREATEST ENVIRONMENTAL CANCER RISK TO THE GENERAL PUBLIC.

The following table shows the grim estimates, both for non-smokers and for smokers. Even at acceptable radon exposure levels (below 4 pCi/l), there is still a relatively high risk. The reason that these exposures are accepted is because they are so common—background indoor levels that you could find in an average home are approximately 1 pCi/l. The goal with radon mitigation is not to completely eliminate it, but rather to get the level down to background.

RADON LUNG CANCER RISK ESTIMATES			
RADON LEVEL (PCI/l)	IF 1,000 PEOPLE WHO NEVER SMOKED WERE EXPOSED FOR A LIFETIME:	IF 1,000 PEOPLE WHO SMOKED WERE EXPOSED FOR A LIFETIME:	WHAT TO DO
20	36 people would get lung cancer	260 people would get lung cancer	Fix your home*
10	18 with lung cancer	150 with lung cancer	Fix your home
4	7 with lung cancer	62 with lung cancer	Fix your home
2	4 with lung cancer	32 with lung cancer	Consider fixing at levels between 2 and 4pCi/l
1.3 (average indoor radon level)	2 with lung cancer	20 with lung cancer	Reducing radon levels below 2pCi/l is not always feasible

Source. USEPA, *Citizen's Guide to Radon*

* Consult the end of this chapter for instructions on how to lower radon levels.

WHERE IS THE PROOF THAT RADON CAUSES LUNG CANCER?

It can be difficult to prove that someone's lung cancer came from their at-home radon exposure. Lung cancer from radon can take over twenty years to develop, and can't easily be distinguished from cancer caused just by cigarette smoke. Since smoking causes eighty to ninety percent of all lung cancers, it can be difficult to pick out the relatively small percentage caused by radon.

The USEPA's cancer estimates for radon are derived from a large number of human epidemiology studies. The early risk estimates were from underground miners who had high-level radon exposure in their work environment. Recently, a number of studies in residential settings have confirmed the underground miners' radon risk. For example, an Iowa study found up to eighty-three percent increased risk for lung cancer in homes with a radon level greater than 4 pCi/l, the current USEPA guideline (Field, 2001). This evidence shows that at-home exposure to elevated radon levels is a real cancer risk.

> **MYTH:** Radon causes asthma and other lung diseases.
>
> **REALITY:** Short-term exposure to radon has no visible effects on your health.

People often assume that since radon is a toxic, radioactive gas, it can cause a host of respiratory ills, from frequent colds to bronchitis to asthma. Fortunately and unfortunately, this is not the case. At the levels present in many homes, radon's damage is very subtle and not noticeable in the short term. Long-term damage to DNA leading to an increased lung cancer risk is the only health effect attributable to radon.

Testing Your Home For Radon

As we said before, although many people hire a professional to test for radon during a real estate transaction, homeowners wishing to do their own test can use simple and reliable do-it-yourself test kits. There are two basic types of devices: short-term charcoal canisters left open in the home for only a few days, and long-term devices left out for up to a year.

Since radon levels in a home can change from day to day and week to week, some feel that longer-term testing is better. However, most people don't want to wait months to a year to determine the radon level in their home. Fortunately, there are ways to get useful information from the short-term (charcoal canister) device. By testing in the winter, when conditions are worst case for radon, you can be assured that you won't overlook a radon problem. If you test in other times of the year (for example, if you are buying a house in the spring), then you may want to retest the following winter. This is particularly true if your warm-weather results are above 1.5 pCi/l, slightly above the background level. If your results are borderline (between 2 and 4 pCi/l), you probably should retest right away to confirm the results. Once you do get final results, keep the report with your house records. (It is usually not necessary to retest a house in future years if the original testing was adequate.)

If you're going the short-term test route, it's a good idea to use two charcoal canisters for testing, one in the basement and one on the first floor or lowest lived-in area of your home. The USEPA's official recommendation is to fix a radon problem if the lived-in-area reading is over 4 pCi/l. However, many people decide to err on the side of caution and base their actions on the basement reading, which almost always is higher. This is a prudent step to take. As the radon table shows, cancer risk does not disappear below 4 pCi/l, so it's best to get your radon level as low as possible.

Remember, if you do have elevated indoor air levels, testing and fixing your water radon level is important. The general rule of thumb is that 10,000 pCi/l of radon in water can add 1 pCi/l to indoor air. Radon-mitigation contractors will often do a water test as part of their work to find sources of indoor air radon.

Lowering Your Home's Radon Level

In most parts of the country, there are many reputable, formally trained contractors who are available to fix radon problems. In some states, radon contractors must be certified. Check with your state health department to see if they have a list of certified radon contractors. The USEPA radon website (www/epa.gov/radon/proficiency.html) also has a list of contractors. These sources also list certified radon inspectors and testing companies.

Once you have selected a contractor (remember to check references!), ask for an outline of how they plan to test and fix your house. The first and most important step is a thorough visual inspection of the basement, looking for obvious radon entry points.

In most cases, the radon solution the contractor provides will involve a "sub-slab suction system." Although this sounds complex, it's actually a simple and inexpensive fix. It usually involves cutting one or more holes in the basement floor and putting 4-inch diameter PVC pipes into each of the openings. The pipes are hooked up to a simple fan that sucks radon gas from under the basement floor, sending it into the outside air and away from your basement. These suction systems are often combined with the sealing of large cracks and other openings such as sump holes. Together, these types of mitigation systems generally cost in the range of $1,000 to $1,500 and are very effective at reducing radon levels, though retesting after the system is installed is a must to assure a proper fix.

Regarding radon in water, the proposed USEPA guideline of 4,000 pCi/l is the starting point for considering whether you should install a water filter. If your test comes back over 20,000 pCi/l, you should definitely treat your water. Levels between 4,000 and 20,000 are a judgment call. The radon level in the air can help you decide: if it is high (>4 pCi/l), then you should probably treat your groundwater as well as your basement. Remember, if you do, the filter should be on the pipe coming into your house, not just at the faucet where you drink. Water treatment devices for radon vary, each with significant pros and cons, so do your homework before selecting a treatment system. For more information, contact your state radon program, which you can find using the resource list at the back of this book.

THE RISK INDEX FOR RADON

In our risk index chart, radon gets a high score for toxicity because it is a potent human carcinogen, and a high score for exposure because millions of homes are likely to have elevated levels. This combination leads to a high overall risk. If you don't already know what the radon level in your home is, you should test. Right away.

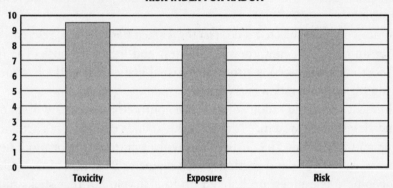

RISK INDEX FOR RADON

RADON CHECKLIST

TEST FOR RADON:
- ❑ **If you are buying a house, make sure the radon test and fix (if necessary) are part of the real estate agreement.**

- ❑ **If you are living in a house that hasn't been tested, conduct the test right away.**
  - ❑ If the result is between 1.5 and 4 pCi/l in the basement, consider retesting to confirm the result.
  - ❑ Also retest in the winter if the current test was in warm-weather months.

IF THERE IS A RADON PROBLEM, FIX IT:
- ❑ **If the level is over 4 pCi/l in the basement, hire a certified radon-mitigation contractor.**

- ❑ **Follow the contractor's advice,** which usually involves installing a sub-slab suction system to remove radon gas before it can enter your house.

- ❑ **Make sure the basement is retested** after the system is installed to demonstrate that it's working properly.

- ❑ **If the radon air level is over 4 pCi/l, test your well water if you have a private well.** If the radon level in your well water is above 4,000 pCi/l, consider installing a treatment system. If it is above 20,000 pCi/l, definitely install a system.

- ❑ **Stop smoking** and help others you live with to stop smoking. This will decrease your lung cancer risk from both radon and your smoking history.

CHAPTER 3

Mold

Mold. Its sight and smell can strike fear in the heart of any brave soul. Given the abundance of news stories and websites dedicated to "toxic mold," one would think it was one of today's most important health issues. Its sudden notoriety might have given you the impression that mold is a new problem.

In reality, mold and the human race have evolved as constant partners. Molds are a natural and vital part of the world; there are thousands of species, and they exist in every nook and cranny. Take a walk outdoors and you are inhaling mold spores with every breath, regardless of whether you are in the woods or the city. In most cases, this kind of casual contact does not make us sick. We usually don't even realize we're sharing our daily lives with these members of the fungus kingdom. However, when our homes or schools become damp for long periods of time, mold can grow beyond normal bounds and present health concerns. The question is not "Is there mold in my home?" but rather "Is there too much mold in my home?"

Molds are plantlike organisms in the fungus kingdom that can grow on many different substances, including wood, paper, clothing, carpet, and, of course, food. This versatility allows them to gain a foothold in many different parts of the home. However, they only actively grow where there is ample moisture, whether in the form of high summertime humidity or in water-damaged materials that result from floods or leaky pipes. In fact, some form of mold is likely to be growing in any part of the house that is chronically warm and damp. Bathrooms are such places, and we've come to expect to see black mold growing on bathroom tile. However, mold growing in other parts of the house is not normal and can present a health risk.

Mold problems are estimated to occur in twenty-five to fifty percent of all homes, with the higher number occurring in places affected by hurricanes and other types of floods (Kowalski, 2000). Approximately ten percent of the U.S. population (twenty million people) is allergic to mold. Beyond allergies, mold colonization of our sinus cavities may contribute to the thirty-seven million chronic sinusitis cases in this country (Ponikau et al., 1999).

In the warmer months, molds grow outside on plants and dead material. They spread via spores, seedlike packets that contain allergens that can cause some of us to sneeze and wheeze. (In fact, some of the seasonal allergies people suffer from are due to outdoor mold rather than tree or ragweed pollen.) After being released into the air, spores can start new colonies if they land on the right surface with the right moisture level. Amazingly, a spore can lie dormant for years, awaiting the proper conditions to grow.

While we can't completely avoid inhaling spores, we should do our best to minimize spore levels in our homes. It is impossible to keep mold completely out, but if you keep your home dry, you can certainly prevent it from gaining a foothold.

There are thousands of mold species, all with different properties that affect where and how they grow. The health threat really has more to do with *how much* mold is present rather than *which* mold is present (IOM, 2004). That's because most species of mold have the ability to cause allergic, irritant, and asthmatic effects as described later in this chapter. The more mold spores in the air, the greater the risk for allergy, irritation, and sinusitis.

▮ MOLD IN THE HOME

TOXIC FILE

Mary and her family have been renting a nice, clean apartment for two years and are generally happy with its condition. The one exception is a patch of dark fuzzy material that started growing at the back of the closet in her baby's room. It looks like mold, and gives off a faint mustiness. She has cleaned the area twice with bleach, but the patch keeps reappearing. Worried about her baby's health, Mary has asked her landlord to test the apartment for toxic mold. He said he would look into it. At the same time, she called her local health department, but their inspector said that since there are no standards for mold, there is nothing they can do about the situation.

Mary's dilemma is typical in the new world of mold. The landlord doesn't really know what to do, and her local government doesn't have much interest or authority in the area. Although Mary's request for testing seems to make sense, what she really needs is a behind-the-wall investigation to find out where the water is coming from. The fact that the mold keeps returning indicates an ongoing source of moisture. Testing the air or the black mold directly will only confirm the obvious fact that mold is growing in the closet. The best solution is to find and stop the source of the water, probably a plumbing leak, then remove and replace the damaged wall board in the closet.

> **MYTH: Mold is a sign of uncleanliness and poor housekeeping.**
>
> **REALITY: Mold will grow wherever it can find moisture.**

Have you ever noticed that mushrooms appear on your lawn after a rainy spell? The spores that produced them were lying dormant in the soil, waiting for the right conditions to hatch. The same thing happens with mold in the home. The spores are tiny and inactive when dry, but they are all around, patiently waiting for moisture to bring them to life as a fuzzy colony. Mold is not a sign of a dirty house, but a sign of one that is too damp.

Toxic Mold: Fact or Fiction?

"Ed McMahon's House Demolished! Toxic Mold the Cause." These days the news is full of stories about houses, office buildings, and schools contaminated with "toxic" or "black" mold. It's true that there are cases when mold is so bad that people have to pack up and leave, and even rare cases where a building is too infested to be salvaged. However, the reality is that mold is not particularly toxic and can usually be removed. The term "toxic mold" is a media creation, one often used to describe a particular species of mold, *Stachybotrys atra*, or "Stachy" for short.

Is there anything that is truly toxic about mold? Yes, many common species of mold produce toxins under the right conditions, but the levels you encounter indoors (even in extremely moldy homes) are too low to be a toxic threat. And yes, mold can produce toxins when present in food, such as the well-known contaminant of moldy peanuts, aflatoxin. Toxins produced by mold, sometimes called mycotoxins, have caused damage in animals who were fed large doses of the purified toxin. But again, there is very little evidence that mold spores contain enough mycotoxin to cause a problem through inhalation, the pathway of concern in moldy homes and workplaces.

Up to this point, we've probably sounded like mold's best friend suggesting it's an overblown myth, and that there's no cause for alarm. Well, now comes the bad news. Mold is bad for you if it has overgrown into visible or odorous colonies in your home, workplace, or child's school. The main concern is the fact that people can become allergic to mold, causing a variety of unpleasant respiratory effects that can look and feel like a cold, sinus infection, asthma, or bronchitis.

THE BEGINNING OF THE TOXIC MOLD SCARE

In 1994, the U.S. Centers for Disease Control (CDC) investigated eight cases of a rare medical condition in Cleveland: infant lung hemorrhage (bleeding in the lungs). The CDC found that the victims lived in water-damaged, moldy apartments that contained a particular black mold, *Stachybotrys atra*, which only grows on porous cellulose surfaces like fiber-based ceiling tiles. This finding was published in a scientific journal and then picked up by the media, which broadcast the story across the country. Suddenly black, toxic mold became a lethal invader. People were finding black mold with alarming frequency, especially in bathrooms, where moisture promotes scary-looking but harmless slimy black growth on tiles and grout. Health departments were flooded with calls, and the media kept fueling a fire that was unfortunately largely based on hype and misunderstanding.

The CDC couldn't substantiate the link between Stachy and infant lung hemorrhage they thought they had found in Cleveland, and in the end had to retract their results. However, the damage had been done—the term "toxic mold" had been coined. The media never went back to correct the story, and it continued to self-perpetuate. Stachy has since been blamed for a wide variety of other symptoms, including memory loss, fatigue, and neuropsychiatric disorders. In 2004, the Institute of Medicine of the National Academies issued a definitive review of the health effects of mold (IOM, 2004). This prestigious body concluded that the literature does not support an association between mold (even Stachy) and toxic effects. Recognizing the uncertainties in their review, they recommended further study.

TOXIC FILE

■ MOLD AND ASTHMA

Six-year-old Julia has had asthma since she was very young. Her parents have taken great care to control her disease by following all instructions from their pediatrician: they removed carpets from most of the house and have not adopted pets. Recently Julia has had a number of asthma attacks as well as more general breathing problems while at home. Noting the timing of her attacks, her parents concluded that something in the house must be affecting Julia's breathing.

The family had converted the basement into a playroom shortly before Julia's symptoms worsened. They occasionally noticed a slightly musty odor, but no more than they would have expected for a basement. However, when they pulled up the carpet in one corner, they found mold growing underneath. They called their pediatrician, who told them mold can trigger asthma attacks. The doctor strongly recommended that Julia not spend time in the basement.

As this Toxic File illustrates, damp homes and mold growth can produce respiratory symptoms, especially in asthmatics and those allergic to mold spores. (Other creatures such as bacteria and dust mites also grow better in damp environments and can contribute to asthma reactions; see Chapter 8). Mold allergies can develop over time, so it's best to get rid of your mold problem sooner rather than later.

It's important to note that by allergy, we do not mean anaphylactic shock, which is a very serious, even life-threatening acute allergic reaction that some people have to bee stings or certain medications. The mold allergy is more like hay fever or other seasonal allergies. It may take the form of a runny nose, congestion, itchy or irritated throat, or sneezing. A mold allergy may appear as a bad head cold or chronic sinus infection, and as we mentioned before, can worsen asthma.

So, how do you differentiate mold allergies from general above-the-neck misery? It often boils down to whether you feel worse when at home (or at work or school, wherever the mold problem is) and better after being away from that environment for a day or two. It also boils down to whether mold is actually present. Mold tends to get blamed for illnesses it has nothing to do with, ranging from arthritis to cancer. Even when respiratory symptoms are present, there is often another cause besides mold. For example, parents often worry that their child is being affected by mold in the classroom. We have to remember that kids come home sick from school all the time, with infections caused by viruses and bacteria spread from child to child. Without clear evidence of a mold problem, you shouldn't be blaming it for your illnesses.

Q *Why are there no standards for mold in indoor air?*

A Setting standards requires solid information on the contaminant levels needed to produce health effects in people. In the case of mold, there is no consistent pattern, because everyone's sensitivity is different. That's compounded by the fact that there are numerous mold species, and that background levels of mold can vary depending upon the time of year and where you live. For those reasons, it's unlikely that government agencies will set a specific numerical standard for mold anytime soon.

So, if there are no standards, and we are not sure whose health will be affected by mold, and we can't say which species are especially bad, how can we protect public health? **The simple bottom line is this: obvious mold growth indoors is not a good thing and should be stopped**. Mold is a crop you do not want to grow. But as you've learned by now, the mere presence of mold is usually not an emergency or reason to panic. Just use common sense and don't overreact.

Testing for Mold

As a general rule, we don't recommend that a home be tested for mold. However, if you see or smell mold, you have a problem that needs to be dealt with. If you think you might have a problem but are not sure, you can hire a mold inspector to come to your house. The inspector should do a thorough walk-through and visual inspection looking for mold in places where it typically grows (e.g., basements, attics, bathrooms) and wherever there has been water damage from leaks in the roof or plumbing. They should not offer to test your house's air for mold without very good cause. Testing would involve taking a sample of the air or contaminated surfaces and sending it off to a lab. Since there are no set standards and mold exists everywhere at some level, testing often produces inconclusive results. Nor do we recommend trying to identify specific species of mold, since it is unlikely such information will affect your cleanup decisions. Any type of obvious mold growth is important to stop.

There are a few borderline cases in which mold testing may be useful. If you have health symptoms consistent with mold (if you're ill at home but better away from it) but there's no obvious growth, an air test may help you to determine whether you are being exposed to an unknown source. Mold growing in hidden areas may be contributing spores to your breathing zone. This kind of growth is not likely to cause a lot of exposure, but highly sensitive individuals may be affected. But if the first thing an inspector or mold contractor tells you is that they need to conduct a mold test (which of course you would pay for), start shopping for another consultant.

Fixing Your Mold Problem

STEP 1: ELIMINATE THE WATER SOURCE

You can't stop the mold problem until you stop the moisture problem. Sometimes the moisture problem is ongoing and chronic—a damp basement or a rising water table from heavy rains. The solution may be as simple as a dehumidifier for the basement in the summertime. However, it may be more complicated if your house was not properly graded or if water from town sewers backs up into the basement during storms. Such chronic problems may need the attention of a waterproofing contractor.

When the water incursion is sudden and unique (e.g., a sudden flood or burst pipe), the rule of thumb is that mold will not grow if you can dry out the area within twenty-four to forty-eight hours. Carpets and furniture should be moved to a dry area to air out. Rooms and hidden areas such as crawl spaces should be ventilated with a fan or dried with a dehumidifier.

Less obvious water sources include small plumbing leaks, roof leaks, window leaks, and condensation around cold windows or plumbing fixtures. The average homeowner or renter will need professional assistance in solving these water problems. However, it's a good rule of thumb to keep humidity in your home relatively low, forty to sixty percent. Check your gutters and other drains and cracks around your windows. Don't ignore small plumbing leaks or any other sign of water incursion.

STEP 2: DECIDE IF YOU CAN CLEAN UP THE MOLD YOURSELF

You need to decide whether you can handle the cleanup yourself or need to hire a professional cleaning contractor. To make this decision, take note of how much mold growth is visible (heavy versus light) and the size of the area impacted. If the area is small (less than three feet by three feet), you should be able to handle the job yourself.

STEP 3: REMOVING MOLD FROM THE AFFECTED AREA

Do-It-Yourself Jobs

- Use protective equipment: N-95 respirators (available at hardware stores; these are inexpensive and disposable respirators similar to surgical masks), gloves, and goggles.

- Isolate the work area. Place plastic sheeting over the doors leading to the rest of the house. Create a negative pressure in the work area by placing a fan in the window facing out so that it pulls air from the room and sends it outside.

- Dry out and clean any materials that seem salvageable (carpets, furniture, books, etc.). If they have been wet for more than forty-eight hours, it may be best to discard them.

- Damp wipe and scrub hard surfaces with water and detergent (diluted bleach may be used, but is not necessary).

- Wet vacuum or HEPA (High Efficiency Particulate Air) vacuum soft or porous materials that are salvageable (e.g., carpets). HEPA vacuums can be rented or purchased.

- Dry out any cleaned items, if wet cleaning methods were used.

- Ventilate and use dehumidifiers in affected areas to remove lingering moisture.

If You Hire a Cleaning Contractor

- Selecting a contractor: find out what formal training they have in mold inspection and removal. Most states do not have a licensing process for mold-removal contractors, so beware of anyone who claims to have official certification.

- Find out if they plan to do any testing. In general, this is an unnecessary expense.

- Monitor the contractor's work, making sure they take precautions to protect themselves and you during the cleanup. This means protective clothing and respirators for the workers, and preventing the release of mold spores into the rest of the house.

- Find out if they plan to use a biocide—a chemical used to kill mold. The effectiveness of this step is unproven. Some biocides can be toxic, so it's important to ventilate the area thoroughly if they are used.

NOT ALL MOLD IS VISIBLE.

TOXIC FACT

In some instances, mold may grow in inaccessible areas of a building, where it can be harder to find and fix. These hidden locations include above the ceiling, inside walls that have been flooded, on the back side of Sheetrock, behind plumbing fixtures such as toilets where condensation occurs, inside ductwork for ventilation/air conditioner systems, in a crawlspace, or in the attic. Mold located in such isolated places may be less of a health hazard, since spores may not easily escape into your breathing zone. However, hidden mold should be investigated and removed. Some spores can find their way into the living area and your lungs, and furthermore, if left unchecked, mold can damage the building structure as it eats the organic material (wood, wallboard) it is living on. Consultants have moisture meters that can test hidden spaces for moisture content. However, if you suspect water damage inside a wall, you may have to open it up to fully inspect and fix it.

THE RISK INDEX FOR MOLD

As we've described, mold is not very toxic, but it is still risky due to its allergic properties. The fact that it is so widespread, both indoors and out, makes it a hazard for those who have asthma or are specifically allergic. Thus the major risk property for mold is not toxicity but allergenicity. Mold's overall risk is high, due to this property, which is reflected in the chart by an extra bar for allergenicity.

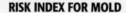

RISK INDEX FOR MOLD

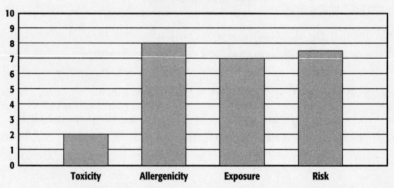

Fortunately, mold is usually easy to recognize and remove. Follow the mold checklist to make sure you are doing what's necessary to safeguard your home.

MOLD CHECKLIST

RECOGNIZING MOLD

❏ Determine if you have a moisture problem somewhere in the building. If so, find the source of moisture.

❏ Look for mold with your eyes and nose. If you see or smell mold, make sure you figure out where it is getting moisture.

❏ Estimate the size of the problem area. A homeowner can handle small cleanups.

❏ Have professionals investigate larger problems.

❏ In most situations, do not test for mold.

REMOVING MOLD

❏ Find and fix the moisture source.

❏ Dry out affected areas and materials.

❏ Throw out porous materials that were damp for more than twenty-four to forty-eight hours.

❏ Clean or scrub mold off hard surfaces.

❏ Don't use biocides in most situations.

❏ If you do the cleanup yourself, use a protective respirator.

KEEPING MOLD FROM RETURNING

❏ Keep areas dry. Use dehumidifiers or air conditioners to cut down on summertime humidity.

❏ Install vents in bathrooms and for appliances (dryers and stoves).

❏ Stop groundwater from entering basement.

❏ Watch for roof leaks and gutter clogging.

❏ Act quickly after a natural or man-made flood.

❏ Increase air movement in the home. Open windows and use fans in problematic areas such as the attic.

❑   Decrease condensation on pipes by covering them with insulation.

❑   Do not use antimicrobial coatings or sealants that are meant to stop mold from regrowing. Their effectiveness is unproven, and the chemicals used may be toxic.

CHAPTER 4

Asbestos

The drop ceiling in your family room. The floor tile in your kitchen. The grayish-white insulation around the pipes in your basement. These common household materials seem innocuous enough. Very few people give them a second thought. Your neighbor would sound like a real worrywart if he said his ceiling tile could cause cancer. However, these are the types of materials that can contain asbestos, especially if your home was built before 1975. Asbestos is a known human carcinogen that can be released from these materials if they are damaged.

Asbestos is a naturally occurring mineral fiber that has been mined and purified because it is light, durable, and fire resistant. There are actually six types of asbestos fibers, with chrysotile, amosite, and crocidolite being the most common still in use. All asbestos fibers are toxic, but unlike other substances, their toxicity is due to physical rather than chemical properties.

The long, microscopically thin asbestos fibers are up to 1,000 times thinner than a strand of hair, so thin and light, they can remain suspended in the air for many hours and freely travel from room to room. The fibers will eventually settle down in dust but can easily become airborne once again by routine activities: walking, vacuuming, opening windows, etc. That's why asbestos can pose an ongoing health threat once it contaminates the home.

There is an even more sinister hazard associated with asbestos's long, thin shape. The tiny, spearlike fibers are skinny enough to pass through the maze of airways that lead to the deep lung after being inhaled. There, they become impaled on cells that line the lung. Asbestos fibers are not only long and thin but also very durable. They remain impaled in the lung, causing an inflammatory reaction. The damaged cells are difficult for the lung to remove and can scar over, causing a loss of lung function. This sets the stage for lung cancer, which can take twenty to thirty years to develop. Asbestosis, an emphysema-like disease caused by asbestos scarring, can also take up to thirty years to develop.

The signature effect of asbestos is a specific type of cancer called mesothelioma, a rare disease for which the only known cause is asbestos. Mesothelioma occurs when asbestos fibers get through the lung lining cells and do their damage to the pleural sac under the lungs. Normally, very few toxins make their way into this sensitive region. However, asbestos's shape and size allow it to enter the sac, instigate inflammation, and eventually cause mesothelioma.

Q *Where was asbestos used in the past?*

A In lots of places, some where you'd least expect it:

- **Boats:** Asbestos insulation was used around boilers and pipes on ships built in the 1930s and '40s. Shipyard workers were exposed to high levels of asbestos and became the first group shown to contract lung cancer and mesothelioma from asbestos exposure.

- **Homes and Schools:** Asbestos was used to insulate heating system pipes and boilers during the 1950s and '60s. It was also sprayed onto ceilings in classrooms; this kind of asbestos became a high concern and was targeted for removal beginning in the 1970s.

- **Commercial Buildings:** Asbestos fireproofing material was sprayed onto many surfaces, including steel girders and decorative and acoustic plaster. When the World Trade Center collapsed during the September 2001 attacks, asbestos fireproofing was released, contaminating much of lower Manhattan.

- **Many types of building products,** including floor and ceiling tiles, joint and caulking compounds, roofing material, textured paints, exterior shingles, and car parts, such as brake pads and linings, clutch facings, and gaskets.

After asbestos was recognized as a health hazard in the early 1970s, it was banned. This ban has been scaled back in recent years, but still applies to fireproofing and insulation, flooring felt, corrugated paper, decorative paints, and sprayed-on decorative materials. The USEPA does not track the sale of products containing asbestos. However, certain asbestos materials such as pipe wrap insulation and floor or ceiling tiles have not made a comeback and thus are uncommon. The most likely products to contain asbestos today are roofing materials and, to a lesser extent, floor tiles manufactured overseas. It is a good idea to ask the store where you are buying materials if any contain asbestos. You should also check the labels.

Since the most common and significant uses of asbestos in the home (fireproofing and insulation) were banned in 1973 and have not come back into use, homes built after that date are not likely to contain asbestos materials. For homes built prior to that date, homeowners should have all suspect materials tested.

> **MYTH: Asbestos has caused cancer in people who have it in their homes.**
>
> **REALITY: While asbestos is a known human lung carcinogen, there are no cases in which homeowner exposure has been shown to produce cancer.**

Asbestos has not caused the type of toxicity around the home that, for example, lead has. In most cases, the asbestos in building materials has not been released at levels high enough to noticeably affect adults or children. Asbestos-related cancer occurs in highly exposed mine workers and their family contacts, not in average households or schools. That said, it is important to treat asbestos with the respect due a potent carcinogen and make sure that it is either removed or kept in check in your home environment.

ASBESTOS AT SCHOOL CAUSES ALARM

Mike came home from school one day with a note from the principal. It grabbed his parents' attention, much more so than the typical meeting notice or fund-raising flyer. The note said that asbestos insulation would be removed from the gymnasium during the school year. Mike's parents had heard of asbestos from legal ads looking for mesothelioma victims as clients. A quick scan of the Internet was pretty alarming—potent human carcinogen, lung damage, takes a long time to clear the lungs. Discovering

TOXIC FILE

that this toxic mineral was present in their child's school made the issue too close for comfort.

Mike's parents could understand why asbestos was put into the school: when it was built in the 1960s, asbestos was the best fire retardant and it also made building materials durable. But, they asked with some outrage, why has it taken so long to address this hazard? Has asbestos been getting spread around the school and affecting kids' health? At a public meeting, a teacher pointed out that a number of school staff have developed cancer during the past decade, and asked if this could be related to the asbestos in the school. Mike's parents asked how the removal would be conducted and how the students' safety would be guaranteed.

A local health official explained that asbestos exposure was only associated with lung cancer and mesothelioma (cancer of the lining of the lungs). Asbestos was not linked to the types of cancers cited by the teacher. The official also noted that the gym ceiling had never been damaged, so there was no reason to worry that asbestos in the ceiling was ever spread around. This removal was just a precaution to make sure the asbestos was never released. The asbestos contractors hired to do the removal would isolate the affected areas during the process. Plastic would be used to line all the walls, doors, and windows. Negative air pressure would be maintained in the cleanup area to ensure that no airborne asbestos fibers could escape to the rest of the building. As an added precaution, air testing would be conducted during the cleanup just outside the removal area to make sure contamination did not spread.

This Toxic File illustrates a fact that surprises many people: asbestos is still present in schools, homes, and office buildings. There is no law requiring asbestos removal; however, schools are required to test all materials that may contain asbestos and then develop a written plan on how they will manage any items that test positive.

Q *My father was a plumber. He worked with asbestos his whole life. He never got sick, and always claimed that asbestos never caused him any problems. How can asbestos make us sick?*

A Your father is lucky that his asbestos exposure did not progress to lung disease or cancer. The longer and more intense the exposure, the more likely asbestos poisoning is. Asbestos workers have five times the risk of lung cancer than the general public. Smoking multiplies that risk, resulting in a rate over fifty times higher than normal. The fact that your father did not become ill from working with asbestos really indicates that he wasn't exposed to high enough levels to cause asbestosis or cancer. We also need to remember that cancer depends on many factors, some of which are host-specific (immune system, lung clearance, repair mechanisms). Therefore, an exposure that might cause cancer in one person may go unnoticed in another.

Everyday Asbestos Exposures

Asbestos-related diseases sound pretty grim. Given the fact that asbestos is present in so many products, should we be worried that there could be an epidemic of asbestosis or cancer?

The answer is no, an epidemic is unlikely. As we've discussed, compared to the exposures that caused cancer in asbestos workers, exposures in most private homes, schools, and other buildings are minor (HEI, 1991). The major exception is for people who live in areas where asbestos mining or manufacturing takes place (see sidebar on Libby, Montana).

We are all exposed to a small amount of asbestos every day. These "background" exposures are the combined result of manufactured and natural sources. Outdoor air contains low levels of asbestos fibers that come from natural deposits in the earth's crust and fibers from automobile brake pads. Most buildings constructed prior to 1975 have a variety of asbestos materials, which can release low levels. For most of us, this background exposure does not result in disease. That's because our lungs have *some* ability to remove the fibers and repair the effects of asbestos before they lead to cancer. Background levels of asbestos fibers in outdoor and indoor air are generally too low to present a serious cancer risk.

The other key factor in the exposure equation is duration. The longer you are exposed to asbestos fibers, the greater your risk. The relationship is thought to be fairly direct. For example, twenty years of exposure is twenty times riskier than one year of exposure. Therefore, brief exposures at home or school will not cause much increase in overall lifetime risk. However, it is important to treat asbestos in your home or school with the respect due a potent carcinogen and keep exposures to a minimum. This means prompt removal of any damaged asbestos-containing materials. See the checklist at the end of the chapter for more information.

WHAT DOES LIBBY, MONTANA, HAVE IN COMMON WITH YOUR ATTIC?

In the late 1990s, officials discovered that the small town of Libby, Montana, had a unique and serious asbestos problem. A vermiculite mining operation running since the 1920s had spread asbestos throughout the town. (The mine had a natural deposit of asbestos that contaminated the vermiculite.)

Mining wastes often contain hazardous materials that need to be carefully managed. Asbestos is a worst-case scenario, because it's so light that it is easily windblown. Libby's case was particularly bad because the mining waste had been used around town as fill material or left in waste piles, from which asbestos blew into people's yards and homes. This led to a high degree of exposure over long periods of time. Health studies in residents have found elevated rates of asbestos-related cancers and asbestosis. A major cleanup is currently taking place, and the mine is now closed.

What does this have to do with your attic? Vermiculite is a mineral that has the unusual property of expanding like popcorn when heated. The expanded vermiculite is very lightweight and is used in many consumer products, including attic insulation and garden soil. Since most vermiculite sold prior to 1990 came from Libby, Montana, most vermiculite insulation from that era has some asbestos in it. (Vermiculite mined today comes from other areas, so it's not contaminated with asbestos.)

Attic insulation with vermiculite is a granular product poured into the spaces between the ceiling joists. It is usually gray to brown in color, and has a coarse texture. Individual pieces can range from not much larger than a grain of sand to over one inch. If you have attic insulation that meets this description, it is best to assume it is vermiculite and that it contains asbestos (see illustrations at www.epa.gov/asbestos/pubs/insulationbrochure2.pdf).

Testing vermiculite for asbestos contamination is not currently recommended by the USEPA. Questions remain about the laboratory analysis of asbestos in vermiculite, and currently there is no guarantee that results will be conclusive. The USEPA is working on developing more reliable test methods, so stay tuned. In the meantime, if you think you have vermiculite insulation in your walls or attic that was installed prior to 1990, take the following precautions:

- Leave it alone as much as possible.
- Decrease the number of visits and time spent in the attic.

- If you decide to remove the insulation, have a professional do the job.
- Plan renovations so that the vermiculite is not disturbed, or have it removed first.
- Seal cracks in ceilings that may allow insulation to leak into living areas.
- This advice may change as new research on vermiculite becomes available. Check the USEPA website on a regular basis.

DOES ASBESTOS STOP THE SALE?

Alice found her dream starter home, a 1950s Cape in mint condition. A home inspector found no major problems, but mentioned that the insulation on the basement pipes looked like asbestos. He also noted that floor tiles in the basement were cracked and might contain asbestos. Alice decided that the presence of cancer-causing asbestos was a definite "no go" on purchasing the home. However, at the urging of her real estate agent, she did a little more research on the issue, with one step being a call to the state health department.

The health officials told her the only way to be sure if the pipe insulation and floor tiles have asbestos is to have them tested by a licensed consultant. They also pointed out that there was no regulation that required removal of asbestos in a home, and that if it's in good condition, it's not a health risk and should be left alone. Alice asked if she should get the air in the basement tested. The health department told her not to test the air, since the results can be highly variable and hard to interpret. Instead, they recommended a physical inspection, which would determine if Alice had asbestos-containing materials and whether they have deteriorated to a point where they could present a hazard.

A consultant for the home seller found that the pipe wrap and floor tiles did contain asbestos. The damaged tiles were carefully removed as a condition of house sale, but the pipe insulation that was in good condition was left undisturbed. Alice moved in, a more educated consumer with a little peace of mind.

As this Toxic File illustrates, asbestos doesn't always need to be removed. It's only a health hazard if the product it is in becomes damaged and releases fibers into the air where they can be inhaled. If the product remains intact with no fibers flaking free, it is not a hazard.

A key term in this regard is "friable." The USEPA defines a friable material as one that can be crumbled with hand pressure (as when products age, dry out, and lose their integrity). An asbestos-containing material that is friable can easily release fibers and should be removed by a licensed contractor. In a typical home where the pipe wrap and boiler insulation are not friable, the best option is to leave the insulation in place. You need to take care not to allow activities in the area that might damage the material. However, if you're planning on renovating, you must properly remove the asbestos material before work begins.

Some people may decide to remove asbestos-containing materials even if they are in good condition. That way, they can be sure asbestos will not become a hazard in the future, particularly in the case of an emergency (e.g., plumbing leak) that would require rapid access to the pipes. Encapsulation, or covering the asbestos, is also an approved process to reduce the potential for fiber release. However, encapsulation involves all the precautions needed for removal, so most people who decide to take action go with removal rather than encapsulation.

Q *What does the government require?*

A Most government regulations cover the inspection and management of asbestos in schools and public buildings. Very few regulations address asbestos in the home unless there is a plan to remove the asbestos or if a home is to be demolished. There is usually not a requirement to test homes for asbestos even at the time of sale. However, most home inspectors will identify suspected asbestos material and some may even test material to assure its content.

The federal 1986 Asbestos Hazard Emergency Response Act (AHERA) requires public and private schools to inspect for asbestos and to develop plans to manage the asbestos-containing materials. The inspections need to be repeated every three years, and teachers and parents must be notified of any changes to the management plan. AHERA has caused most schools to inspect and remove damaged asbestos over the past twenty years. There is generally little asbestos left in schools to worry about—what might remain is generally in good condition and not an immediate hazard. However, it needs to be inspected regularly.

Q *My child's school is planning to have some asbestos materials removed. We are afraid that due to low budgets, they will have the school janitor do the removal after hours when no one is around. Is this illegal?*

A Yes. A licensed contractor must conduct any asbestos removal in a school or other building. These removals are subject to very strict precautions: the removal area must be sealed off from the rest of the building with plastic sheeting. Large air filters must also be placed within the enclosed work area. These filters draw air from inside the enclosed work area and capture floating asbestos fibers, in addition to creating a negative pressure within the work area. A negative pressure ensures that air (and fibers) will not flow out of the work area toward the rest of the building. In schools, air testing is required during and after the asbestos removal to assure that the rest of the building has not been contaminated.

The USEPA has established clearance levels for asbestos-removal projects. The asbestos air levels must be less than 0.01 fibers per cubic centimeter, or less than the background level measured outside. Air monitoring is only recommended during and after abatements and is not normally used to evaluate buildings before removal begins. That may seem contrary to common sense. Why would you not want to do an air test to see if an asbestos problem exists in your home or school? The answer is, because fibers settle out of the air within twenty-four to forty-eight hours. Any air-test result is dependent on how much activity occurred in an area before and during the air test. Air tests on an unoccupied room may provide a false negative result, since all the asbestos had settled out of the air and into the dust.

Neither is dust testing normally used to evaluate the level of asbestos hazard. No standards currently exist for asbestos in dust, making results very hard to interpret. A thorough visual inspection, combined with "bulk" testing to identify the presence of asbestos in building materials, is still the primary method to decide if an asbestos abatement is needed.

Q *The house I want to buy has some old-looking asbestos pipe insulation in one area of the basement. Some of it has fallen on the floor. The seller is willing to have it removed as a condition of the house sale. Shouldn't I be* *worried that the fibers may have spread throughout the rest of the house?*

A That's a good question, and a tough one to answer. Damaged asbestos insulation may have sent fibers through the rest of the basement, and although unlikely, possibly into the other floors of the house. Rather than testing, the best answer is to ask the seller to have the house thoroughly cleaned by a professional service that uses a special vacuum cleaner (HEPA vacuum). The HEPA will collect any fibers that might have traveled to other parts of the house. In addition, simple wet cleaning methods like mopping will do a good job of reducing fiber levels on hard surfaces throughout the house.

Various professional services are involved in the testing, inspection and removal of asbestos. It is not a good idea to hire the same consultant to inspect and remove asbestos. You want an independent inspector who can provide oversight of the removal company. Government agencies and trade associations sponsor training courses for asbestos professionals. Most states have a listing of approved asbestos contractors.

To find a list of certified professionals in your area, contact your regional USEPA office or state asbestos program (USEPA Asbestos Hotline: 800-471-7127). The USEPA website www.epa.gov/asbestos also lists regional and state contacts.

THE RISK INDEX FOR ASBESTOS

Our message on asbestos can be summed up simply: "Don't overreact." The word asbestos has become almost synonymous with mesothelioma and lung cancer. While it's true that asbestos is a known human carcinogen and has cut short the lives of workers who received high-level exposures, there is little evidence of disease in the general public with lower-level exposures. The following risk index illustrates this fact, showing high toxicity but low exposure, leading to a fairly modest overall risk. Of course, people exposed under unusual circumstances, such as in Libby, Montana, are at much higher risk.

This modest risk level for the general public does not mean that asbestos

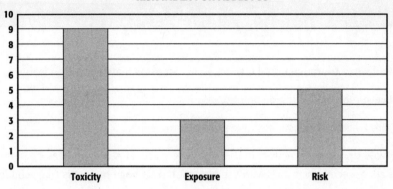

should be ignored. Living, working, or attending school in buildings that harbor damaged asbestos materials carries a theoretical increased cancer risk. All sources of exposure should be properly inspected and removed, if damaged. For home owners and home buyers, this begins with simple visual inspections that can bring you safety and piece of mind.

ASBESTOS CHECKLIST

DO:

❏   Perform a thorough visual inspection for asbestos material in your home.

❏   Leave materials in good condition alone.

❏   Hire a licensed consultant to test suspect materials.

❏   Avoid unnecessary activity in the area where asbestos material has been identified, especially activities with the potential to damage materials (e.g., children's recreation, construction).

❏   Check asbestos materials regularly for new wear or damage. Make sure they have not aged to the point where they have become friable.

❏   Hire a licensed professional to do a removal if material is damaged or renovations are planned in the area.

❏   Consider placing a new floor over asbestos floor tiles.

❏   Check the credentials of all professionals hired.

DON'T:

❏   Assume all asbestos is a major health hazard.

❏   Disturb materials containing asbestos if they are in good condition.

❏   Dust or vacuum debris that may contain asbestos (only licensed professionals should handle this type of cleanup).

❏   Hire the same consultant to do testing and cleanup.

❏   Have yourself or your family tested for asbestos exposure (medical testing is never needed).

SECTION 2

Toxics in What We Eat, Drink, and Buy at the Store

CHAPTER 5

Food Toxics

Food toxicology is in many ways a Pandora's box—when we open the lid, a legion of chemicals spill out into the light of day, and we can't stuff them back inside. Toxics like mercury, PCBs, dioxin, acrylamide, phthalates, polycyclic hydrocarbons, pesticides, and perchlorate grab headlines and make consumers nervous. After all, we are talking about the basic elements of life, what we put into our bodies every day. If that's contaminated, then we're contaminated.

What is the health effect of all this food contamination? The answer to that question can seem elusive and complex. Public health toxicologists often tread lightly on the subject because of the lack of concrete answers, and because many of the questions we raise challenge the choices we're used to making as consumers and as a society. Furthermore, the Food and Drug Administration (FDA) technically has responsibility for food safety, so it's sometimes convenient to refer the tough questions to them. Safeguarding America's food supply is a difficult job, especially since certain contaminants are pretty much unavoidable. It seems as if every night, a new finding is jumping right off the data sheet and onto the six o'clock news. Some would say these are false issues, Pandora's fantasies and illusions. Certain chemicals are at such trace levels that no one should be concerned—they've been in food for many years, and only now that we have the technology to detect such tiny amounts do we even know about them. We'd be foolish to get caught up in every novel chemical detected in our food supply. That said, we'd be remiss if we completely ignored them.

This chapter will address some of the major risks raised by toxics in food. This Pandora's box is quite large; the more you peer in, the more you find. The Milky Way is a reasonable analogy: the further you gaze toward the blackness of space, the more stars you see that blend into the background. Similarly, many chemicals in food are in tiny quantities and smear together to create an ingredient list that is far too complex to take apart and analyze one by one. We have chosen to focus on the major and most avoidable food chemical risks.

This chapter is broken into three parts: Boomerang Toxics (we throw them out, and they come right back), Intentional Additives to Our Diet (including pesticides, dietary hormones, and animal antibiotics), and Containers and Cookware in Our Diet (chemicals that leach from cookware and packaging).

Boomerang Toxics

The word "boomerang" is intended to be descriptive, not fanciful. Industrial societies have been throwing these persistent chemicals out into the environment for many years, and like boomerangs, they have been coming right back to us. But unlike boomerangs, these chemicals go out in one form (smoky plumes or oozing sludge) and come back hidden in our beef, fish, and dairy. Telecommunications have made our planet a smaller place in a positive way, allowing people to exchange ideas across the globe, but boomerang chemicals have shrunk the planet in a negative way. Their globetrotting behavior sends them from one pole to the other and everywhere in between. My throwaway chemical may be your food contaminant, even if we live five thousand miles apart and you are a polar bear.

In this section, we're going to talk about four major boomerang toxics: mercury, dioxin, PCBs, and persistent pesticides.

MERCURY

Mercury is probably the most familiar of all food toxics. The silvery bead of mercury in your thermometer seems innocuous enough. However, this heavy metal is a master of disguise, changing physical state from liquid to gas, and from gas to fish contaminant. Mercury moves in mysterious but dangerous ways, multiplying in concentration as it makes its way up the food chain to our dinner table.

Why is mercury hazardous? Because it is a highly mobile and reactive metal that attacks cellular proteins. It stays in the body a long time, especially if it manages to get into the brain. This is a particular concern for babies: there is a barrier that protects the brain from toxics in the blood (the blood/brain barrier), but it's not well developed in the fetus and infants. Therefore, mercury exposure during pregnancy can more easily reach the brain and cause damage during critical stages of development. At high doses, this can translate into fetal death and birth defects. At lower doses, mercury causes more subtle effects on brain development. Epidemiology studies show that mothers who had higher mercury exposure during pregnancy (from fish consumption) had children who performed below average on standard neurological tests and were slower learners in school (Grandjean et al., 1997). The study proves that exposure in utero can have long-term consequences on learning and behavior. There is also a chance that mercury may be related to the development of attention deficit disorder (ADD) and autism (Mutter et al., 2005).

Mercury is also toxic to the nervous system of adults, although it appears that these risks are about three times greater in the fetus. Therefore, it is important for everyone to watch out for mercury exposure, but especially so for pregnant women and young children.

FISH CONSUMPTION IS THE PRIMARY SOURCE OF MERCURY EXPOSURE.

Most of our exposure to mercury comes from our diet, in fact, a particular part of our diet: fish. How did it get there? Through a great example of the boomerang effect we were talking about earlier.

Mercury has been present in the trash, medical waste, and fuels we've been burning for hundreds of years. But burning doesn't destroy mercury—you can't destroy an element. It only liberates it, sending it up the smokestack and out into the environment in the form of a gas or tiny particles that can travel long distances and fall out into bodies of water. Once in water, mercury settles to the bottom, where it is changed by bacteria to a form that is particularly good at bioaccumulating in fish: methyl mercury. This gets ingested by little fish, and as bigger fish eat little ones, they accumulate methyl mercury in their flesh, too. As top-of-the-chain predators, every time we eat fish we ingest a mercury dose that has accumulated over many fish generations and species. Contamination is usually greatest in the largest and oldest fish—just the kind we like to eat.

People often worry that the bodies of water that have fish with high mercury levels are too contaminated for swimming. This is rarely the case. The levels in fish are thousands of times higher than the levels in water. However, it is always a good idea to check with your town's health director to make sure the water is safe to swim in.

> **MYTH:** Mercury contamination of fish is the worst from water bodies in urban and industrial areas.
>
> **REALITY:** Mercury in fish is often just as much of a problem in remote areas as in the areas where the chemical was initially put into the air.

You might think the urban and industrial areas that are the sources of mercury release would have the highest mercury contamination. That expectation was shattered when data from across the northeastern United States started coming in during the late 1980s. The data showed that lakes in rural Maine, far away from industrial incinerators, were as heavily contaminated as lakes in New Jersey. In fact, mercury levels were fairly uniform throughout the whole Northeast. We learned that mercury is both a regional and a local issue: what comes into your region from upwind incinerators is as important as what is emitted locally.

To avoid mercury-contaminated freshwater fish (fish from rivers and lakes), you can't simply go to a different pond—it's just as likely to be dangerous. That's why approximately twenty states have blanket warnings for the entire state against consuming too much of captured large predator fish like bass, walleye, and pickerel. How about going to a different state? Be careful—just because a state doesn't have an advisory doesn't mean its fish are cleaner. Not all states have the resources to test for fish contaminants or interpret the data, and some don't have advisory boards at all. That's why it's so important to ask questions of state or local officials before eating fish from a particular locale. Have they tested the fish? Do they know how many fish can be eaten safely by pregnant women and young children? Do they know which are the safest water bodies and cleanest species of fish? You can get a general idea about fish advisories in a particular state by going to the USEPA's National Listing of Fish Advisories at http://www .epa.gov/waterscience/fish/advisories/index.html.

Something else to keep in mind is that fish in rivers tend to have lower contaminant concentrations than fish in lakes. Mercury that deposits in a lake can accumulate over time, while rivers are always recharging with fresh water and sediment. So, you can eat a little more fish from rivers and streams than from lakes, unless the river has been the site of a mercury spill.

TOXIC FACT

FISH FROM THE SUPERMARKET CAN ALSO BE HIGH IN MERCURY.

Keeping mercury off your shopping list requires being aware of the mercury content of market fish. For most of us, what's in the fish we buy is more important that what's in local waterways because we spend a lot more time standing in the check-out line than on the pier with our fishing rod. To make matters more complicated, most fish sold in markets don't come from local waters but from fish farms or the ocean. Fortunately, most of what is sold commercially are marine species that tend to be lower in mercury than fish from rivers and lakes. However, certain species, most notably swordfish and shark, can have high levels of mercury, and should be avoided by the high-risk groups: pregnant women, women of child-bearing age (who might become pregnant), nursing mothers, and young children.

Canned tuna has low to moderate levels of mercury, and isn't a concern if eaten occasionally, once or twice a week. However, eating canned tuna more frequently can push a pregnant woman over the recommended mercury exposure limit, especially if she's combining it with other types of fish (e.g., tuna for lunch and sushi for dinner). Canned "light" or "chunk light" tuna has lower mercury levels than "white" tuna, and should be chosen more often. The advice for fish-eaters in general is that the high-risk group should only eat two meals per week, regardless of the type of fish and source.

Q *I've been having trouble getting pregnant and have had two miscarriages. Among other things, I've had a blood mercury test done. The doctors said the result was high (70 ug/L). Is this the reason I can't get pregnant? Should I even be trying to get pregnant?*

A Your level of mercury is high compared to most people, but it is still low compared to the levels that can cause serious problems during pregnancy. Levels high enough to affect fertility are usually high enough to cause other symptoms, such as disorders of the nervous system. You would have noticed these symptoms if your mercury exposure was high enough to cause your miscarriages. So, there's likely some other explanation for your inability to maintain a pregnancy.

Your second question, about whether you should even be trying to get pregnant, takes more thought. Your current blood level is in the range where some effects on brain development in your child are probable. Ideally, your blood concentration would be ten times lower when you become pregnant.

You probably have high levels of mercury because you are a frequent consumer of fish that contain the metal. We recommend that you moderate your fish consumption and switch to species with lower amounts of mercury (see the listing at the end of the chapter for more information). The time it takes for half of the accumulated mercury to be removed from your body by natural processes (the half-life) is roughly two months. That means your blood level can be expected to drop from 70 to 35 ug/L in two months if you stop ingesting mercury now. Since you're starting from such a high level, you should wait three half-lives (six months) before getting pregnant. If you can't wait that long, still switch to fish low in mercury as soon as you can.

CONTROLLING MERCURY IN FISH

The debate over mercury in fish has heated up as more and more states have started testing for mercury and finding it in fish at potentially risky levels. This is compounded by the fact that recent human studies have found learning deficits in children born to women who had only moderate exposure during pregnancy (NAS, 2000). All in an era when fish is being promoted as a healthy alternative to red meat! Eat more, eat less, eat only certain fish—the message can be confusing. What everyone agrees on is, the less mercury entering the environment from this time forward, the better.

Strides have been made on three fronts in the attempt to decrease the amount of mercury released into the environment. 1) Mercury has been phased out of many consumer products such as thermometers, batteries, paint, and flashing sneakers. 2) A number of mercury-containing products are now collected at town hazardous waste sites rather than with the garbage, which keeps more mercury out of incinerators. 3) Incinerators are now required to implement better mercury controls.

Future efforts to control mercury releases will hopefully go farther. However, it will likely be decades before we see improvement in fish contaminant levels because of the large pool of mercury already in the environment.

THE RISK INDEX FOR MERCURY

Exactly how risky are the contaminants in fish? The exposure factor for mercury is high, because millions of Americans ingest the toxin in fish. The National Academy of Sciences report on mercury (NAS, 2000) estimated that 60,000 women of childbearing age have enough mercury in their blood for their babies to be at risk for developmental problems. Other studies indicate that the levels of PCBs and dioxins in certain fish can be a reproductive and cancer risk (see later sections in this chapter). Therefore, the overall risk index for fish contaminants is high, which underscores the importance of heeding fish-consumption warnings.

RISK INDEX FOR MERCURY

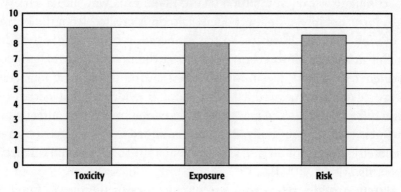

WHAT ABOUT MERCURY IN DENTAL AMALGAMS?

You are also exposed to mercury if you, like millions of Americans, are walking around with dental amalgam tooth fillings. Until recently, this silver-based filling, which contains significant quantities of mercury, was the most commonly used material for fixing cavities. Fortunately, most of this mercury remains in your mouth, but small amounts do get out of the filling and enter your blood. Studies indicate that people with mercury amalgam fillings have higher mercury blood levels than people with none—those with eight or more fillings had a level that was sixty percent higher than the no-amalgam group (Becker et al., 2002). However, their total level of mercury was below the level of concern for reproductive and other types of health risks, the kind most commonly caused by fish consumption. The bottom line is, it's best to not let your dentist install new mercury amalgam into your mouth, but it's not worth the effort to rip out the amalgam that's already there.

DIOXIN: THE ENVIRONMENTAL HORMONE

Another boomerang chemical, dioxin is one of the most feared environmental toxics. Like mercury, dioxin doesn't break down, but instead bioaccumulates through the food chain, making its way into a variety of foods, most notably animal products. Dioxin is created from the burning of chlorine-containing wastes, so the incineration of plastics (which contain chlorine) in trash-to-energy plants over the past fifty years has added to the environmental dioxin load. Recent efforts to improve incinerator capture of dioxins has helped, and there is evidence of a decrease in dioxin in human tissues in recent years. However, most of us already have high levels stored in our body. Because continued exposure may be an important risk factor, modifying your eating habits to a "low-dioxin diet" is a good idea (NAS, 2003).

Dioxin actually refers to a specific member of the dioxin family of chemicals, 2,3,7,8-TCDD. This specific dioxin has just the right shape to fit into a protein (the dioxin receptor) that is normally floating in the cells of our body. When TCDD binds to its receptor, it unlocks the door to the cell's nucleus, allowing it access to the information code that governs how a cell looks and behaves: its DNA. That's a lot like how natural hormones work, except the body tightly controls when hormones are released and how they can affect genes. TCDD is an unnatural hormone-like agent; when it interacts with DNA, it turns on many genes inappropriately. Once TCDD starts hacking, the readout of the DNA can become deranged, turning on genes that should be quiet and causing toxicity and cancer.

Among dioxin's effects in animals and in at least some human studies are cancer, endometriosis, diabetes, immune disorders, altered blood lipids leading to cardiovascular disease, learning disorders, and impaired male reproductive function (ATSDR, 1998). Animal studies indicate that TCDD is the most potent carcinogen ever discovered. There is debate as to whether it is so exquisitely potent in people—even if it isn't, it would still be potent enough to warrant dietary changes.

Can TCDD cause these effects at the exposure levels typical in food? Before we start blaming dioxin for all of our medical ills, we have to keep in mind that doses in the general population are generally lower than what has been shown to cause disease. However, we cannot rule out the possibility that our accumulation of dioxin, along with other long-lived organochlorines (e.g., PCBs; see the next section), is contributing to the high frequency of some illnesses. Since we can't metabolize or excrete TCDD very well, even a small amount every day can build up over time. This can lead to a chronic effect on the way that genes are expressed and how they control our nervous, endocrine, and immune systems.

Estimates by USEPA and the National Academy of Science indicate that the average American's body burden of dioxin is already in the range where effects can occur. In other words, the less dioxin we are exposed to from here on out, the better. We can't chelate or otherwise scrub dioxin out of our systems—it's a long, slow clearance process. If you stopped all dioxin intake right now, it would take five to ten years to get rid of only half of what's in your body.

While decreasing dioxin ingestion in adults is a worthwhile goal, it's especially important in children, early in their years of accumulation. It's possible to stop the chain of passing dioxin along to the next generation. A major goal for the next generation of nursing moms should be to not have to worry about things like dioxin, PCBs, and persistent pesticides in their breast milk.

OUR MAIN EXPOSURE TO DIOXIN IS FROM HIGH-FAT ANIMAL PRODUCTS AND FARM-RAISED FISH.

A wide array of foods have trace levels of dioxin, but dioxin deposits are greatest in the fatty tissues of animals, and is stored there until a higher predator consumes the animal and makes it part of its own fatty tissue. In this way, dioxin moves up the food chain, becoming more concentrated as it goes. When we eat fatty animal products—including beef and dairy items such as whole-fat ice cream, butter, cheese, milk, and yogurt, dioxin is a hidden and unavoidable part of the meal (Jensen and Bolger, 2001).

Farm-raised fish are another source of dietary dioxin. Although they're portrayed as being grown in carefully controlled environments, and thus clear of contaminants, the diet of farm-raised fish is not so carefully controlled. Dioxin and several persistent pesticides are present in the fish oil which is used to supplement the diet of growing salmon (Hites, et al., 2004), which is why farm-raised salmon have recently been in the news for their dioxin, PCBs, and pesticide content. These toxics are considerably higher in farm-raised as compared to wild salmon (Hites et al., 2004; Foran et al., 2005), and to a lesser degree in farm-raised catfish (Jensen and Bolger et al., 2001). There is not enough data on other farm-raised fish to know whether dioxin is an issue in them as well. The bottom line is, farm-raised as opposed to wild-marine fish can be the major source of dioxin in your diet.

THE RISK INDEX FOR DIETARY DIOXIN

The chart reflects the fact that dioxin is far more potent at producing cancer, immunologic, neurologic, and developmental effects than other chemicals, even in humans. While some have argued that dioxin is somewhat less potent in humans than in test animals, the potency is so high in animals that dioxin is still the the most dangerous carcinogenic threat we face. Dioxin exposure ranking is also high, since dioxin is present in many foods. Based upon how much dioxin we have in our bodies, we can say that our typical exposure is high—high enough to put us on the precipice for toxic effects. The unfortunate reality is, no matter who you are, your dioxin risk is high, and the less exposure the better.

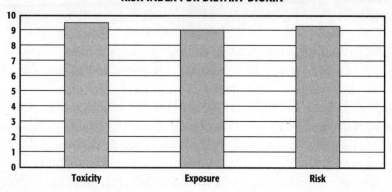

RISK INDEX FOR DIETARY DIOXIN

PREVENTING DIOXIN EXPOSURE

When most people think of dioxin, they think of trash-to-energy inciner-ators. But the reality is, our major exposure is from food, not from living near incinerators. For beef and dairy, the dioxin avoidance message is sim-ple: eat leaner meat and low-fat or skim dairy products (NAS, 2003). That advice has been promoted by health officials for years for a totally differ-ent reason—low-fat diets decrease the risk of heart disease and cancer. So, we're not saying anything new regarding the meat and dairy in your diet, just giving you another reason to eat lean. Poultry is also a good alterna-tive, as dioxin levels in chicken and eggs are well below that in beef and dairy (NAS, 2003). (An outbreak of higher levels of dioxin in chickens was found in 1997 and was traced to contaminated feed. It appears to have been an isolated problem.)

As we've discussed, the message regarding farm-raised fish is more complicated, because there is a health benefit to eating oily fish like salmon and the omega-3 fatty acids they contain. However, your dioxin exposure from farm-raised fish can easily exceed that from meat and dairy. It's smart to limit your consumption of farm-raised fish to no more than one meal per week. This will still grant you the benefits of eating fish without giving you unnecessarily high dioxin exposures.

PCBS

Polychlorinated biphenyls (PCBs), actually part of the dioxin family, are a mixture of large, bulky molecules that are oily in nature and very slow to break down. Like dioxin, they deposit in the fat of animals and move up the food chain, becoming more concentrated in each higher predator, with humans receiving the greatest exposure and health risk. Certain types of PCBs can even bind to the dioxin receptor: these PCBs may cause cancer and other toxicity by collaborating with dioxin in its mischievous mission to foul up DNA readout. However, there are important differences between PCBs and dioxins. Dioxins are released into the environment from burning and so are sprinkled primarily over land. In contrast, PCBs are released as an oily waste into the ground or directly into waterways, eventually oozing into groundwater and surface water. So, while the main dietary source of dioxins is food produced on land (meat and dairy) or farmed fish (salmon, catfish), a key source of PCBs is oceanic fish.

In contrast to dioxin, which serves no purpose in the production, packaging, or preparation of food or food products, PCBs actually had a very important industrial use: they were the main dielectric fluid used in electrical transformers for approximately fifty years, until they were banned in the late 1970s. During that period, millions of gallons of PCBs were released into the environment through sloppy disposal practices. Our ghastly environmental mistake started dawning on us during the 1970s when PCBs accidentally got into Japanese rice oil (Yusho), causing severe toxicity and birth defects in those who were unlucky enough to have used it. These findings prompted increasingly detailed animal testing, which showed PCB toxicity at low doses. Environmental sampling found PCBs liberally spread throughout river and lake sediments, with alarmingly high levels in fish, leading to a ban on this oily toxin. Even though PCBs have been banned for decades, water bodies can still become contaminated as the toxins continue to slowly ooze from old spills, moving through the soil to find rivers and lakes.

PCBS CAN AFFECT HORMONE STATUS DURING PREGNANCY AND FETAL BRAIN DEVELOPMENT.

Dioxin is generally much more toxic than PCBs, but our exposure to PCBs, especially in those who eat fatty fish, can be thousands of times higher. The most worrisome health effect of PCBs is their ability to interfere with fetal brain development, likely due to their inhibition of the mother's thyroid gland. Normally, thyroid hormone crosses the placenta and stimulates the baby's nervous system during critical periods of brain growth. But PCBs interfere with the mother's production of thyroid hormone, leaving less available for the fetus. Like dioxin, PCBs linger in the body for a long time, so it's best to keep PCBs to a minimum for the years before one becomes pregnant, ideally starting in childhood. The other toxic effects of PCBs, including cancer and damage to the immune system and skin, can occur across the board, so it's important that everyone limit their dietary exposure to PCBs.

The good news is, most fish you catch or buy will be low in PCBs. The bad news is, some very popular species, bluefish and striped bass in particular, tend to be high in PCBs due to their high fat content. These marine fish travel long distances and can pick up PCBs at many locations along the way. Cleaning up one waterway may only make a small difference for such far-ranging fish. Other fish species can be high in PCBs due to local contamination problems—you should always check with state or local officials for a specific waterbody before deciding to eat your catch.

As mentioned above, farm-raised salmon has been shown to be higher in PCBs than wild salmon. However, the levels detected thus far in farm-raised salmon are still relatively low, approximately 100 times below the levels in striped bass. PCBs are not the main reason to limit consumption of farm-raised fish, dioxins are.

THE RISK INDEX FOR PCBS

The risk index shows that PCBs are a legitimate health concern, having both relatively high toxicity and exposure potential levels. Avoiding the risks from PCBs means following the fish-consumption advice described at the end of this section. This means limiting your consumption of striped bass, bluefish, and any other fish from local waterbodies that are known to have PCB contamination.

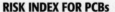

RISK INDEX FOR PCBs

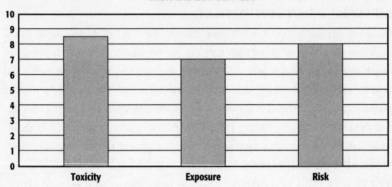

GOOD FISH, BAD FISH: THE DO'S AND DON'TS OF FISH CONSUMPTION

Our experience in health departments taught us that simple messages work best. The simplest message in this case would be to tell pregnant women to not eat fish for nine months. But we can't do that: fish have important nutritional benefits, especially during pregnancy. It is an inexpensive protein-rich food that is also low in saturated fat. It's also rich in polyunsaturated fatty acids (omega-3s) that promote brain development.

Instead, our message is slightly modified: keep eating fish, but be moderate in your fish consumption (no more than twice per week for pregnant women and other high-risk individuals) and select fish that are low in contaminants. The following Healthy Fish Consumption chart outlines how to eat fish safely. Note that this chart was constructed not only for mercury-safe fish consumption, but represents a unified approach to also prevent exposure to PCBs and dioxins.

HEALTHY FISH CONSUMPTION

The following consumption guidelines are based upon test data reported by FDA (2005) and various state agencies.

In General, Choose the Following Fish Most Often

- Haddock
- Pollack
- Cod
- Flounder
- Perch
- Herring
- Sole
- Sardines
- Trout
- Tilapia
- Shellfish

Women and children:[1] Up to two meals per week
General Public: No limits (daily is OK)

Advice for Specific Fish

Swordfish, Shark, Tilefish, King Mackerel (contain mercury):
Women and children:[1] Do not eat
General public: One meal per week

Canned Tuna (contains mercury): Choose "light" instead of "white" for lower mercury content
Women and children:[1] Up to two meals per week
General public: No limits (daily is OK)

Farm-raised Salmon and Catfish (contain dioxin and other toxics):
Women and children:[1] One meal per week
General public: One to two meals per week

Tuna Steak/Sushi (contains mercury):
Women and children:[1] Two meals per month
General public: Two meals per week

Striped Bass and Large Bluefish (> 25″) (contain PCBs):
Women and children[1]: Do not eat
General public: One meal every two months

Locally Caught Fish from Lakes, Rivers, and Streams

Follow local advisories issued by state and local health departments. In general, large predator fish in lakes such as **bass, trout, pickerel,** and

---

[1] Refers to pregnant women, women of child-bearing age, nursing mothers, and children less than six years of age.

walleye tend to be higher in mercury than panfish such as **perch** and **sunfish**.

TRIMMING FATTY FISH

PCBs and dioxins are concentrated in the fat of the fish, while mercury is in the fillet (muscle). Sometimes the fatty portions are obvious and can be trimmed away. These include the dark meat found along the mid-line of some fillets and the lining of the belly flap. The skin also contains fat, and should be trimmed away in most cases. Note that these trimming practices will cut down on your exposure to PCBs and dioxin, but will not affect mercury.

PERSISTENT PESTICIDES

Dieldrin, DDT, chlordane, and toxaphene. These chlorine-rich pesticides persist in the environment so long that, even though they were banned decades ago, they still find their way to our dinner table. We woke up to the serious problems posed by these pesticides in the 1960s and '70s with the revelation of their ability to move through the food chain and bio-magnify as big species eat smaller ones. DDT was the focus of Rachel Carson's book *Silent Spring*, an exposé that sparked a highly influential environmental movement. DDT was shown to move from the soil where it was sprayed into earthworms. The birds that ate the worms accumulated high levels of DDT and couldn't reproduce because their egg shells were too thin, and cracked open prematurely. This led to Ms. Carson's description of a "silent spring"—a spring without the song of birds.

The book led to extensive field research, which found DDT and its organochlorine cousins widespread in soil and wildlife. And now, thirty years after these contaminants have been banned, we are still dealing with trace levels in our diet and environment. It's also worth noting that DDT is still used in some tropical countries to kill mosquitoes and thus cut down on malaria. Durable and mobile, the DDT sprayed in faraway lands can find its way into our soil and local food supply.

TOXIC FACT

PERSISTENT PESTICIDES HAVE SIMILAR RISKS AS DIOXIN AND PCBS.

These pesticides have a generally similar organochlorine structure as dioxin and PCBs, which allow them the same exposure pathways (high-fat animal products, farm-raised fish). They cause cancer, can disrupt the endocrine system, and have been shown to disrupt reproduction and development in animals. In fact, DDT was the main pesticide associated with shrunken alligator genitalia in a contaminated Florida lake (Semenza et al., 1997).

THE RISK INDEX FOR PERSISTENT PESTICIDES

These persistent pesticides get a high toxicity rating because they are carcinogens and endocrine disruptors. While exposure is widespread, the levels have come down, so the overall risk is moderate. Since it takes years for these chemicals to be cleared from our body, the less exposure the better. These chemicals tend to travel in the same circles as dioxin and PCBs, so if you follow the fish, meat, and dairy advice described in this section, you'll also be protected from these organochlorines.

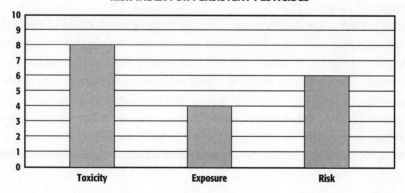

RISK INDEX FOR PERSISTENT PESTICIDES

BIOMAGNIFICATION: WHERE ARE YOU ON THE CONTAMINATED FOOD PYRAMID?

You've probably heard about food pyramids from nutritionists trying to get us to eat better. But we're talking about another pyramid: the contaminated food pyramid, which demonstrates how persistent contaminants such as mercury, PCBs, dioxin, and pesticides get to our dinner table. The technical term is biomagnification, which refers to the increasing levels of contaminants as you go up the food chain.

At the bottom of the pyramid is a wide diversity of plant and animal species, all having tiny amounts of contaminants. The next level of the pyramid are feeders, grazing on the plants and smaller animals. They are fewer in number but higher in contaminant level, because what had been spread out amongst many creatures has now been concentrated into the few. Humans are at the top of the food pyramid, the top predator, getting the biggest dose of persistent chemicals.

One of the arguments for being vegetarian is that by eating lower on the food chain, you won't get nearly as much exposure to things like DDT, PCBs, and mercury. While that is generally true, vegetarians can still get some exposure to persistent contaminants via full-fat dairy products. And we can't forget about the nonpersistent pesticides that are present in many fruits and vegetables. While these pesticides are generally not as worrisome as the persistent chemicals, they are not without some risk and uncertainty.

The bottom line is that it's better to not be on top of the contaminant pyramid all the time, but instead to eat a wide diversity of foods, liberally choosing those from the bottom of the pyramid (vegetables, fruits, grains, beans). If you do eat foods from the higher end of the food chain, choose fish that have fewer contaminants and eat low-fat or skim dairy products. This is especially important for children because they accumulate contaminants over their entire lifespan, building up levels that may be unhealthy to pass along to their children, with some effects not realized until later in life.

Intentional Additives to Our Diet

In this section, we'll address two kinds of Intentional Additives: those added to the final product we consume, and those left over from the production of the product. In the former category are colorants; in the latter are today's pesticides, dietary hormones, and animal antibiotics.

TODAY'S PESTICIDES

In the chemical aftermath of the green revolution, farmers continue to apply millions of pounds of pesticides to the crops we eat. These chemicals are used to kill a variety of pests: insecticides for beetles, borers, and other insects, herbicides for weeds, and fungicides for mold, in addition to the hormonal agents used to enhance the growth of the crop (plant growth regulators). Agri-business can lead to substantial human exposure to toxic chemicals, most notably in those whose job it is to apply the pesticides. But by far the most common exposure is via diet, as millions of Americans ingest pesticide residues in fruits and vegetables on a daily basis.

Modern pesticides are much less persistent than the banned pesticides of the 1950s, 1960s, and 1970s, yet they last long enough to make it to your shopping basket and dinner table. The USEPA sets the level of pesticide that can remain in food at the time of harvest, also called the food tolerance. The FDA's job is to enforce those tolerances by testing for pesticides and seizing foods that exceed the limits. Recognizing that it's impossible to test everything sold, as an added safety measure, farmers are required to wait a certain number of days after spraying a pesticide before harvesting the crop. This ensures that pesticide residues will be low when the produce goes to market.

The regulation of pesticides is intended to instill confidence in the safety of our food supply, but not everyone is convinced. Consider the sheer number of pesticides that we may ingest even in a single meal. Common fruits like peaches, strawberries, and apples can have up to nine different pesticides on a single piece of fruit. Of the vegetables, spinach, celery, and bell peppers tend to have the greatest number of pesticides—up to ten per item (EWG, 2003).

Assuming these pesticides are all below their respective tolerances, federal regulators would conclude that a peach or celery stalk is safe to eat. But do we really know the effect of adding trace levels of one pesticide with another on the same piece of fruit? Or how the nine pesticides on peaches interact with the ten on celery? No, we don't—historically, the tolerance for one pesticide was determined in isolation without considering interactions with other chemicals. There is some comfort in the fact that pesticides often act differently from one another. In other words, their effects won't necessarily be additive. However, there are special cases where pesticides may interact with each other and lead to additive $(1+1=2)$ or even synergistic $(1+1=5)$ effects.

Congress recognized the problem of poly-pesticides (numerous pesticides simultaneously being ingested) and passed the Food Quality Protection Act of 1996, which requires the USEPA to evaluate the cumulative risks from pesticides that act in a similar manner. The agency must then set tolerances low enough so pesticides with the same mechanism cannot add up to a level that will cause the "pesticide cup" to overflow. This act has led to the tightening of regulations on certain pesticides (the organophosphates such as malathion, chlorpyrifos, diazinon), but it cannot hope to encompass all the combinations of pesticides in our diet.

MYTH: The pesticides farmers use today get into our diet and cause widespread illness.

REALITY: Modern pesticides are much less toxic and persistent than in the past, so risks are lower. While they still get into our diet, it's unlikely that these pesticides cause widespread health effects.

This is an easy myth to fall prey to. Pesticides are designed to be toxic, even lethal. Farmworkers spraying pesticides need to wear protective equipment and can still be poisoned. While these pesticides sound risky, they are at low levels in the diet, making them less worrisome than other dietary risks. Pesticides in food, not only on produce but also in dairy, meat, and other types of foods, are regularly tested. In general, the levels are well below the tolerance levels, which are set in a reasonably health-protective manner. Of course, the FDA does not come close to testing every crate of produce; in 2002, the FDA tested 2,100 market samples of produce grown in the United States and over 4,600 samples that came in from out of the country (FDA, 2003). The imported results were mixed: the majority showed no pesticide residue, but out of those that did have a detection, approximately four percent were greater than the tolerance. This suggests that imported produce is generally fine but that there are isolated cases of improper pesticide use. Less than one percent of the produce samples from the United States had residues of potential concern.

Since pesticides are usually present at levels that are well below the tolerance, it is unlikely that they will be able to interact with each other. There is just too little for each to have its own effect, much less alter how a pesticide cousin would act. But this is still an active area of research, and it is still possible that certain dietary pesticides can combine to be a health risk. Thus, it is always a good idea to eat less pesticide.

So where did the big pesticide scare originate? Primarily from a few controversies in the past, one having to do with watermelons, another with apples.

TEMIK IN WATERMELONS

The Temik poisonings of July 1985 gave the U.S. consumer a reason to be scared of pesticides. Temik is a highly toxic carbamate insecticide that poisons the nervous system of insects and, at high enough doses, people as well. It was never supposed to be used on watermelon, but apparently some grower(s) felt that it would give them the edge in the war against bugs and that no one would be the wiser. This illegal use had never been tested, so when the melons hit the market in the western United States and Canada, the consumer was the guinea pig. It turns out that enough Temik remained in watermelons to sicken over 1,000 people with stomach ailments, heart arrhythmia, loss of consciousness, and convulsions. A total of seventeen were hospitalized (MMWR, 1986). These illness totals would have undoubtedly been higher had it not been for public health officials seizing watermelons in affected regions of the country. Although Temik is one of the most toxic pesticides still used, in most cases it is not a health risk. The one crop where there was lingering concern about high residue, potatoes, saw Temik use end in 1990.

Temik is a good example of why extensive toxicity testing and market-based sampling are needed to ensure the safety of the food supply. The FDA and the USEPA appear to be doing a reasonable job along these lines. Furthermore, the pesticides being developed today are less toxic than Temik and are generally not persistent in the environment, helping alleviate the concerns over pesticides in our food supply.

ALAR IN APPLES

When learning the "ABCs" of pesticide risks, the "A" has to stand for Alar. That's because it was the largest pesticide controversy of its day, perhaps of any day, and taught us a number of important lessons. At the root of the Alar story was a huge mistake by government regulators, which allowed Alar to remain on the market for fifteen years without adequate testing. Alar was a plant hormone used extensively on fruiting crops to keep them on the tree/vine longer, allowing for more uniform ripening. This made harvesting easier, with fewer drops and better long-term storage in the cold room. Apple production molded itself to Alar's properties, so the industry was up in arms when claims began surfacing about the carcinogenicity of the plant growth regulator.

In 1977, a decade before the controversy began, a scientific paper was published in a well-respected journal that should have raised a big red flag. It showed that daminozide (aka Alar) caused a fairly rare blood vessel tumor in mice (Toth et al., 1977). The USEPA and the industrial maker of Alar knew about the study, but failed to follow up, even though an adverse finding of that magnitude normally merits an investigation of the chemical's database and new testing if necessary. Instead, the question of Alar's carcinogenicity remained open while it continued to be heavily used. Its residues were not only in apples, but also in baby food and apple juice.

The Alar cancer study became an item of public notice and then alarm as the chemical went through its normal regulatory review in the mid-1980s. As the positive cancer study rose to the top of the data pile, environmental groups initiated a campaign to ban this "apple carcinogen" before any more children were put at risk. Anti-Alar protests were staged at supermarkets and in the media, featuring actress Meryl Streep decrying how we are exposing the next generation to carcinogens.

As the exaggerated anti-Alar ads were swirling, industry and government inspectors got in gear and paid a visit to the lab where a decade earlier Alar had caused tumors in mice. They uncovered enough irregularities to raise serious doubts about the study, but of course by that time, the die had been cast, and Alar was "voluntarily" pulled from the market. Follow-up testing showed that Alar was not particularly carcinogenic, but that a breakdown product (UDMH) that could form when heating apples, to make things like apple sauce, apple juice, and likely also apple pie, was. In the end, it was a good thing that Alar was removed from the market, but in reality the risks were only moderately elevated, certainly not worthy of the level of fear and panic brought on by the anti-pesticide groups. The lesson the USEPA learned was that years of inaction let the issue slip away from the regulatory process, and allowed it to be tried by media rather than by science.

Overall, the current news about pesticide testing is encouraging. The results suggest that the imposed wait period before a crop can be taken to market really does keep a lid on how much gets to the consumer. The poly-pesticide question will always be debated, because you can't test the complex mixture of contaminants present in our food supply in an animal study. However, given the low levels usually found, the potential for serious interaction is less likely. Further, since 1996, the USEPA has been evaluating the potential for cumulative effects across chemicals, which seems to be helpful in decreasing the potential for unexpected interactions.

THE RISK INDEX FOR TODAY'S PESTICIDES

Our overall rating of the risk from pesticides used in produce today is low. As shown in the chart below, even though there is extensive exposure, the levels are low enough to make toxicity and risk relatively minor concerns, especially compared to the other food contaminants discussed in this chapter. There are still uncertainties with regard to how all the different pesticides will combine in your body, and you can never be sure that you won't receive one of the few pieces of imported produce that is above the tolerance. That's why eating less pesticide is a good idea.

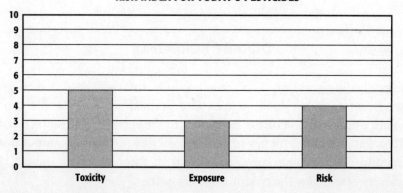

RISK INDEX FOR TODAY'S PESTICIDES

AVOIDING TODAY'S PESTICIDES

Here are some of the main ways you can avoid pesticide consumption:

- Buy organic produce: people buy organic for many good reasons, including the desire to eat fewer pesticides and to support a form of agriculture that is less toxic to farmworkers and that won't contaminate groundwater. While the quality and quantity of organic produce at supermarkets has improved in recent years, it is still an expensive choice. The hope is that as more people buy organic, the more it will be produced, making it affordable to people of all means.

- Peel vegetables: certain pesticides are highest in the peel, especially of root crops such as carrots and potatoes. These vegetables are often peeled anyway for aesthetic reasons. You should be aware that peeling vegetables has the tradeoff of losing some vitamins and fiber.

- Wash produce: while this practice can't hurt and may give you the sense that you are doing all you can to fight pesticides, the reality is that most produce is pre-washed to get it cleaned up for market. Your kitchen wash probably won't do that much more. Further, many pesticides are "systemic," meaning they are taken up into the peel or edible portion of the vegetable—no amount of washing will remove them. A gentle but thorough rinse prior to food preparation is always a good idea to make sure that the food has been washed; however, produce washing is not worth a huge effort or the use of special cleaning solutions.

DIETARY HORMONES

Just as chemicals are used to grow produce, they are also used to grow animals for meat production. And like pesticide residues, there can be residues of growth-enhancing hormones in the cuts of meat we pick out at the market. Extra hormones in our diet may affect the way our children grow and develop, mature sexually, and in the case of estrogenic hormones, may increase the risk of breast cancer.

There are six hormones that are commonly given to cattle in the United States to get them to bulk up faster at a lower cost: the natural sex steroids estradiol, progesterone, and testosterone, and their synthetic forms zeranol, melengestrol acetate, and trenbolone acetate. These hormones can add muscle and fat to beef cattle the way they do to professional atheletes bulking up with illegal locker room steroids. The hormones are bundled in an ear patch, which slowly releases the growth mixture to the animal. The concern for human health stems from the possibility that the hormones are still present in the parts of the animal we eat.

The controversy over growth hormones is heightened by the fact that countries cannot agree on how they should be regulated. The United States has allowed cattle farmers to use hormones for the past forty years; this affects approximately ninety percent of our beef. This is in stark contrast to Europe and Canada: in 1988, several European countries made the initial determination that hormones should not be used in beef production because of public health concerns. Over the past fifteen years, under pressure by other countries to reverse that decision, the European Union has revisited the issue several times, conducting laboratory research to address what it felt were key uncertainties. Studies completed in 2000 and 2001 confirmed that hormone supplementation in cattle is a potential health risk (Associated Press, 2002), showing that standard hormone dosing led to as much as a seven-fold increase in estrogen levels in cattle, and a twenty-fold increase in the levels of lipoidal ester, a fatty form of estrogen (SCVPH, 2001). Supplementary studies, in which the hormones were applied in ways that are technically illegal but likely to occur in actual cattle production, showed even larger hormone increases in edible beef. Combined with studies showing that the hormones and their metabolites in beef can be toxic and mutagenic, the new evidence has led to the continued ban of hormone-dosed meat in Europe and Canada. That means no imports of U.S.-grown beef, a policy that creates a barrier to free trade and considerable political angst.

The FDA disagrees with Europe and Canada, and states there is no evidence that shows that hormones in beef, in the amounts they are currently used, will actually cause effects in humans. Technically, they're correct: there is no smoking gun. However, there is enough suggestive evidence to have caused other governments to ban the hormone treatments.

CHILDREN MAY BE MOST SENSITIVE TO ANIMAL HORMONES IN THEIR DIET.

Children's sex hormone levels are naturally low, so an extra source may cause accelerated or unusual sexual maturation. However, there have been very few studies evaluating whether eating hormones in meat actually affects development. Clusters of cases of early puberty in Puerto Rico and gynecomastia (breast development in males) in Italy were evaluated to see whether dietary hormones might be responsible, but the results were inconclusive. The increasing phenomenon of girls reaching puberty before the age of nine is still largely unexplored (Herman-Giddens et al., 1997)—a disturbing fact, considering that it increases breast cancer risk later in life. The leading theory has more to do with weight than hormones (it is known that obese girls mature more quickly than thin girls). However, we cannot rule out the possibility that the intake of dietary hormones increases the chance that early puberty will occur.

Bottom line: While we don't have direct evidence that beef from hormone-dosed cattle is a health risk, we also don't have studies to refute the possibility. In this case, it's best to use a general precautionary principle: where there is a plausible risk, and where certain governments have acted to remove the risk (but your government hasn't), the individual may want to take steps to decrease exposure just in case the risk is real. Right now, it's most important that children follow this until better information is available.

Q *Are these hormones also in dairy?*

A No, the hormones described above are not approved for use in dairy cows. However, another hormone, bovine growth hormone (BGH), is approved in dairy cows. Approximately thirty percent of dairy cows receive BGH treatment in the United States, which can increase their milk production by ten percent. The hormone is naturally present in milk, but appears at much higher levels in those cows given the booster treatment.

BGH is not known to have adverse effects in people. However, the treatment can cause lactational problems in cows leading to inflammation and infection (Dohoo et al., 2003). These problems might necessitate treating the cow with an antibiotic that may well end up in the milk you buy. It's also possible that BGH alters the natural composition of milk, but the effects of these alterations on humans aren't well understood.

REDUCING YOUR HORMONE INTAKE

One simple method is to eat less beef by switching to other sources of protein like fish, ham, poultry, eggs, beans, and grains. Chicken and pigs are not fed hormones. Another alternative is to buy meat that is sold as "certified organic." Organic animals can only be given one hundred percent–organic feed without antibiotics or growth hormones. Finally, you can look for meat from Europe or Canada, which will be free of hormones.

If you want to avoid the issues associated with BGH in dairy, you can find milk in most supermarkets that is certified organic and thus hormone-free. However, it may be difficult to find cheese, yogurt, and other dairy products that bear an organic label. While low-fat or skim dairy products are a good way to avoid other types of contaminants, keep in mind that option will not help you cut out BGH and its related issues.

THE RISK INDEX FOR DIETARY HORMONES

The hormones we ingest in beef have the potential to modify endocrine development in children and so are given a high toxicity rating. The amount of exposure is uncertain, but not expected to be very high. This leads to a moderate risk level, one that warrants diet modifications. The hormones in dairy (BGH) are less of a direct health threat, but still raise some important concerns (antibiotics, modified milk composition).

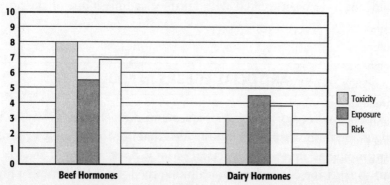

RISK INDEX FOR DIETARY HORMONES

ANTIBIOTICS IN FARM ANIMALS

There's a lot more to the story of antibiotics in food production than just the effects of BGH. No one argues about treating sick cows with antibiotics—controversy arises when a large percentage of the twenty-two million pounds of antibiotics used in meat production each year are to treat *healthy* animals. Dosing otherwise healthy animals allows farmers to crowd them into tighter quarters without risking the spread of infections. This space- and money-saving scheme has a large drawback: wanton use of antibiotics causes antibiotic-resistant strains of bacteria to emerge. Antibiotics wipe out most but not all of the bacteria. Those left behind become resistant to the drug and overgrow because the competition (all the other types of bacteria) has been removed, allowing the resistant bacteria to spread to other animals and possibly also people. Ironically, the main worry is not human consumption of antibiotics, but rather the consumption of the hardy bacteria that overgrow from antibiotic mismanagement on the farm.

The medical community is very concerned that its major weapon against infection, antibiotic drugs, is becoming less useful, and have lobbied the meat industry to stop giving antibiotics to healthy animals. The campaign has done some good; in 2003, McDonald's announced that all beef used in its stores must be from animals that don't receive extra antibiotics. It was a promising development, though unfortunately there are still many cows and cattle subject to antibiotic overuse.

Since antibiotic use in beef and dairy is not a toxics issue per se, we have not developed a risk index chart. However, it is still advisable to decrease consumption of such animals. Certified organic beef and dairy are again a good option for consumers. Animals raised organically should not have been treated with antibiotics unless one of the animals fell ill.

ARTIFICIAL COLORS IN FOOD

We Americans readily accept hair dyes and cosmetics as a way to look younger and more attractive. But the idea that our food supply needs similar primping is more controversial. Many have argued that dyes are meant to trick the consumer into thinking the food is fresher or of higher quality than it actually is. For example, since meat is supposed to look red, processed meats like cold cuts, hot dogs, and beef jerky are dyed red to make them look fresh. Artificially colored candy and cereals are more fun and enticing to children, and thus have a marketing advantage.

The backlash against artificial colors has been led by those who see them as false advertising. However, we should be concerned with another food-dye issue: food coloring was one of the earliest hot-button toxic issues plaguing the FDA.

Food dyes had been used for over a century without much thought to testing and safety. In 1938, the Food, Drug and Cosmetic Act created a system of numerical designations (e.g., ethryosine became FD&C Red No. 3, tartrazine became FD&C No. 5) and also required certification, which involved safety testing. By the 1950s, evidence was building that certain dyes were toxic and carcinogenic in rats and dogs, in some cases at doses that weren't that much higher than those allowed in food. Around that time, there were several incidents in which the overuse of colors in candy and popcorn was associated with diarrhea in children. Suddenly, everyone realized that the colors millions had been eating for decades were actually a health risk. In 1958, the Delaney Clause was passed, requiring the FDA to ban any additive from the food supply if it was a known carcinogen. Several yellow and red colors were banned from food on this basis, though others survived despite evidence of carcinogenicity. That's because in 1960, FDA was given the discretion to either set a tolerance for food additives (an amount FDA deemed was safe) or allow it to remain in food temporarily until more studies were done.

Today nine artificial colors are approved for food use: three reds, one orange, two yellows, one green, and two blues. Combinations of these basic colors produce the rainbow of colors found in candies, ice cream, soft drinks, cereal, and other foods (like processed meats) that get touched up to be more marketable. There is still some concern about Red No. 3—it was found to cause thyroid tumors in rats and so was removed from certain uses (cosmetics, drugs), but is curiously still allowed in food. FDA has plans to rescind food uses of Red No. 3, but so far it hasn't happened. Fortunately, the main red dye in use, Red No. 40, has not caused cancer in animal studies, although a recent test found that it can cause genetic damage in mice (Tsuda et al., 2001). In fact, all three red dyes were subjected to genetic testing and produced some positive results, but not enough to prove a cancer risk.

FOOD COLORING AND HYPERACTIVITY

In the late 1970s and '80s, reports surfaced that colorants and other food additives were associated with hyperactivity in children. Putting children on "elimination diets" that were low in food additives seemed to help control their hyperactivity disorders. However, the evidence was weak and contradictory. There is really no basis for a widespread advisory against food colors in children, though there may be some benefit from such elimination diets in the small percentage of children who are hyperactive and have food allergies (IFIC, 2005).

Perhaps the main issue with food colors is the potential for allergic reactions to Yellow No. 5. There's evidence that the lemon yellow color can cause reactions such as hives in a small percentage of people. Given its widespread use—it's the most widely used yellow colorant—that could mean hundreds to thousands of people across the country are at risk of allergic reactions. Yellow No. 5 hasn't been banned, but like other food colors, it must be specifically identified on the ingredient list if present in a particular food item. In theory, this gives people who know they are allergic to Yellow No. 5 the chance to avoid it, although you usually don't ask for the ingredients list when ordering a scoop of ice cream.

THE RISK INDEX FOR ARTIFICIAL COLORS IN FOOD

In general, we don't need to avoid food colors, as they are not a large public health risk. Cancer risks are low, especially since the most blatant bad dyes have already been taken off the market. Compared to the other carcinogens in our diet, including PCBs, dioxin, banned pesticides, arsenic, and polycyclic aromatic hydrocarbons, the cancer risk posed by food colors is low. People allergic to food colors appear to represent a small percentage of the population. The chart below reflects the fact that the overall risk from food color is not very high, although we can't say that there is no risk at all.

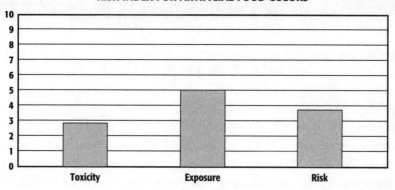

AVOIDING ARTIFICIAL FOOD COLORS

Some people may choose to limit their family's intake of artificial food color. It is worth noting that there are no regulatory limits on how much artificial color can be used in a food—it is up to the food industry to self-regulate. A food with excessive food coloring may have risks that haven't been adequately tested, as evidenced by the diarrhea outbreak in children in the 1950s. It can be hard to cut back on artificial food color because so many food items are colored to one degree or another. However, if you pay attention, you can moderate how many brightly colored items you and your children eat every day.

You should also be aware that there are many natural colors derived from things like beets, carrots, and spices, which means you can have an "all natural" food item that is also colored. These natural colors are considered safe because they are derived from common dietary items, but are less commonly used because they are more expensive, less stable, and can impart a taste or texture to the food. People looking to eat less artificial color can read labels and select products that use the natural agents instead.

Containers and Cookware in Our Diet

PLASTICS AND PLASTICIZERS

From sleds to soda bottles, car bumpers to credit cards, plastics have given us lightweight, durable, and inexpensive consumer goods. Most of us look past the fact that they create dioxin when burned, never biodegrade, and use large amounts of natural resources. Modern society has accepted plastics on a grand scale, surrounding itself with more and more of this industrial art form. However, when plastic not only surrounds but also turns up inside of us, it's time to take a closer look at what's going on.

Plasticizers are chemicals that add flexibility and durability to plastic, making it adaptable to many different uses. The main type of plasticizer is a group of chemicals called phthalates—primarily in a type of plastic known as polyvinyl chloride (PVC). PVC is used in a wide variety of household items including shower curtains, floorings and wall coverings, baby toys, teething rings, food packaging, medical tubing, and storage containers (those with the "Number 3" recycling designation). Phthalates in these products are not tightly bound and can come off in a baby's mouth or the food stored in the container.

Phthalates are moderately toxic chemicals with some carcinogenic potential, as seen in high-dose animal studies. However, the main concern with phthalates is their endocrine disruption effect. A recent epidemiology study found that phthalate levels typical of the U.S. population were associated with adverse outcomes in newborn male babies. In the study (Swann et al., 2005), eighty-five women were analyzed during pregnancy; the amount of phthalates in their bodies correlated with how well their baby boys developed in utero, specifically with respect to reproductive organs. In other words, the mother's intake of phthalates appears to have correlated with impaired male fetal development.

These data are consistent with a large body of animal testing showing that phthalates are strongly anti-androgenic—they combat male hormones. The fetal period seems to be particularly sensitive. The boy fetus is in a female environment where there is a prevalence of female hormones, thus the default trend is feminization. However, there are carefully timed signals for the immature male gonad to release testosterone and trigger the development of male characteristics. It appears that phthalates can interfere with these "become male" signals, affecting things like penis size and the descension of testicles. These early life effects may have consequences for males in adulthood.

The limited data currently available make it difficult to draw firm conclusions about the level of risk to the general public. We expect much more will be known in coming years. Since the data so far suggest that pregnant women are exposed to levels of phthalates that can make a difference in utero (Swann et al., 2005), it's important for us to better understand where our phthalate exposure comes from.

> **MYTH:** Most of our phthalate exposure comes from food packaging.
>
> **REALITY:** Most food containers are not made out of PVC, but from other types of plastic that don't contain phthalates.

It's true that storing food—or worse yet, microwaving it—in PVC containers is a good way to get exposed to phthalates. However, today's food packaging industry relies primarily on non-PVC containers, so the leaching of phthalates into your food isn't a big concern. It's still prudent to make sure that any food storage containers you have around the house are not PVC—make sure the recycling symbol on the bottom does not bear the number 3. Additionally, you should only microwave food in microwave-approved plastic or glass containers that won't degrade or release other chemicals into the food when heated to a high temperature. Plastic cling wrap can leach a different kind of plasticizer into your food. To be on the safe side, don't microwave with plastic wrap, or if you do, keep the wrap suspended above the food. This will keep the moisture in the food and the plasticizer out.

MOST OF OUR PHTHALATE EXPOSURE IS NOT FROM FOOD PACKAGING, BUT FROM PERSONAL CARE PRODUCTS.

TOXIC FACT

A study by the Centers for Disease Control found phthalates in nearly all of the 2,500 people sampled, young and old alike (Silva et al., 2004). If food packaging isn't a major threat, then where is this widespread exposure coming from? The main culprit appears to be cosmetics and personal care products, discussed in more detail in Chapter 7. The types of phthalates that show up in our blood most closely match the kind used in these products. House dust is another possible source, due to the widespread use of PVC (and thus phthalates) in floors, walls, and other household products. Phthalate levels are also high in hospital bags and medical tubing; anyone receiving an intravenous (IV) infusion is getting a dose of plasticizer. The main source of exposure for infants is likely their soft "vinyl" toys and teething rings.

Q *Do baby bottles contain phthalates?*

A Fortunately, phthalates are not found in polycarbonate, the type of plastic commonly used for baby bottles. But there is another ingredient of concern in polycarbonate, bisphenol A, which can leach into formula (*Consumer Reports*, 2000). This chemical behaves like estrogen in the body, and thus has the potential to upset hormonal balance and development in early life. Because bisphenol A is much less estrogenic than the natural hormone and is consumed in trace amounts in formula, it shouldn't have a large "feminizing" influence. However, we can't rule out that it could have some effect, especially since babies would be getting a daily exposure to a hormonally active agent. Fortunately, there are ways to avoid feeding phthalates and bisphenol A to your baby.

AVOIDING PHTHALATES AND BISPHENOL A

Though we don't have enough information to construct a risk index for plasticizers in your diet, we can give you some advice about how to avoid these potential risks:

- Pregnant women and women planning to become pregnant should heed the advice concerning cosmetics presented in Chapter 7.

- Do not use PVC ("Number 3" plastic) for storing or microwaving food. In fact, only use microwave-safe plasticware or glass for heating up food.

- Do not let cling wrap come in contact with food that is being heated in the microwave.

- Try to use glass baby bottles. If you can't, reasonable alternatives to glass are polyethylene or polypropylene, which shouldn't leach phthalates or bisphenol A into formula. Look for plastic baby bottles with a Number 1, 2, or 5 symbol on the bottom.

- If you have an infant, look for toys that are labeled as "PVC-free" and choose wood toys over plastic whenever possible.

TEFLON

One of the breakthrough chemicals in our modern kitchen is Teflon, the coating that makes frying pans nonstick and pancakes a cinch to flip. Recently, the discovery that pet birds can be sickened and killed by Teflon fumes made us take a close look at this kitchen convenience. Based upon the experience of our feathered friends, we shouldn't be surprised to learn that the fluoropolymer ingredients in Teflon cause a variety of toxic effects in test animals, including cancer and reproductive and developmental effects. And here's another eye opener: the Teflon fluoropolymers are present in most people's blood, not just in adults but in young children as well.

Frying food at high temperatures can release these potentially harmful chemicals into your breathing zone. The chemicals we are referring to, of course, are the Teflon polymer cousins PFOS and PFOA, which stand for perfluorooctanoate sulfonate (PFOS) and perfluorooctanoic acid (PFOA). As the bad news started coming in on Teflon, the USEPA conducted an expedited review of one of the polymers, PFOS. They found that it was persistent in the environment, bioaccumulative, and toxic in a variety of ways. As a result, in 2000, the industry began to voluntarily phase PFOS out of cookware and other consumer products. Now, the focus is on PFOA as the major fluorinated polymer on the market. New research suggests that the average person is exposed to one hundred to one thousand times less PFOA than what was found to be a toxic level in rats (USEPA, 2005). That's good news, though there are some important points to remember: for one, rats can clear PFOA out of their body in a matter of days, while humans take years. No one has uncovered the reason for this difference or how it may ultimately affect risk. As of now, we know of no serious human illnesses caused by Teflon fumes, but the chemicals have been linked to eye and respiratory inflammation and other flu-like symptoms. Day-in and day-out exposure to Teflon could lead to cumulative health effects. And there's no denying that PFOA is an animal carcinogen, so we might not want to tolerate anything but the most miniscule exposures in our food supply and surroundings.

Perhaps the most troubling aspect of the PFOS/PFOA story is that we're really not certain where the chemicals come from. It's not just Teflon pans—these polymers are in numerous consumer products, wherever a stain-resistant coating can be found. Upholstery and carpeting are treated with products containing PFOA, as is some stain-resistant clothing such as Gore-Tex. The grease-resistant food packaging you bring leftovers and fast food home in may well contain these polymers. Even babies get some from mom, packaged in breast milk.

How much of our exposure comes from each source is unknown, but is currently being researched. At this point, we can't tell you to get rid of your Teflon pan. Although Teflon pans were the first suspect in the PFOS/PFOA exposure mystery, they may not be a particularly large source unless you routinely overheat the pan. It's not likely that your typical bacon and egg breakfast will get hot enough to cause much PFOA to go airborne. In general, the lower the temperature you fry at, the better.

It's disconcerting that there has not been a proper risk assessment on a chemical that has been running loose in consumer products (and our bodies) over the past twenty years. Could USEPA have predicted that these persistent, toxic chemicals might find their way out of pans and carpeting and into our bodies? One would think so, or at least hope that current and future chemicals would be tested more thoroughly and used more judiciously. In the meantime, there are a few things you can do to decrease your exposure. Everyone is exposed to PFOS/PFOA to a small degree—the key is to not take in any more than necessary.

- Teflon pan cooking: Avoid excessive temperatures by minimal preheating of the pan. If the pan overheats and smoke develops, leave the house immediately while leaving exhaust fans turned on. Take birds outside with you. Discard any food that may have been in the overheated pan. Consider replacing old pans with new ones that are formulated without PFOS.

- Fast food containers: Don't store leftovers from the restaurant in coated cardboard containers, and certainly don't reheat food in these containers in the microwave.

Unfortunately, we can't give you any more advice than this right now. Further recommendations will have to wait for the results of exposure testing that is now under way.

BREAST-FEEDING AND TOXICS

Up until now we have pretty much focused upon store-bought food. However, one of the most important sources of nutrition for babies is home grown—breast milk. Breast-feeding is strongly encouraged because of the antibodies and nutrients mom can pass along to her baby. However, mom can also pass along toxic chemicals she has ingested and that have gotten transferred into breast milk. The chemicals most likely to get packaged in breast milk are those mom has the hardest time clearing from her own system: PCBs, dioxin, and persistent pesticides. A new class of breast milk contaminants, polybrominated diphenyl ethers (PBDEs), are similar to PCBs in structure and possibly also in toxicity. The compound is a flame retardant that makes consumer products such as foam cushions and computer monitors resistant to fire. The rapid rise in PBDE levels in breast milk over the last decade has prompted worldwide research to understand how these chemicals get into people and what health risks they pose. (While the worst forms of PBDE have been phased out of consumer products, debate continues over the PBDEs that remain on the market.) The chemicals that concentrate in breast milk are fat seekers—they dissolve into the body's fatty tissues and into milk fat. Nursing leads to greater doses in the infant than the mother (on a body weight basis), at a time when the child's organs are rapidly developing and thus possibly more sensitive.

Given that all women have these chemicals in breast milk to some extent, the obvious question is whether women should discontinue breast-feeding altogether. The answer is a resounding NO! Breast milk has such important nutrients that its benefits outweigh its risks. Women should nurse their children, but also do their best to avoid the persistent toxicants that can get into breast milk, not only during the nursing period but also beforehand, so they can cut down on their chemical burden before starting nursing. Eating less PCBs, dioxin, and banned pesticides generally involves eating lower and leaner on the food pyramid—low-fat or skim dairy products, lean cuts of meat, and consumption of poultry and meat alternatives at least some of the time. Farm-raised salmon makes a substantial contribution to our load of dioxin, so women should limit themselves to no more than one meal per week.

Breast-feeding is still better, even in our modern contaminant-filled world. Breast-feeding can be best if nursing moms avoid these persistent chemicals.

Food Contaminant Summary

The range of food contaminants described in this chapter was probably enough to make your head spin and your stomach turn. How can you follow all this advice and still find something to eat? Well, take heart and pick up your fork, because there are many foods that are low in contaminants. Lean protein sources (minimal animal fat) are generally low in contaminants like dioxin, pesticides, and hormones. These foods include poultry, eggs, ham, vegetarian sources (beans/grains), and certain fish (see fish listing earlier in chapter).

The following chart pulls this information together by ranking the risk level associated with each type of contaminant discussed in this chapter. You should follow the "avoid exposure" options for the high- and moderate-risk contaminants. Avoidance of low-risk contaminants is not essential, but presented for those who want to be extra careful. Where we have indicated a risk is plausible but uncertain, we can't be any more precise at the present time, so some caution is warranted.

CONTAMINANT OR ISSUE	LEVEL OF RISK	OPTIONS TO AVOID EXPOSURE
BOOMERANG TOXICANTS		
Fish Contaminants	High	Eat no more than 2 fish meals/week Select fish low in mercury Trim away fat to remove PCBs No more than 1 meal of farm-raised fish/week
Persistent Pesticides and Dioxin	Moderate to High	Eat lean meat, and low-fat dairy Follow fish consumption advice above
INTENTIONAL ADDITIVES		
Modern Pesticides	Low	Eat organic produce Peel vegetables, especially root crops Wash vegetables in water
Food Colors	Low	Moderate how many colored items eaten in a day Choose foods with natural over artificial colors
Hormones in meat	Plausible but Uncertain	Eat less meat Eat certified organic meat Choose protein that is hormone-free: eggs, poultry, fish, ham, vegetarian sources Eat meat from Europe or Canada
Hormones in dairy	Low	Consume certified organic milk and milk products
Antibiotics in meat/dairy	Low	Consume certified organic products
CONTAINERS/COOKWARE		
Plasticizers	Plausible but Uncertain	Use microwave-safe ceramic, glass, or plastic cookware Use glass baby bottles; certain plastics are also OK Keep cling wrap above food in microwave Look for phthalate-free baby toys See Chapter 7 on cosmetics during pregnancy
Teflon / PFOA	Plausible but Uncertain	Do not overheat nonstick fry pans

CHAPTER 6

Water Pollutants

In a complex world where very little is what it seems, the purity of water is a refreshing change. After all, nothing could be simpler chemically than just hydrogen and oxygen, a simplicity reflected in water's freedom from color, odor, and taste. Water quenches the thirst of all life, provides us with our most basic sustenance, raining down upon us as a gift, magically collecting in lakes and groundwater, awaiting our turning of the faucet. We drink, wash, swim, cool off, and even give birth in it. We, like our planet, are approximately two-thirds water, a fact that reminds us what is outside is also inside.

Our relationship with the life-giving properties of water borders on the sacred. Perhaps that's why water contamination seems to be a higher offense than other forms of pollution. We don't have to be told that whatever is in our water besides hydrogen and oxygen will also end up in us, changing our body's chemistry. Unfortunately, this most basic nutrient often does contain other ingredients, some potentially harmful. Which brings us to the complex world of water safety: risk assessment, safety standards, water filters, bottled water, and trade-offs between the benefits of killing bacteria and the risks of toxic disinfectants.

We drink water from a wide range of sources, from the water that comes out of our home tap to the water at work to what we may encounter when traveling. Of course, there's the ubiquitous bottled water that's in every convenience store cooler, the water we inadvertently drink when we're swimming, and even the water our kids ingest when taking a bath.

But amidst all that water consumption, the central question is where our at-home tap water comes from. For most of us, the house tap is our most important source of drinking water. Chances are you're either on a public water system or have a private well. The following are brief descriptions of public and private water supplies.

Public Water Systems: A water company has the rights to large quantities of water, which it sells to the public. Often called "city water," public water is distributed all over town via pipes that bring it into each home—all you have to do is turn on the faucet and pay the bill. Public systems vary in size from those that supply millions to those that serve only a few people. Small systems are those that supply twenty-five to 3,300 people, moderate systems supply 3,300 to 50,000 people, and large systems supply over 50,000. Large systems typically rely on above-ground reservoirs, groundwater, or a mixture of the two.

All types of public systems treat the raw water before sending it out to homes and businesses. The treatment consists of filters to remove sediment and some biological contaminants, water softeners to deal with hard water (high mineral content), pH adjustments, and chlorine to kill bacteria.

Private Wells: You might be blessed with a plentiful supply of potable groundwater. If your house does have its own supply, all you need is a well that pumps the water from deep under ground up to the faucets in your house. There are no water bills to pay, so the water is basically free after the initial cost of installing the well, and no added chemicals—whatever is in the groundwater is what you drink and bathe in. That may or may not be a good thing, as biological and chemical contaminants can sometimes make their way into wells. Of course, you can install a filter to remove the contaminants, but no one is going to test your water for you. If you don't do it yourself, you won't know what contaminants may be lurking in that pitcher of ice water. And of course, there's always the risk of copper or lead leaching out of your pipes—a problem that affects both private wells and public systems.

> **MYTH:** At least natural water from springs and groundwater is free of contaminants.
>
> **REALITY:** We don't have to look very far to start finding water contaminants. Even underground water from the purest spring will have coursed through layers of bedrock and soil, drawing out elements and salts including sodium, magnesium, aluminum, and calcium. These minerals and salts give water properties of hardness or softness, change its pH from neutral to acidic or basic, and can impart a taste. It would be very difficult to find natural water that didn't have at least some amount of dissolved minerals. But we usually don't consider this water to be "contaminated," in the toxic sense of the word. It's still natural, and its extra ingredients are nontoxic.
>
> All that changes when natural water picks up contaminants like sulfur, which has a rotten egg odor and taste; iron, which gives a rusty look to water; manganese, which stains porcelain and is toxic to the nervous system; arsenic, a carcinogen; uranium, a radioactive kidney toxicant; or radon, a radioactive carcinogen. These elements also dissolve out of bedrock and soil, but their presence is noticeable in taste or toxicity or both. It is not unusual for groundwater to be tainted by such "natural" contaminants, and what you may be exposed to depends on the type of water system you use.

Public Water System Pollutants

The vast majority of U.S. households, approximately 230 million people, drink from a public water system. Public water supplies—reservoirs and groundwater—can become contaminated from landfill runoff or by chemicals that have been spilled by businesses or industry, many of which have the ability to seep down through layers of soil and pollute groundwater. Reservoirs are usually less at risk, but can still receive chemicals dumped into the rivers or groundwater sources that feed them. Both large and small public systems must test their water, but the federal requirements vary depending upon the size of the system, the type of contaminant, and the number of local requirements. The USEPA has created a broad list of contaminants that water companies must test for, and has established a safe level for each chemical in drinking water, called the Maximum Contaminant Level (MCL). If contamination is found above the MCL, then the water company must lower the level, either by blending in water from a different supply or by filtering the water to remove the contamination.

Even if a contaminant is present below the MCL, there are still repercussions—the water company must test more frequently.

The testing and reporting requirements required of public water companies provide us some reassurance that "city water" is fine for drinking and bathing. Companies must not only meet the MCLs for chemical contaminants, but also ensure that their water is free of bacteria and bears a pH that is near neutral, not acidic or basic. As discussed in Chapter 1, maintaining pH is essential to making sure the metals in your pipes (e.g., lead, copper) don't leach into your drinking water.

CHLORINE

We take for granted the high water quality of our public supplies. That wasn't always the case–in fact, drinking water used to be an enormous risk factor for the spread of deadly diseases. At the dawn of the industrial revolution, population in cities swelled; overcrowding and poor sanitation brought about waterborne epidemics such as typhoid and cholera. Safeguarding water supplies from human and animal wastes became a critical step forward in fighting these diseases. One of the key safeguards, a stalwart in the defense against waterborne illness, is a double-edged sword that goes by the name chlorine.

Chlorine is a highly reactive element that destroys bacteria on contact. A powerful disinfectant, it is the basic ingredient in bleach and other common household cleansers. It is used at much lower concentrations in drinking water, concentrations that balance the need to kill bacteria with the desire to have good-tasting, safe water. (No one wants to drink water that tastes like the neighborhood pool!) Chlorine itself can be somewhat irritating and toxic to the stomach, so it's doubly important to keep chlorine levels to a minimum.

Fortunately, water companies are usually able to handle chlorine properly and deliver bacteria-free water that tastes reasonably good. But there's a fly in the ointment—the problem with chlorine is that it reacts with organic materials always present in natural waters to form trihalomethanes (THMs). These chlorine byproducts are not only toxic, but also carcinogenic. The most famous THM is chloroform—yes, the chemical that was used as a general anesthetic until safer anesthetics were developed. THMs are present in virtually all water supplies that use chlorine as a disinfectant (AWWA, 2006).

There are federal standards, MCLs, for how many THMs can be safely consumed in drinking water. The limit is 80 ppb, not as stringent as one might like, given the toxic nature of these chemicals. Some epidemiology studies suggest increased cancer and reproductive risks from drinking THMs at concentrations near the MCL (Villanueva et al., 2004; King and Marrett, 1996; Bove et al., 2002). For example, women who regularly drank tap water from public supplies in California had an elevated risk for spontaneous abortion (miscarriage) at THM levels as low as 75 ppb. Evidence linking bladder and colorectal cancer to THMs has appeared in a number of studies, and the USEPA estimates that three in 10,000 people would get cancer if the MCL were 100 ppb, where it formerly was (OK DEQ, 2005). The USEPA dropped the MCL to 80 ppb in 2002, a very small decrease that still leaves us with at least ten times more cancer risk than what regulators normally target to protect public health. THMs are allowed at such levels because they are unavoidable when water is chlorinated, and because it would be expensive for systems to filter them out to more protective levels. However, you as the consumer of public water have the option to filter THMs out of your own household water.

If your water system has THM levels above 10 ppb, you should look into getting a filter. Later in this chapter we'll tell you how to learn about the contaminants in your water supply, and what types of filters you should buy.

Small Public Water Systems

The idea of country living conjures up images of fresh air and open space. But chances are pretty good you'll be drinking water from a small public water system. There are no large systems in rural areas, so homes—as well as businesses, schools, and restaurants—are either on private wells or are hooked into small public systems tapped from nearby groundwater supplies. Compared to the large supplies you'll find in cities or suburbs, are you better off on a small public supply? The answer is no.

Small water systems are more vulnerable to water contaminants for several reasons. Large systems pull water from a large area. If contamination is getting into the system from a point source (like a gas station), it has a good chance of getting diluted out. However, small systems don't have this diluting capacity and may be unlucky enough to pull water directly from a hotspot of contamination into your condominium unit. On top of this, the monitoring requirements for small systems are generally less stringent than for large systems. Since there are many small water systems scattered across the map, they don't form a coherent network, which makes it harder for state and local authorities to keep track of their water quality. Some small systems may not even be on the books— even if they do undertake the bare minimum testing, they may well report nothing to the state.

TOXIC FILE

CONTAMINANTS IN A SMALL PUBLIC WATER SUPPLY

Janice awoke one morning, stumbled half-asleep into the shower, and turned on the water nice and hot. The pulsating spray got her senses going just in time to catch a whiff of some off odor. She had a flash of being in a gas station refilling her car, only in this case she was trapped in her little shower stall. Janice panicked and turned off the water immediately. The odor quickly passed but she skipped the shower, grabbed a cup of coffee, and headed off to work. Over the next several days these "gasoline whiffs" became routine when she was running hot water for laundry or taking a shower. She asked her neighbors if they ever smelled anything funny, but they said they didn't. Finally, Janice called her landlord; she was renting a condominium from the owner, who lived on the other side of town. He told her to talk to the condo association, which was responsible for all the utilities. The condo association told her there was very little chance of a problem because the water was regularly tested and had never shown a problem. They told her that they hadn't had other complaints, and that the odors were probably coming from cars parked outside.

This explanation did little to calm her fears. She had become nauseous and dizzy from the water, and was breaking out in a rash. Convinced that she was being poisoned, Janice took matters into her own hands. She called a lab that could test her water. They sent her a sealed bottle and told her to fill it with a sample of her tap water the next time *the smell returned. She happily paid the $125 fee to get to the bottom of the problem, and felt vindicated when the results came back: toluene: 37 ppb; benzene: 8 ppb; methyl-t-butyl ether (MTBE): 302 ppb. The levels in her water were considerably higher than the numbers in the column labeled "Federal or State Standards." She immediately called her health department. They told her she might be at some risk, and said she should stop using the water until they could confirm the tests. The health department came out to sample her water; their tests confirmed the initial results. The state environmental unit sent out investigators, and after a period of months, was able to show that a nearby gas station had affected one of three wells that supplied the condominium complex—the well that supplied Janice's unit and two others. It turned out that one of the units was vacant and the other was occupied by an elderly couple who didn't notice the smell.*

The condominium association was required to take the bad well offline until a treatment system was put in place to remove the contaminants. Janice asked how the condominium association's tests could have missed her problem. She learned that the condominium's wells got tested for organic chemicals once every three years, not frequently enough in Janice's case.

This Toxic File story points out the problem of limited monitoring of small public systems. To some extent, this is a resource issue: the government does not want to overburden small systems with hefty testing requirements. Large systems have much more income and resources to conduct frequent testing (and there is more at stake in large systems, as many more people are drinking the water). However, if you are the one drinking water from a small system, then you, too, have a lot at stake.

Water contamination may suddenly appear due to a new spill; it's also possible for an old spill to move long distances in groundwater, and then all at once appear in your well. Infrequent testing could be years behind the pollution. Fortunately in Janice's case, the chemicals had an odor, which led to the discovery of the problem. Many contaminants don't have such warning properties.

MTBE AS PUBLIC ENEMY #1?

MTBE, or methyl tertiary butyl ether, is a chemical that's been used as a fuel additive in gasoline since the late 1970s, designed to replace lead as an octane enhancer. MTBE raises the level of oxygen, helping gas burn more cleanly and efficiently, thus creating less air pollution. MTBE has gotten itself into trouble, not so much because of health risks, but because it is a widespread contaminant, appearing in wells far from where it was spilled. Millions of pounds of MTBE were packaged into gasoline, shipped off to gas stations, and put into underground tanks beneath gas pumps. Unfortunately, many of these tanks leaked, releasing MTBE and other, more toxic chemicals (like benzene) into groundwater. Once there, MTBE travels faster and farther than other gasoline chemicals—in many cases, the only chemical reaching a well will be MTBE, tainting the water and creating the need for filters and ongoing monitoring. In fact, MTBE is the most common groundwater contaminant, for both public and private systems, with millions of Americans drinking low levels on a daily basis. And while low levels (<5 ppb) are common, people living close to gas stations (like our friend Janice) or with fuel spills in their yard, can have hundreds or thousands of ppb in their water.

The good news is, at the low levels of exposure typical in groundwater, there is no appreciable cancer risk. Some people may begin to notice its pungent odor or a taste difference in the water beginning at about 50 ppb, but most people need several hundred ppbs in the water to notice an odor or taste. (At those relatively high levels, there is an increased risk for kidney toxicity and cancer.) There is no federal MCL at this time, and state standards vary across the country from about 10 to 100 ppb. As we said, if you can smell or taste it in your water, you are probably exposed to too much and should stop drinking your water until the problem is fixed.

FLUORIDE

Public water supplies have another double-edged sword, another element added to drinking water that provides some benefits and some risks: fluoride. Unlike chlorine, fluoride doesn't make the water any safer; in fact, many public supplies, especially outside of the United States, do not fluoridate the water. Rather than killing bacteria in water, fluoride is intended to protect our teeth from the bacteria in our mouth by depositing in tooth enamel and hardening it against the acidic decay wrought by bacteria. Good oral hygiene (meaning less sweets and frequent brushing) will prevent bacteria and tooth decay, decreasing the need for fluoride. However, government regulators and water companies agreed half a century ago that we Americans can't be trusted to practice good oral hygiene on our own, so they introduced fluoride.

Some baby boomer parents who see fewer cavities in their children's teeth than in their own are thankful for this intervention. However, others harbor a lot of ill will toward fluoride, not to mention the questionable science behind it. Some object to the mass dosing of a population with a druglike substance without their informed consent, and even worse, without having determined all the risks. It's hard to blame them for being skeptical and feeling like guinea pigs.

The key questions in the debate haven't changed in fifty years: does a personal hygiene issue that does *not* spread in epidemic fashion need a massive societal intervention? Is fluoride so effective in fending off cavities that everyone should be taking it regardless of its risks? Is fluoride in tap water safe for adults and children, old people, and newborns? At least we've progressed past the question: Is water fluoridation a Communist plot aimed at taking over the country? That one was actually circulated by right-wing conspiracy theorists during the Cold War. Nevertheless, there's still plenty of hyperbole on both sides of the debate.

MYTH: Fluoride has been put into public water supplies for the past fifty years because it is known to be safe and effective at preventing cavities.

REALITY: While over one hundred million Americans drink fluoridated water, the debate over the safety and effectiveness of fluoride in public water rages on. Many health authorities, including the American Dental Association (ADA), the Centers for Disease Control (CDC), and water industry groups, are pro-fluoridation. In contrast, numerous scientists, advocacy groups, state and local governments, and much of Europe are more cautious or downright against fluoridation. The debate boils down to the benefit of fighting cavities versus the risk of causing cancer.

THE BENEFITS OF WATER FLUORIDATION

Fluoride prevents cavities, cutting down their number by as much as half. That may seem like a public health victory for water fluoridation, but keep in mind, at about the same time, dentistry changed to accommodate fluoride, introducing it into toothpaste, mouth rinses, and drops. There's been an overall drop-off in cavities, even in those who never drank fluoridated water—about the same decline in fluoridated and nonfluoridated areas (Hileman, 1989). A common argument for fluoridation is that not everyone has access to good dental care. Putting fluoride in the water guarantees this preventive measure reaches all people, especially children.

THE RISKS OF WATER FLUORIDATION

Fluorosis

The spotty, lacy white discoloration of teeth in children caused by excess fluoride is called fluorosis. In mild forms, fluorosis is a simple discoloration that doesn't affect the integrity of the teeth. Severe fluorosis causes pitted enamel that is prone to wear and fracture, but fortunately is pretty rare. While statistics for the mild form are somewhat inexact, kids who drink fluoridated water appear to have a greater risk of getting at least some tooth discoloration (Cochrane et al., 2004), and since fluorosis often occurs in the permanent teeth, it's a lifelong condition. Misuse of fluoride rinses and drops and ingestion of fluoride toothpaste can also lead to fluorosis.

It seems that it's relatively easy to overdo fluoride intake; kids on public water already have a head start in that direction (Whelton et al., 2004). Regardless of the type of drinking water they have, it's important for parents to make sure their children are not eating toothpaste or swallowing the rinse. For those on well water, it's important to find out how much natural fluoride is already present before agreeing to give your children any fluoride products, and to make sure these products (rinses, drops) are used properly. It's true that fluorosis is more of a cosmetic issue than a health risk, but it's important to realize that once you have it, you have it forever.

Bone Cancer

Of much greater health concern is the chance that fluoride ingestion causes bone cancer. When we drink fluoride, it has to go from our stomachs via the bloodstream to our teeth, where it can do its job. But this circuitous path also exposes our bones to fluoride, where it can accumulate and, some have theorized, cause abnormal bone growth and cancer. This issue has been studied extensively in animals and in community epidemiology studies. In the majority of cases, fluoride was not associated with bone or any other type of cancer, even at the high doses used in animal studies. However, there was one dose group in a rat cancer test that had an increased rate of osteosarcoma, a rare bone cancer, which is unlikely to have happened by chance (ATSDR, 2003). That test gave fluoride the label of possible animal carcinogen.

In terms of human data, the fluoridated versus nonfluoridated studies have mostly failed to find an association with bone cancer. However, a recent Harvard University study raises new questions. The study, which featured an improved design to find osteosarcoma during critical, early life periods, found a link between water fluoridation and osteosarcoma in boys but not girls, and has created a swirl of controversy. The study has not been published in the open literature; it has appeared only as a Harvard Ph.D. dissertation (Woffinden, 2005), and therefore, has not been rigorously peer-reviewed. Nevertheless, its findings, as tentative as they may be, have been widely broadcast and used to strengthen the anti-fluoride side of the debate.

The National Academy of Sciences recently completed a review of water fluoridation (NAS, 2006). The nation's leading scientific review board found that fluoride can cause severe fluorosis of the teeth and weaker bones at the USEPA's MCL of 4 ppm. However, the NAS did not determine a safe level, or comment on whether the amount of fluoride typically put into public supplies—1 ppm—is safe. Therefore, the debate will likely rage on.

Q *What can we conclude about water fluoridation?*

A After fifty years of widespread use and study, there is still no smoking gun for a serious health effect, which suggests that those who are on a fluoridated supply don't need to take evasive action. If you are careful about how much extra fluoride your kids are getting from toothpaste or from overzealous dentists, you can prevent fluorosis and minimize any bone cancer risk that may theoretically exist. There is generally no need to use water filters to remove fluoride from your supply or drink bottled water.

Those who would rather not deal with the uncertainty can avail themselves of filters or bottled water to avoid fluoride. If you choose this path, you should realize that your kids might need extra help fighting cavities—good hygienic practices, dental sealants, or some form of fluoride supplementation under dentist supervision.

HOW DID A LETHAL AGENT GET LOOSE IN MILWAUKEE'S WATER SUPPLY?

Even in modern times there is still a risk for the spread of waterborne infection as seen in Milwaukee in 1993. A protozoan parasite called cryptosporidium sickened over 400,000 people with stomach symptoms (diarrhea). The sick and elderly had the most trouble fending off the parasite: some 4,400 were hospitalized and 111 died (Corso et al., 2003). You might be wondering how a public water supply let a toxic organism slip by. Although chlorine kills bacteria, it doesn't stop parasites like cryptosporidium. Heavy spring rains overburdened Milwaukee's water treatment plants and allowed the protozoan to get flushed past filtration systems and into everyone's water. The problem goes further than Milwaukee: that same year authorities identified twenty-nine other outbreaks of cryptosporidium affecting nearly 2,400 people (fortunately, in those cases, there were very few hospitalizations and no deaths). The key is not to overburden the water system. Waterborne parasites can strike anywhere, but outbreaks are unlikely to occur if the system is running at adequate filtration capacity. And if they do occur, these outbreaks are typically mild. However, Milwaukee's experience shows us there is potential for serious illness. You should see your doctor if you have a bout of unexplained diarrhea or other stomach symptoms that lasts a week or more. It also may be wise to report your condition to your local health department. They can investigate if there is a local outbreak that can be traced to the water supply or some other source (e.g., contaminated food from a local market or restaurant).

TOXIC FILE

THE RISK INDEX FOR PUBLIC WATER SUPPLIES

The following chart presents risk rankings for the major chemicals in public water supplies, some of which are intentionally added (chlorine, THMs, and fluoride) and some of which are environmental pollutants (MTBE, benzene, pesticides, inorganics, biological agents). The risk for THMs is relatively high because they have important toxic effects like cancer and reproductive toxicity; there is a high likelihood of exposure; and the levels in public supplies can be of public health concern. For fluoride, the risk index is uncertain due to questions about the toxicology (bone cancer) studies, although at this time, the risks do not appear to be a major public health threat. Regarding environmental pollutants, given the requirements of public systems to monitor for and remove these contaminants, most consumers of public water are safeguarded and the risks are low. However, safety is somewhat less guaranteed for small systems that test less often. And as shown by the cryptosporidium outbreak in Milwaukee, even big systems can be vulnerable to an occasional biological risk.

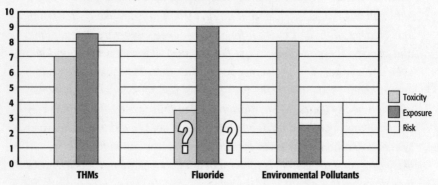

Safety Tips for Those on a Public Supply

1. READ THE REPORT CARD

The Safe Drinking Water Act requires water companies to tell their customers what contaminants are in their water. The report card is officially called the "Consumer Confidence Report," which gives the impression that its main purpose is to convince you your drinking water is safe. However, it does contain key water-quality testing information. The report card is typically sent out with the midsummer water company bill. Any contaminants in the water must be reported, even if they are lower than the MCLs. Various websites provide guidance on how to read these reports (see the resource list at end of the book). In general, you should look to see if your drinking water contains any of the six major types of contaminants described in the table at the end of the chapter. If any contaminants are one-half or more of the MCL, your water is approaching a health risk. This indicates a need for follow-up testing, especially since water contaminant levels can fluctuate over time. Find out if your water supplier is doing the extra testing. If a certain contaminant was above the MCL, make sure the water company fixed the problem and has data to document that the chemical was decreased to a safe level.

Pay particular attention to the levels of THMs reported. Technically, a violation of the MCL occurs only if the level is above 80 ppb; however, there's a risk of cancer, miscarriage, and other reproductive effects at levels above 10 ppb. The higher the THM level above 10 ppb, the greater the risk. The best solution for THMs is filtration; a simple carbon filter will effectively absorb the contaminant out of the water.

2. FIND OUT HOW MUCH TESTING IS BEING DONE

There's no guarantee that your water company is doing an adequate job of testing your water. This is an especially important question for small and even moderate-sized systems, since their requirements can be more lenient. Systems that test less than once per year may be questionable, and should have to explain the low frequency—if they claim their testing meets state requirements, then get in touch with the state public water people. There may be a good reason for infrequent testing (such as a lack of detections or contaminant sources in the area), but then again, there may not be.

3. CONSIDER YOUR OWN TESTING

Most people start thinking about their water quality *after* they become ill, either with cancer or some other disorder. It's natural to assume your drinking water is safe until something bad happens, especially if you're on a public system that already does some testing. However, as we pointed out above, that may not be sufficient to guarantee safety. If you test on your own, you can increase the frequency and number of chemicals you're testing for. But be careful—testing your own water is not cheap, so it's important to be smart about what to test and when. Refer to the chart at the end of the chapter to learn about which contaminants are more likely to affect your water supply; the guidelines presented for private wells in the next section are reasonable for small public supplies. Certainly, if you smell or taste anything unusual in your water, you should talk to your water supplier and consider your own testing if you don't get satisfying answers.

Private Well Pollutants

These days, relatively few of us drink from private wells. The number has dropped over the years as suburbs have grown, replete with the modern conveniences of shopping malls, trash pickup, sewers, and city water. It's a little harder to generalize about water quality from individual as compared to public supplies. For one thing, each well is unique, drilled to the precise depth necessary to reach an ample water supply. The pollution risk factors surrounding each well are also unique, in terms of proximity of sources and direction of groundwater flow. There is no one type of contaminant (like THMs and fluoride for public supplies) that is common to all private wells.

The biggest difference is that, if you're on a private well, there is no one to safeguard the supply for you—no outside party to test your water or make sure a neighbor isn't dumping chemicals that will show up in your well. Public water supplies have watershed protection regulations that create buffer zones around reservoirs, where it's illegal to spray nasty pesticides or dispose of wastes. There are no such regulations for private wells, nothing to stop a gas station from moving in near you and installing tanks that may someday leak gasoline into your supply. If you drink from a private well, you are responsible for the safety of your water.

Safety Tips for People on Private Wells

Although all wells are unique, there are four basic principles for keeping your private well water safe. The first tip is **don't do anything to contaminate your well**. This is the environmental equivalent of shooting yourself in the foot. It seems like common sense, but unfortunately, the situation does occur.

CONTAMINATING YOUR OWN WELL

Mike loved working on cars, and decided he didn't want a desk job. After college he was determined to start his own auto repair shop, so he got a job at a garage in town and lived at home to save up. His parents were happy to see him being so industrious and looked the other way when he started bringing his friends' cars home in the evenings to earn some extra cash. Things were going smoothly until Mike's aunt came to stay for a few days. After her first night in the house, she declared that someone was trying to poison her—she claimed that the water smelled and tasted bad, gave her nightmares, and was toxic. Mike's dad decided to humor his sister and send a water sample off for a test. To their surprise, the water was contaminated with VOCs (volatile organic compounds) and hydrocarbons, the kind that can make you dizzy, nauseated, and irritable. They immediately called the health department, who said that they should stop drinking the water, even not to use it to wash the car.

Mike's family was very thankful for the aunt's acute nose. The health department official told them that the odor may have come on gradually and so might have been hard to notice. However, a newcomer to the house could have picked it up right away. The state sent someone out to investigate. It didn't take long to find the problem: the dirt driveway had dark stains where Mike had been doing his mechanical moonlighting. He admitted to being a little sloppy with gasoline and used motor oil, saying "some" had spilled on the ground in recent months. Mike might have gotten away with his sloppiness if not for the fact that his makeshift business was only twenty feet away from their well.

The state issued Mike's family an order to clean up the contaminated soil so it wouldn't spread to other wells. It was an expensive procedure, as they needed to hire an environmental contractor to remove the contaminated soil, test the remaining soil, and submit a report to the state. They were able to salvage their own well by filtering the water with activated carbon, which was also complicated, as the filter needed regular changing and the water needed ongoing testing to make sure the filter was working. They were told that eventually the groundwater would flush itself out and the filters would no longer be needed.

As our Toxic File makes very clear, you should never dump gasoline, fuel oil, paint, varnish, pesticides, or other chemical-bearing products into soil—regardless of whether you are on public water or a private well. One way or another, some of what you put in the ground will find its way back up to the surface. The general rule is don't put anything into the ground that you wouldn't want to end up drinking.

Q *What about pesticides designed specifically for residential yards (as opposed to the agricultural pesticides we talked about earlier in this chapter)? How do those pesticides affect well water?*

A It turns out they're a fairly minor concern. Modern pesticides are biodegradable, and so will likely break down too quickly to reach substantial levels in groundwater. However, it's always a good idea to minimize pesticide use (Chapter 12) and in so doing, add extra assurance that your well is protected.

The second tip is **be aware of groundwater risk factors in your neighborhood**. Pollution from industries, landfills, gas stations, waste sites, farms, and other agricultural businesses (e.g., garden shops) can travel in groundwater and land in your well. Even if the actual polluting industry is long gone, its lot overgrown with weeds, soil and groundwater pollution may be left in its wake. (Chapter 15, "Pollution from Below," fully describes these sources and the risks they present.) Local and state agencies will investigate groundwater contamination if alerted to it. But be aware, in many cases these agencies cannot find and intercept groundwater pollution before it gets to private wells. In fact, it may be your well test or odor complaint that tips them off to a groundwater problem in the neighborhood.

Third, **test your well at least once every few years:** more often if you live close (within a quarter mile) to possible sources of pollution or if you or your neighbors have had problems in the past, less often if you are in a low-risk area. Testing is expensive, with the most basic of water tests running about $50 and a full scan upwards of $300. You don't want to test too often or for more chemicals than you need. If you know what you are looking for (e.g., industrial solvents because you live near a metal parts factory, or gasoline because of a gas station), you can narrow down the testing and save yourself money. However, most contaminants are worth testing for at least once if you are on a private well (refer to the table at the end of the chapter for a complete listing of the contaminants you should be on the lookout for).

A good general testing plan for private wells follows:

- Get a full scan when you move into a new house, and definitely before you start drinking the water. Maybe the former owners or their neighbors misused pesticides, dumped gasoline, or had leaks in their heating oil tank. Maybe there is an old industrial site up the road that twenty years ago released solvent into the ground. You can try to make this testing a responsibility of the sellers when entering into your purchase agreement.

- Retest annually for the chemicals most likely to be in your neighborhood from man-made sources. Volatile organic compounds (VOCs), pesticides, nitrate, certain metals (chromium, nickel, cadmium), and biologicals may fluctuate due to changes in chemical use at nearby sources, or because an underground load of contaminant finally reaches your well. However, you only need follow-up testing for chemicals that have a reason to be in the ground near you. For example, if you don't live near a farm or garden shop and your initial water testing found no pesticides, there isn't much reason to retest for pesticides. Disinfection byproducts are normally a public water supply issue, and so are not usually tested for in private wells after the initial scan.

- Natural contaminants like arsenic, manganese, and the radiologics are typically from bedrock rather than from industry or landfills, and fluctuate less over time. If they are well below the MCL in the first test round, you can stop testing for them. If they are within one-half of their respective MCLs, however, annual testing is a good idea.

- The so-called Leached Metals—lead and copper. If you live in post-1985 housing, it's very unlikely you have lead in your pipes, so testing for lead more than once is probably not necessary. For pre-1985 houses, you should test for lead annually for several years to make sure it's not leaching from the pipes—the pH in your groundwater may vary over time, which can affect lead leaching. Copper is much less toxic than lead and does not need frequent testing, unless someone in your home has Wilson's disease. This rare genetic deficiency impairs one's ability to excrete copper.

INTERPRETING YOUR WATER TESTING RESULTS

Contrary to popular belief, you don't actually need a toxicologist to interpret your water test results.

The water quality report from the lab is pretty basic and easy to understand, and you should be able to quickly tell if there is anything present over a health standard level. However, you may need to talk to an expert to see what elevated results mean to your health.

Here are some tips for interpreting your water test report and for taking follow-up action, if needed:

- If the result is undetectable or far below the standard: it's a no-brainer. You don't have to worry about that chemical.
- If the result is within one-half of but still below the standard: there may be a specific contaminant source near you. You can keep drinking the water, but retest within a few months. If the result is stable or decreases, you can reduce your test schedule to once per year. However, start investigating possible sources as described in this chapter and also in Chapter 15. Let your local health department know and ask your neighbors if they're experiencing the same type of contamination.
- If the result is over the federal or state standard: stop using the water for drinking or cooking. Immediately call your local health department and ask for their help in investigating the problem. They may bring in your state's environmental agency to test groundwater in the neighborhood. Find out how to treat your water with filters, in case the contamination can't be quickly resolved.

In the third scenario you might need that toxicologist to answer some key questions like: Can I still use the water for other purposes (baths, showers, laundry, dishes)? What health risks have I been accumulating over the past years while using this water? Should I go to the doctor to get tested for toxic effects? Are my children going to be OK? This is where toxicologists really earn their salary. Every situation will be different, but there are a few general principles we follow in answering these questions. The most important is what we call "defusing the bright line syndrome," one of the most basic rules in risk communication, no matter what the issue. The general public lives with the myth that there is a "bright line" or absolute standard above which there is rampant toxicity and death, and below which is safety.

Public health toxicology doesn't work like that: from the start, we set standards that are *well below* where toxic effects have been seen in test animals or people. We set the standards so low so we can be sure the public is protected and because we realize everyone is unique: we cannot test chemical X on every person to know his or her susceptibility. We take what the animal test results show and build in uncertainty factors that cover the possibility that people are more sensitive than animals, and that you may be more sensitive than I am.

What does this mean to you and your over-the-MCL water test result? Often the detected level is still below the amount known to be toxic or carcinogenic. When you are above the MCL but below the known toxic level, you are in a gray area where we can't guarantee safety, although we can't point to a case where anyone has been harmed. It means stop drinking the water and fix the problem, but at the same time, don't worry about the years of drinking the contaminated water. A test result above the MCL isn't an immediate "Ah ha!"—now I know why my family has health problems or why Rover died so young. However, if the result is high enough above the MCL and the chemical is nasty enough, maybe there is a link. That's why you would want to discuss this with your local health department, who may triage you to the state toxicologist.

The fourth private well safety tip is this: **consider using a water filter.** If testing has found contaminants at levels of concern in your supply, what are your options? If you are on public water, get on the phone immediately with your water company to find out why the result is so high and what they are doing about it. If the answer is "not much," you need to talk with the state agency that regulates water companies. (Note: if your concern is a THM reading of, for example, 60 ppb, the water company and state official are unlikely to help you, because the result is below the MCL of 80 ppb. In this case, you may want to take your own action and install a water filter.) If you are on a private well, the steps described previously are a good start. Ultimately, you may need to install a water filter so you don't have to keep buying bottled water. Fortunately, water filters work pretty well for most contaminants, although there is no one filter that can handle all types. The following table gives you basic information on the type of filter you need for different chemicals, along with the MCL for each chemical.

CONTAMINANTS AND THEIR WATER FILTERS

CONTAMINANT	MCL[1]	TYPE OF FILTER
Arsenic	0.01 mg/L	Reverse Osmosis, Distillation
Atrazine	0.003 mg/l	Carbon Adsorption
Benzene	0.005 mg/l	Carbon Adsorption
Ethylene dibromide	0.00005 mg/l	Carbon Adsorption
Fluoride	4 mg/l	Reverse Osmosis, Distillation
Hardness	Not applicable	Cation exchange softener
Lead	0.015 mg/l	Carbon Adsorption, Reverse Osmosis, Distillation
Manganese	0.05–0.5 mg/l	Greensand Adsorption or Ion Exchange
MTBE	0.01–0.1 mg/l	Carbon Adsorption
Nitrate	10 mg/l	Reverse Osmosis
PCBs, Persistent Pesticides[2]	Depends upon contaminant	Carbon Adsorption
Perchlorate	0.001–0.02 mg/l	Reverse Osmosis
Radon	> 4,000 pCi/l[3]	Adsorption, Aeration
Sulfides	Not applicable	Carbon Adsorption
Trichloroethylene	0.005 mg/l	Carbon Adsorption
Trihalomethanes	0.08 mg/l	Carbon Adsorption

Table extracted from National Sanitation Foundation (NSF) website (www.NSF.org)

[1] In most cases, the federal MCL is shown; in some cases where there is no federal MCL, a range of state drinking water guidelines is shown (e.g., manganese, MTBE).

[2] Examples of persistent pesticides you may encounter in your well are chlordane, dieldrin, DDT.

[3] Radon in water should be treated if level is above 4,000 pCi/l and radon in air is high—see Chapter 2.

THE PROS AND CONS OF THE COMMON FILTERS

As the table indicates, the most common and versatile filters are carbon adsorption and reverse osmosis. In carbon adsorption, water is forced through a block of activated carbon, which binds up a wide variety of contaminants. The contaminants are left behind on the filter, and the water that exits is much cleaner. Carbon filters can produce large volumes of purified water, with the cost in the $100 to $300 range depending upon the size of the system purchased. Be aware, the carbon filter will eventually become saturated with contaminant, at which point you must replace it— an overused, saturated filter can experience a "break-through" where some of the built-up contaminant breaks free of the filter and passes into your drinking water. This can lead to much higher contaminant levels than if you didn't use a filter at all. Avoid the problem by simply replacing the filter on schedule, or a little ahead of schedule to play it safe. The specifications for the unit you buy should tell you approximately how many gallons the filter is good for.

A drawback for the carbon filter is that it can be a breeding ground for bacteria accumulating in water that sits in the filter for long periods of time. You can solve this problem by flushing water through the filter if it hasn't been used in a while. Before you draw a glass of drinking water first thing in the morning or after being out all day, run your water for ten to twenty seconds. To avoid wasting water, consider filling a gallon jug (or more) after you initially flush the filter—that way you'll know the entire gallon is good. Leave whatever you don't use immediately in the refrigerator to keep it fresh.

Reverse osmosis is a more complex process involving a membrane that allows tap water to flow through, but holds back contaminants based upon differences in pressure on the two sides of the membrane. The reverse osmosis unit requires a certain level of water pressure, which it attains by running a pump to push water through the system at high pressure, and features a number of other filters that keep the membrane in good shape. The unit runs in a manner similar to your hot water heater, in that it stores up a reservoir of filtered water in a tank so you don't have to wait around for a glass—when the tank level is reduced, the unit kicks in to fill it back up. The systems are expensive ($300 to $3,000, plus installation) and not very efficient, producing only two to ten gallons per day and wasting five or ten times that amount. The membrane needs to be replaced according to the manufacturer's schedule, so there are ongoing costs. However, all of these down sides may be worth it to get contaminant-free tap water without the hassle of buying bottled water, which in itself is no guarantee of contaminant-free water (see the next page).

TOXIC FACT

BOTTLED WATER IS GENERALLY NO LESS CONTAMINATED THAN PUBLIC OR PRIVATE SUPPLIES.

Bottled water has become a booming business over the past two decades, with the number of brands and the amount they are selling still increasing. It's hard to go to a public event, food outlet, or vending machine without running into this ubiquitous convenience. The benefit of all this bottled water is that people are choosing to quench their thirst with something that isn't loaded with calories or caffeine. However, bottled water is no panacea of good health, and isn't necessarily any better than plain old tap water.

MYTH: Bottled water typically comes from mountain streams or fresh springs.

REALITY: The bottled water industry paints many nice images of where their product comes from. However, some of the most popular brands are simply tap water from public supplies (city water) that have been treated to remove chlorine and THMs. Other brands come from groundwater that is comparable to anyone else's private well, complete with the issues described earlier. The reality is far from the marketing hype used to sell this product.

You may recall the bottled water scare of 1990, in which low levels of benzene were found in bottles of Perrier, that sparked a huge (70 million bottle) recall and also led to much closer scrutiny of the industry. Nonetheless, bottled water is regulated less stringently than tap water, with fewer testing requirements. Testing done by environmental and consumer groups have generally found bottled water to be relatively free of contamination issues (NRDC, 1999). A few brands harbored bacteria that wouldn't have been allowed in public water, and which may have been a risk to people with weak immune systems. In sporadic cases, levels of VOCs were detected that, even though they were within drinking water standards, still shouldn't have been in an unblemished supply. A natural question is whether the bottle itself adds chemicals (plasticizers, Chapter 5) to the water. This does not appear to be a common problem, especially since the kind of plastic used for bottled water does not contain plasticizer chemicals.

Generally, as long as bottled water is not in some way contaminated, there's really nothing wrong with drinking it. But there's no guarantee of purity or even an improvement on regular old tap water. You can fill a bottle at home, keep it cold in a little insulated pouch, and avoid spending money on this over-hyped product.

Q *Should we filter all the water in the house, or only the water we drink?*

A This is an excellent question whose answer depends upon the specific contaminant(s) you are confronting. Here are some general rules:

- **Drinking Water:** Filter to remove all contaminants of concern. You should ideally have a filter set up wherever you drink tap water, including the kitchen and bathroom(s). For the kitchen, you can use a countertop filtration system that diverts the water you want to drink away from the regular tap via a hose to the filter unit (which are quite effective). For the bathroom, you may want to install a smaller, simpler faucet-mount unit that attaches right to the faucet head and has a diverter, so that only the water you want to drink is filtered. These units are small and cannot handle the drinking water demands of the kitchen.

- **Cooking Water:** Filter to remove all contaminants except VOCs, THMs, and ethylene dibromide (EDB). These contaminants are volatile (can readily leave water and form a gas) and will escape from your boiling tea or pot of soup as you cook it. Keep the exhaust fan on the stove going to vent the contaminants out of the kitchen.

- **Bath and Shower:** Filter to remove only the VOCs, THMs, EDB, and other pesticides. These chemicals are volatile and can be inhaled during a shower or bath, and some can also penetrate the skin—studies have shown that you take more THMs into your body during a ten-minute shower than from drinking a quart of water (Betts, 2002). The inorganic contaminants are not volatile and in general don't penetrate the skin fast enough to worry about. If you decide you need a filter for bathing, you will have to put in a whole-house filter, installed right where your water enters the house plumbing. You'll have the advantage of having all the water in your house filtered, and only one filter to worry about changing. However, whole house units are more expensive and require a plumber to install.

DON'T COOK WITH HOT TAP WATER

You might be tempted to cook your stew or soup with hot water from the tap, assuming it would be quicker to cook with water that's already hot. We have very simple advice for you: DON'T DO IT. Hot water is not necessarily fresh or clean—it sits around in a hot water tank for hours or days at a time at high temperatures, in an environment that may not be completely clean or sterile. It's fine for bathing and washing chores; you can also use hot tap water to thaw frozen foods as long as it doesn't directly contact the food. However, you shouldn't cook with or ingest water from the hot tap.

THE RISK INDEX FOR PRIVATE WELLS

People on private wells don't usually have THMs and fluoride to worry about—just a long list of other contaminants, as shown in the table immediately following this chart. These contaminants are more of a worry for people on private wells, because there's no outside testing agency and no one to remove them if they are present. The absence of this safety net makes private wells riskier. The chart below shows that the toxicity of these contaminants can be high and exposure moderate (high for some people but low for most). The net result is a moderately high overall risk index for private wells, one that calls for proactive testing and water filtration, if necessary.

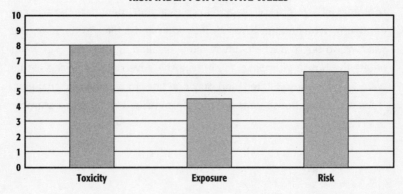

RISK INDEX FOR PRIVATE WELLS

SUMMARY OF COMMON WATER CONTAMINANTS

CONTAMINANT TYPE	CONTAMINANT NAME	LIKELY SOURCE	HEALTH RISKS	SHOULD I TEST FOR IT?[1]
Biological	E. Coli	Human/animal waste	Infection, stomach illness, death if immunity is poor	Private well—yes Public water—no
Biological	Cryptosporidium	Human/animal waste	Same as E. Coli	No
VOCs	MTBE	Spilled gasoline	Liver, Kidney	Yes
VOCs	Benzene	Spilled gasoline	Carcinogen	Yes
VOCs	Toluene	Spilled gasoline	Nervous system damage	Yes
VOCs	Ethylbenzene	Spilled gasoline	Nervous system damage	Yes
VOCs	Xylene	Spilled gasoline	Nervous system damage	Yes
VOCs	Perchloroethylene (PERC)	Dry cleaners or metals industries	Kidney, cancer	Yes, if near stores, industries
VOCs	Trichloroethylene (TCE)	Metals industries	Kidney, cancer	Yes, if near current or former industry
Disinfection By-product	Trihalomethanes (THMs) such as Chloroform	Chlorine used in public water supply	Cancer, adverse birth outcomes	Private well—no[2] Public water—no
Inorganic	Nitrate	Fertilizer, landfill, human/animal waste	Blood toxicity in babies	Yes

[1] A simple yes or no refers to homeowners on either a private well or small public water supply only. In some cases, the advice is different depending upon type of water supply, as indicated.

[2] If you recently sterilized your well with chlorine, you should test for disinfection byproducts.
Proximity: by near, we mean within one-quarter mile.

CONTAMINANT TYPE	CONTAMINANT NAME	LIKELY SOURCE	HEALTH RISKS	SHOULD I TEST FOR IT?
Inorganic	Perchlorate	Munitions, blasting sites, military waste, fireworks	Thyroid, brain development	Yes
Inorganic (metal)	Arsenic	Bedrock	Cancer	Private well—yes Public water—no
Inorganic (metal)	Copper	Household plumbing	Upset stomach; toxic to liver in Wilson's disease	Yes
Inorganic (metal)	Lead	Household plumbing	Brain development	Yes, if plumbing is from before 1985
Inorganic (metal)	Manganese	Bedrock	Toxic to brain	Yes
Inorganic (metal)	Chromium, Nickel, Cadmium	Metals industries	Variety of effects	Yes, if well is near an industrial area
Persistent Pesticide (banned)	Ethylene dibromide (EDB)	Old farmland	Cancer	Yes, if well is near current or former farmland
Persistent Pesticide (banned)	Organochlorines (DDT, chlordane, dieldrin, etc.)	Old farmland, use of chlordane around home in the past	Cancer, liver toxicity	Yes, if well is near farmland or if used chlordane in past
Pesticide (current)	Organophosphates, pyrethroids	Current farmland, greenhouse/garden shop	Nervous system	Yes, if well is near farmland or greenhouse
Radiological	Radon	Bedrock	Lung cancer	Yes, if radon in air is high
Radiological	Uranium	Bedrock	Kidney	Yes
Radiological	Gross Alpha	Bedrock	Cancer	Yes

The preceding table provides a summary of the major contaminants you might find in public and private water supplies. It is divided into six broad groups: biological agents, volatile organic chemicals (VOCs), disinfection byproducts (THMs), inorganics, pesticides, and radiologics. The last column is directed to those people on private wells and small public systems—it provides general guidance on whether the contaminant is worth testing for. If you are on a large public supply, you don't have to do any of your own testing as your company should test often enough already.

This chapter's basic message is that you have to pay attention to your drinking water quality, no matter what type of supply you are on. However, our advice differs somewhat depending upon whether you drink from a private well or public supply and whether that public supply is large or small. Therefore, our safe drinking water checklist is organized around the type of water system that serves your house.

SAFE DRINKING WATER CHECKLIST

PUBLIC SUPPLY–LARGE SYSTEM (> 50,000 PEOPLE SERVED)

❑ Read your water company's report card.

❑ Determine the level of total THMs (reported as TTHMs).

❑ Consider using a carbon filter to remove TTHMs if level is above 10 ppb.

❑ Decide whether whole house or only drinking water filtration is desired (whole house prevents exposures while bathing/showering, but is more expensive).

❑ Determine from the report card whether other contaminants are in your water; if present, ask water supplier why they are there, whether levels are going up or down over time, and how often they are monitoring.

❑ If your home was built before 1990, test your tap water for lead at least once.

❑ There's no need to remove fluoride from your drinking water, but make sure other sources of fluoride exposure in children (e.g., toothpaste ingestion, fluoride rinses) are minimized.

PUBLIC SUPPLY–SMALL (< 3,300 PEOPLE) OR MODERATE SIZED (3,300 TO 50,000) SYSTEM

Follow the suggestions above for large systems but add:

❑ Ask your water company how often they test for each type of contaminant.

❑ Consider doing your own testing for contaminants that are not tested for at least once per year if:
  ❑ these contaminants have been detected in your water supply in the most recent report, even if below the MCL.
  ❑ these contaminants might logically come from industries or pollution sources located near your public supply well (a small supply well is likely to be near your home, but may not be).

❑ Consider using a water filter if your test results are high.

PRIVATE WELLS

❑ Run a full set of water tests when you first move into the house: VOCs, THMs, pesticides, inorganics, radiologicals, bacteria, nitrate. Filter out any contaminants that are above the MCL.

❑   Retest the well annually for any contaminants that are within one-half of the MCL, and for contaminants that might plausibly be present in groundwater due to nearby sources (e.g., farms, landfills, gas stations, industry).

❑   Retest for contaminants if conditions change:
    ❑   Neighbors have contamination problems in their well—find out what and test accordingly.
    ❑   You accidentally spill fuel oil or gasoline into the ground—test for VOCs.
    ❑   You notice an unusual taste or odor from the water—start with VOC testing, but you may have to go to full scan to find the problem.
    ❑   You disinfect the well with chlorine tablets to address a bacteriological problem—test for chlorine and THMs.

❑   Test annually for lead if your home is pre-1985. After several years of good results, you can decrease the frequency of lead testing.

CHAPTER 7

Consumer Products

Chemists have helped fill the marketplace with wondrous products that get clothing whiter, nails longer, floors shinier, carpets cleaner, as well as kill ants, glue things back together, and decorate our homes. Amidst heavy advertising and skillful labeling, consumers purchase these items and try them out, never dreaming that they might contain toxic chemicals that can get into our bodies and have unintended effects. For most people and most products, there's not enough exposure to cause alarm. However, it's generally a good idea to minimize our exposure to toxic chemicals, especially since we don't know how they will interact inside of us. Minimizing exposure is especially important if you are sensitive to chemicals or have young children—not only might kids be more sensitive, but also more curious and they might decide to taste the product. Keeping consumer products, especially the more toxic ones discussed in this chapter, away from young children is a cornerstone of family safety.

We cannot hope to cover the entire marketplace of toxics in one chapter. In fact, our coverage of consumer products spills over into the chapters on indoor air (Chapter 8, carpets, furniture, unvented gas appliances, air purifiers); yard and garden (Chapter 12, pesticides); school (Chapter 10, art supplies); lead (Chapter 1, glassware, pottery, hair dyes); and food (Chapter 5). The current chapter focuses on chemicals contained in products that we use to clean our houses (cleansers and disinfectants); that we use to protect our walls, floors, and furniture (paint and waxes); that come in handy when we need to make a home repair (coatings and adhesives); that we apply to protect our home from insects (household pesticides); or that we apply to look and smell attractive (cosmetics and personal care). In some cases, the misuse of these products has put thousands of people in the hospital each year from unintentional (typically accidental, non-suicidal) exposures (TESS, 2002). For example, there are approximately 200,000 overexposures reported to poison control centers each year for household cleaners alone.

Many of the products described in this chapter contain VOCs. These chemicals readily become airborne when used, making inhalation exposure unavoidable. Other chemicals can present hazards to the skin and eyes (e.g., harsh cleaners) or can be absorbed through the skin to present an internal risk (e.g., cosmetics).

MYTH: There are state and federal agencies that test consumer products and don't allow anything on the market that isn't safe.

REALITY: Unfortunately, that's far from the truth. The federal agency responsible for testing, the Consumer Product Safety Commission (CPSC), is swamped by an abundance of products and brands in the marketplace. It has to deal with physical hazards ranging from baby swings to circular saws, fire hazards, and the safety of tires, cars, and boats. Chemicals in consumer products are certainly on their radar, but no one agency is able to review or test every type of product. There is nothing to stop a company from using known carcinogens such as benzene and trichloroethylene in glues and cleaners. It's really up to the companies that make, repackage, and sell these products to ensure safety, because if their product is dangerous and people are harmed, they will be sued. So, in large measure, it's the fear of toxic tort cases that keeps the worst chemicals out of consumer products.

TOXIC FACT

WARNING LABELS ARE NOT THE ANSWER.

CPSC may not prevent a chemical from being in a product, but it is mandated with the task of reviewing product labels to make sure they contain appropriate warnings. The public is thrown a bone of safety information, which would be a good thing if it weren't for three factors: 1) the warnings are usually in tiny letters, much smaller than the promotional language; 2) many types of chemicals are exempt from labeling requirements (see fragrances and phthalates later in this chapter); 3) consumers are not educated to pay attention to warning labels, instead assuming that if a product is in the store, it must be safe to use. That's part of the reason California developed Proposition 65, a product-labeling law that requires the listing of any carcinogenic or reproductive hazards. In addition to informing (in some instances scaring) the consumer, it also provides an incentive for industry to remove toxic chemicals from their product—obviously, a product whose label has a carcinogen warning looks worse to the consumer than one that has no warning. Unfortunately, so many products merit labeling under Proposition 65 due to toxic ingredients that it's difficult for the consumer to sort out a serious risk from "just another cancer warning." This and a number of other reasons have kept the Proposition 65 concept from spreading to other states.

The bottom line is that the public cannot be guaranteed of the safety of consumer products. Labeling is typically inadequate, and toxic chemicals can be present without oversight by government authorities.

Cleansers and Disinfectants

Household cleaning products span a range from harsh chemicals, which make you run for rubber gloves and fresh air, to more subtle versions that are less concentrated but can still pack a punch. Simple cleansers like soaps, detergents, and scouring powders are fairly innocuous, causing chapped hands from overexposure and having fragrances that may be bothersome to some. Products that also disinfect are usually harsher because their mission is not only to clean but also to kill germs, which requires more powerful "antimicrobial" chemicals that destroy bacteria, viruses, and mold on contact. While those who work in hospitals are familiar with chemical disinfectants containing iodine and alcohol, our focus is on the chemicals more commonly used in household cleaning products. For example, the hazardous nature of harsh cleansers is evidenced by the 50,000 overexposure cases per year that are attributed to bleach alone (TESS, 2002). Of the total number for cleaning products (a staggering 212,000 cases), 35,000 people needed medical attention and 9,000 people had moderate or severe effects. In 2002, 32 people died from household cleaners.

We're also including carpet spot removers and drain uncloggers in this section as cleaning products that sometimes involve very different chemistry and potential for risk.

THE COMMON HOUSEHOLD CLEANERS AMMONIA AND BLEACH ARE LIKELY THE MOST HAZARDOUS PRODUCTS IN YOUR HOME.

If you want to clean your toilet with something that is guaranteed to kill everything on contact, ammonia or bleach are the natural first choices. Ammonia has a high pH, and nothing can survive under such extreme basic (as opposed to acidic) conditions. The pungent ammonia smell jumps out of the bottle when you unscrew the cap, unable to be masked by the lemon scent usually thrown in for good measure. Many who clean bathrooms have gotten used to ammonia and so tolerate the eye, nose, and throat irritation it causes, as long as it remains mild. However, using ammonia, even diluted in extra water, in a closed-in environment such as a shower stall is not recommended, as you can be exposed to higher vapor concentrations and experience more irritation. Those with asthma or other types of respiratory problems or chemical sensitivity should avoid exposure to ammonia altogether. Of course, everyone should handle this chemical with care, as accidental splashing into the eyes or on the skin can cause permanent damage. Ammonia will cause damage to the gastrointestinal tract if ingested by young children, and can be fatal if enough goes down. Bottom line, although it's a useful and inexpensive product, ammonia can be so harsh on the body that it may not be worth the risks.

Bleach is not much different—it's as irritating and hazardous as ammonia, but has a distinct swimming-pool odor. That's because chlorine, or more precisely, sodium hypochlorite, a very reactive form of chlorine, is bleach's main ingredient. Bleach is excellent at killing bacteria and mold on contact, but will also leach away the color of your clothing, or even your skin, causing damage to both. It should be diluted for most uses, as it is more powerful than necessary straight out of the bottle. Bleach is one of the leading causes of child poisoning, which is surprising because it has a strong, irritating odor that you'd hope would keep kids from imbibing.

Adverse effects from bleach or ammonia are usually reversible, as long as you don't ingest or splash the chemicals into your eyes. However, the same cannot be said if, for some reason, you mix the two together, as the following Toxic File shows.

BAD CHEMISTRY IN THE BATHROOM

Jane was late for her morning workout class and had to drop the kids off to preschool on the way. The last thing she needed was a clogged bathroom drain. Not finding any drain unclogger under the sink, she grabbed at the bottle of ammonia, figuring it would burn through any hair balls stuck down there. But it didn't work very well. After the ammonia had finished slowly draining out of the sink, she reached for the other part of her chemical arsenal, bleach, which she poured down the drain while putting on some makeup. Within a minute she started gagging, choking, and experiencing a stinging eye and nose irritation. She lunged out of the bathroom and pulled the door shut behind her, leaving the mess for later. After her workout, she went to the market for some things and figured she would pick up some drain cleaner. She called her husband, Dave, to ask his advice on what to buy and told him about her morning run-in with the drain. He gasped as he heard his wife's description of the two chemicals and then the horrible feeling in her throat. He realized the ammonia was probably still in the drain when the bleach went down, and that the two chemicals probably mixed. He made her hold on while he checked the Internet for more information. Sure enough, he quickly found red flags about never mixing ammonia and bleach together: they form chlorine gas and chloramines, which are highly toxic to the lungs and can cause irreversible damage. People have died from chlorine gas; it was even used as a chemical warfare agent during World War I.

Reassured that his wife felt OK, he was still worried about the house. He asked his wife if the bathroom window had been open, and she confirmed it hadn't. He also established that the ceiling exhaust fan hadn't been on. All of that meant chlorine gas had probably been building up in the bathroom all day. He blurted out: "Don't go in the house until I get there." On his last click before exiting, he noticed a website talking about explosions caused by mixing ammonia and bleach in the wrong proportions. Would his house even still be there? He decided to take no chances and called the police department, who instructed him to call the fire department, the designated hazmat (hazardous materials) responder in his town. They were equipped with the proper gas masks to deal with chlorine and anything else that may have been brewing in his bathroom. The fire chief was duly concerned, and offered to send a truck over right away.

Jane and Dave were greeted by the sight of a fire truck with sirens blaring as they turned onto their street. Embarrassed by the attention but relieved to see the house still standing, they opened the front door for the firemen, who were wearing full protective gear. They carefully went upstairs and slowly opened the bathroom door, opened the window, and turned on the ceiling fan, wiped down the bathroom surfaces with a neutralizing agent, and told Jane and Dave that in an hour it would be safe to go back upstairs.

However, chlorine gas had built up to such a high level, the porcelain sink and chrome fixture were pitted and ruined. Jane and Dave were glad that it was only hardware and not the soft tissue of their lungs that had been damaged by the corrosive gas.

As the Toxic File makes clear, using bleach and ammonia products in the same bathroom is a disaster waiting to happen. They won't interact if they're simply stored near each other, but if mixed, they can create a toxic train wreck (a purposeful analogy, since chlorine gas leaks into communities are most common from derailed trains). Never mix ammonia and chlorine. Also, be aware that bleach can mix with regular drain cleaner and form chlorine gas, as well.

You need to read the labels of your bathroom cleaners to see if they have ammonia or bleach (sodium hypochlorite) in them. These harsh chemicals can be hidden as one of several ingredients in a disinfectant cleaner and again, you want to be absolutely sure that you don't use an ammonia and a bleach product at the same time. The simplest solution is to only use one product for a given cleanup job. If it doesn't work to your satisfaction, thoroughly rinse and try a second product—that way, there is very little chance of the second product interacting with the first.

Two other under-the-sink bottles you should pay special attention to are drain unclogger and toilet bowl cleaner. These are often formulated with sodium hypochlorite (bleach) or other highly irritating chemicals (e.g., hydrochloric acid), and thus show up in poison control records as leading causes of household poisoning. Mixing these products with ammonia can release the toxic gases we just described. They must be handled with a tremendous amount of toxic respect, which includes wearing gloves, taking care to avoid splashing in the eyes; using in a well-ventilated area; keeping them far away from children; and never using them in conjunction with other cleaners. Consider whether cleaning products that require so much vigilance are worth the effort. Get good at using a plunger and snake if your drain gets clogged. Look for milder and "greener" toilet bowl cleaners that avoid the use of bleach or strong acids.

MILD DISINFECTANTS

Most other kitchen and bathroom cleaners (e.g., Comet, Spic and Span, Formula 409, and Lysol) are less irritating, and contain a disinfectant either in the glycol ether or quaternary amine class. These disinfectants are not particularly irritating and are not highly volatile (don't readily form a gas), which means exposures and risks are typically not very high. However, some people may be particularly sensitive to chemicals in general or these in particular; in addition, there are people who react to the fragrances in such products.

A good rule of thumb is to minimize exposure by avoiding the spray products and sticking to liquids that are poured from the bottle. To clean a surface there is no need to make the chemical airborne—judiciously pouring small quantities onto the surface that needs cleaning, spreading with a sponge, and wiping up the residue will clean and disinfect. You'd also be smart to wear rubber gloves to minimize your chances of skin irritation.

You should also keep in mind that disinfectants are not needed for many cleanup jobs: removing dirt and grease from floors, walls, and counters only requires a good scrubbing with soap or detergent. Disinfectants are only needed to kill germs (bacteria, viruses) that may be lingering in bathrooms or on surfaces that people with a respiratory infection have contacted. Just take your dishes as an example. Soap and hot water prevents us from transmitting colds or the flu from our dinner dishes. You can do the same for most of the cleanup jobs around the home, and not worry about spreading germs.

Finally, as with all household products, look for brands that are free of fragrances if you are prone to allergy.

TOXIC FACT

CARPET CLEANERS CAN HAVE POWERFUL SOLVENTS THAT YOU END UP INHALING.

Cleaning hard-to-remove spots out of carpets involves chemicals different from anything else in your cleaning arsenal. Rather than cleaning with detergent, these products dissolve dirt and grease using powerful solvents like glycol ethers, perchloroethylene (PERC) or trichloroethylene (TCE); some even contain extra solvents such as petroleum distillates and isobutene. The solvents in carpet cleaners are volatile so that, by applying them to the carpet, you are also introducing them into your home's air and into your body, where they can produce effects on the nervous system (headache, dizziness, drowsiness) as well as irritation to the eyes and respiratory tract if exposure levels are high. TCE is a well-known carcinogen that used to be in liquid paper and a variety of other consumer products (ATSDR, 1997). While it has been phased out of most products, you may still find it in degreasing products and spot remover available at the hardware store. PERC also affects the nervous system and is a carcinogen (ATSDR, 1997b); it's also the cleaning chemical used at the dry cleaners. You should avoid exposure to both solvents by looking for spot removers that are TCE- and PERC-free.

PERC IN DRY-CLEANED CLOTHES

You expose your clothing to the dry-cleaning solvent PERC every time you go to the cleaners. Unfortunately, not only do your clothes get exposed, but so do you, as PERC takes a while to fully vent from garments. A simple solution is to air out clothes you have just picked up. Take your clothing out of its plastic coverings and let it air out in a well-ventilated area outside the house, such as a porch. The exact time needed to totally air out all the PERC is not certain, but a minimum of two days is a good rule of thumb.

USEPA has recently targeted dry cleaners, trying to get them to decrease their air emissions of PERC. This has helped spawn greener dry-cleaning technology that does not involve toxic solvents, but instead things like carbon dioxide, silicone, or a computer-controlled wet wash (*Consumer Reports*, 2003). To find an establishment offering these greener cleaning technologies, you can start with the USEPA listing (http://www.epa.gov/dfe/pubs/garment/gcrg/cleanguide.pdf).

THE RISK INDEX FOR HOUSEHOLD CLEANSERS

The following chart summarizes the risks from cleaning products discussed in this chapter. Harsh cleansers, including bleach, ammonia, toilet bowl cleaners, drain unclogger, and oven cleaner, contain toxic liquids and all have a reasonably good chance for human exposure at levels that may cause symptoms or even serious health effects. The potential for toxic gases from improper mixing of these chemicals adds to their risk. The milder cleansers are commonly used, so their exposure level is high, but due to their low toxicity, the risks are moderate and mostly apply to those who have chemical or fragrance sensitivity. Carpet cleaners can contain toxic chemicals, but the amount used and level of exposure tends to be low, so the overall risk is low to moderate.

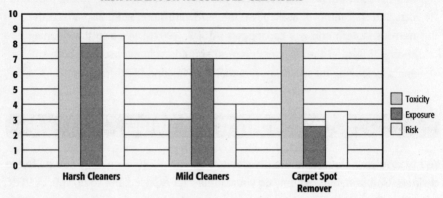

RISK INDEX FOR HOUSEHOLD CLEANSERS

DECREASING YOUR EXPOSURE TO CHEMICALS IN CLEANING PRODUCTS

The following points are useful to remember when purchasing or using a cleaning product:

- Never mix ammonia and bleach, or products containing ammonia and bleach. To avoid the chance for an unsafe mixture, use one cleaning product at a time, and thoroughly rinse to make sure there isn't a residue of one left when using the second product.

- Avoid harsh cleansers; instead opt for milder disinfectants and soaps.

- Select carpet cleaners and other products that are free of VOCs such as PERC or TCE. Increase ventilation with fans in area where spot remover is used to speed drying and removal of VOCs from carpet.

- Use a pourable liquid rather than a spray cleaner to decrease exposure to the lungs and eyes. This is especially important when cleaning enclosed areas such as a shower stall.

- Keep cleaning products away from young children.

Paints, Varnishes, and Waxes

Sprucing up around the house often involves reaching for a can of paint, stain, or shellac. What you may not know is that the act of protecting and beautifying walls, woodwork, and floors can create the largest exposures to toxic chemicals in the house. Paints, varnishes, and waxes are used in large quantities and can have high levels of VOCs. The VOCs used in such products are usually the most cost effective and least toxic alternatives available. That does not mean they are completely safe. Volatile chemicals are needed because the coating has to "cure" or dry out quickly once it has been applied—the longer the drying time, the longer people have to be kept out of the area, and the less they'll want to use the product. Volatile chemicals easily evaporate into a gas, leaving behind the pigment and other solids to cure on the wall. Without evaporation of VOCs, paints as we know them would not exist.

The flip side of all this is that, once evaporated, the chemicals remain in our household air, waiting to be drawn into our lungs. For many years these ingredients were thought of as inert (inactive) ingredients, just carriers for the pigment and binder in the coating. However, studies of painters led to the coining of "Painter's Syndrome," a grouping of neurotoxic effects that occurs in painters (see next section).

There has been a major push to lower VOC levels in consumer products, in part due to the health effects they cause, but also because VOC emissions indoors get outdoors and contribute to the formation of ozone (Chapter 11). Nevertheless, VOCs are still abundant in paints and other coatings and are a major source of indoor air pollution. This is no surprise to anyone who walks into a house whose interior is being painted. That classic paint smell is the VOCs leaving the walls and hitting you in the nose.

TOXIC FACT

OIL-BASED PAINT EMITS MORE VOCS THAN WATER-BASED PAINT.

Oil or water—both professional and amateur house painters are commonly confronted with the choice. Oil-based paint coats certain surfaces better, lasts longer, and provides a more desirable look; water-based paint dries faster and is easier to clean up. But you should also consider how they differ in terms of odor and chemical exposure.

Oil-based paint has a much different composition than water-based paint. The alkyd resin in oil-based paint requires a high concentration of petroleum-based VOCs (mineral spirits, toluene, xylenes, 1,1,1-trichloroethane) to keep the resin liquid and spreadable. Oil paint hangs on to VOCs longer, resulting in slower drying. Water-based paints have acrylic (or other) resins—these VOCs are more water soluble, and include an array of alcohols, aldehydes, and esters. Therefore, water-based paint emits much fewer VOCs into the air, and the VOCs it does emit are less toxic.

In addition to paints, paint remover and paint thinner such as turpentine have a high VOC content. Some of these VOCs are the same as those found in paints, and others are not, most notably the relatively toxic methylene chloride used in furniture stripper and paint remover.

"Painters Syndrome" was discovered in a study of European painters who had nervous system toxicity because of their extensive exposure to VOCs (Lindberg and Lindberg, 1988). The syndrome is primarily a concern for those using oil-based paints on a regular basis. However, nervous system effects, including headache, dizziness, memory loss, and lethargy, can occur even in those who are just painting their own home without proper ventilation. Other types of health effects, notably asthma, are also possible.

▌TOXIC FILE ▌ MOVING BACK IN TOO SOON

Charlotte and Dan decided that the upstairs of their house needed a fresh coat of paint, but were hesitant to paint it because of Sammy. Their two-year-old had a very active case of asthma, and outdoor air pollution and indoor factors such as pet dander, perfumes, and soaps were among the things that triggered his attacks. They hoped he would grow out of this condition, but in the meantime, they delayed projects such as house painting. However, when Charlotte's mom convinced her to come out to the West Coast with Sammy, Charlotte and Dan saw their chance to give the house a facelift without Sammy being there. Dan oversaw the painting project, choosing only water-based paints and making sure the house was aired out. Since it was only early October, he was able to keep the windows open. Charlotte and Sammy stayed in California for ten days, five days for the painting to be completed and five extra days for the house to air out.

Charlotte and Sammy came home to fresh, vibrant colors and a house put neatly back together by Dan. There was no obvious paint smell, although Charlotte thought she picked up a hint of an odor. She attributed it to parental anxiety and decided not to worry, but also to keep a close watch on Sammy. That night was chilly and the windows in the house were closed. The next morning, Sammy woke up coughing and wheezing—not too badly, not a reason to rush off to the doctor, certainly manageable with Sammy's inhaler medication. However, Charlotte and Dan were concerned and talked about whether it could be a reaction to the paint. The next few days seemed fairly normal. Then a cold front came through, dropping the temperature fifteen degrees and causing Charlotte and Dan to use the heat for the first time that fall. Sammy woke up at 1 A.M. gasping for air, seemingly immune to his inhaler. They quickly dressed and headed for the emergency room. Sammy was treated with stronger medications and kept under surveillance for several days. Eventually, his asthma came under control, and his dosage was scaled back.

Sammy's lung doctor asked the family about possible household triggers. He told Charlotte and Dan that they were very smart to have Sammy away from the house during and after the painting project—however, he cautioned, it may have been too soon to bring him back home. Paint can give off VOCs for several weeks, and with the added element of turning on the heat, there may have been an extra dose. Charlotte and Sammy didn't go back home from the hospital. They stayed with relatives in a nearby town for two more months before they dared trust their house again. At that point, the heat had been running for several months and the paint had finished giving off VOCs.

The fact that Sammy's problem with painted walls occurred a week after painting was done shows the impact VOCs can have on sensitive individuals. Even after the paint feels dry to the touch, it may still emit an odor and VOCs. Emission off the wall increases with higher temperature until all the VOCs have evaporated. For most people, the only noticeable effect is an annoying odor, but asthmatics and other sensitive individuals may need to keep away from paint and its vapors for weeks after the paint job is over.

VARNISH, POLYURETHANE, AND WAXES ARE ALSO HIGH IN VOCS.

TOXIC FACT

Polyurethane varnish is similar to oil-based paint, with a high petroleum-based VOC content that can lead to a strong odor, irritation, headache, dizziness, and potential worsening of asthma. Both oil-based and more health-friendly water-based varieties of polyurethanes are available. Water-based polyurethane has fewer VOCs, and these (glycol ethers, methylpyrrolidone), are somewhat less toxic than the VOCs in oil-based products. However, these VOCs are still a health concern if there is a lot of exposure during coating or curing operations (irritation, nervous system effects).

Another group of products containing high levels of VOCs are the polishes and waxes we spread onto furniture and floors to protect the finish.

These products can have a VOC content of fifty to ninety percent or more, guaranteeing a hefty dose for those applying the products or those having to live with the treated furniture or floor. Many people coat their dining room table with a furniture wax, and then eat off the same table later that day; others allow their infants to crawl around on recently waxed floors, which emit VOCs right in the baby's breathing zone.

Adhesives

You should also be careful with the array of adhesives on the market, everything from the simple glues used to fix broken pottery, to rubber cement used in artwork, to the adhesives used to put down linoleum and carpets. Your workbench is turned into a chemistry lab as irritating and toxic chemicals squeezed from the tube interact to form a substance that will tightly bond two surfaces together. If you get some on your skin, it can become part of the chemical reaction and become bonded as well—as you may know all too well, you may have to grow some new skin. Some glues come from a single tube, and start bonding as soon as they hit the air; the other type, epoxy resins, requires the mixing of two separate tubes to cause a bonding polymer to take shape. In both cases, you can get a fairly concentrated exposure to VOCs (styrene, toluene, ethylbenzene), along with some highly toxic and irritating chemicals (acrylonitrile, cyanates). These chemicals are involved in a chain reaction that makes the glue rapidly convert from liquid to solid and bond two surfaces together. However, not all of the chemicals are consumed in the reaction—some are left over for you to inhale or get on your skin. Strong irritation reactions are possible from inhalation, the most worrisome effect being an asthmatic attack. While the amount of adhesive used is typically small compared to paint or varnish, its components should make you handle these products with a healthy dose of respect and caution.

Other products that are likely to give off toxic gas into your home are caulking, sealants, patch/repair kits, and other hardware store items that are squeezed out of tubes and need to cure. In some cases, manufacturers have done indoor air good by making patching and spackle compounds with low VOC formulations for indoor use. However, the outdoor version, which needs to be sturdier, is still laden with VOCs. It is important for those doing home repairs to adhere to label instructions on whether to use a product indoors or out. That commonsense recommendation, along with others listed in the next section, should help you minimize your exposure to VOCs.

THE RISK INDEX FOR COATINGS AND ADHESIVES

The following chart highlights the fact that oil- or solvent-based paints and wood finishes have high VOC contents that give off gas upon application, leading to substantial exposure around the house. These relatively risky coatings contrast with water-based products, which are much lower in VOCs; furthermore, the VOCs present in water-based products are less toxic, leading to relatively low risk for most people. Finally, adhesives and bonding agents can have highly toxic chemicals, but since exposure is generally limited to the specific area in which the material has been applied, their overall risk is only moderately high. Minimizing exposures to the chemicals in these products is both prudent and feasible.

RISK INDEX FOR COATINGS AND ADHESIVES

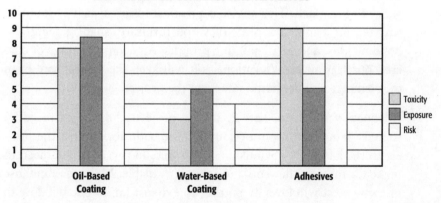

AVOIDING VOCS FROM COATINGS, ADHESIVES, WAXES, AND OTHER PRODUCTS

The following general guidelines are intended to increase your ability to use VOC-containing products safely.

- The first golden rule: read and follow label directions. Even if the print is small, persevere. The instructions will usually tell you how to handle the product safely, including recommended protective clothing (e.g., gloves, goggles), need for proper ventilation, and other use or storage issues (e.g., keep away from flame or heat source).

- Stop using any product that is immediately irritating to your nose, throat, or eyes, or that you find has an objectionable odor. It's better to look for a "greener," less toxic alternative.

- Choose low-VOC and "green" household products when you can. There are a variety of companies and websites that offer green product alternatives to common household products (see www.thegreen guide.com). For paints and wood coatings, the typical water-based products in your hardware store are much lower in VOCs than oil- or solvent-based products—choose those coatings whenever possible. If a green solution is not available, be sure to adhere to the following recommendations.

- Adequate ventilation, Part 1: Go outdoors if possible. The first choice is to move the project outside, or to an enclosed shed or garage that has a large opening. Keep the coated or glued material outside until it is dry to the touch. This advice is practical for jobs such as staining, waxing, or stripping a piece of wood furniture, small glueing and bonding jobs, and small painting projects. An open-air garage or covered porch is an ideal location, as it will keep the project safe from the elements and the home safe from the project.

- Adequate ventilation, Part 2: Indoor projects. For larger projects, such as painting a room or caulking the bathtub, moving the project to the garage is obviously not possible. In this case, you need to make the most of the ventilation that is available. Make maximal use of the nearest windows by putting an exhaust fan in one window to draw contaminated air out of the work zone and fresh air in from a second window. Further reduce your own exposure by leaving the work zone every now and then so that VOC levels do not build up inside your body. A ten-minute break for every hour of coating work is prudent.

- Keep children and other family members out of the work area until the coating or glue is dry and the odor has dissipated. This could take anywhere from one day to several weeks.

- Consider taking on the project in warm-weather months—higher temperatures will cause the coating to cure faster, and you'll be able to open lots of windows. Try to plan the project for low-humidity stretches of weather for the fastest drying time.

- Do not expect dust masks to help. The only kind of respirator that works against VOCs is one that is tight-fitting and equipped with a charcoal filter to purify the air you take in. The standard dust mask the hardware store sells does not stop VOCs and normally doesn't fit well enough to prevent what it was designed for—dust.

- If you must use oil-based paint, consider hiring a painter to do the work and vacating the premises until the paint has thoroughly cured.

- Reseal any unused portion of glue, varnish, or paint in its container and ideally store it in a shed or garage that is not attached to the house. This will keep the VOCs that inevitably escape from used containers from getting into your home.

Household Pesticides

No homeowner or apartment dweller is happy to see the springtime parade of ants in the windowsill, winding across the countertop and into the pantry. The same goes for the moth infestations that come with a bad batch of grain and never seem to leave. Pesticide companies and exterminators have a straightforward solution: spray with toxic chemicals. Using bug killer is convenient, and if you're persistent, you can poison a goodly number of invaders like a gunslinger going after outlaws in the kitchen. However, these chemicals are not magic bullets, and inevitably result in health risks for people.

TOXIC FACT

THREE-FOURTHS OF U.S. HOUSEHOLDS USE PESTICIDES. THE TOTAL AMOUNT USED TOPPED 100 MILLION POUNDS IN 2001.

Not all pesticides are created equal, with some being more toxic or persistent than others. The most highly persistent and toxic pesticides have, for the most part, been banned. Just recently, the major pesticides on the market, the organophosphates, were phased out of indoor homeowner use. These insecticides are not persistent—their big problem is that, as cousins of powerful nerve gas agents developed during World War II, they can be highly toxic to the nervous system. While we should be grateful that we are left with safer alternatives, it is still discomforting to know that for decades homeowners were using pesticides that were too unsafe to be used by the public.

Today the main ingredient in your typical can of bug spray is a pyrethroid-type insecticide. This class of chemical was developed based upon a natural pesticide in chrysanthemums, and functions by scrambling an insect's primitive nervous system, causing overstimulation and death. Humans are more resistant because we're bigger, and our nervous system is better able to handle an acute chemical assault. However, pyrethroids can cause a variety of toxic effects in people: sensitization and allergy, which can appear as skin rash or breathing difficulty or asthma, numbness and tingling from getting the pesticide on your skin, and the potential to overstimulate the central nervous system (behavior changes, tremors, convulsions) at high doses. Animal evidence suggests that the young are particularly sensitive. In other words, the less you use them around the house, the better.

That's not so easy to do. Pyrethroids show up in numerous household products, including all-purpose bug sprays, flea/tick treatments for your pets, anti-lice shampoos for your kids, and sprays for houseplants. Recent biomonitoring surveys show that most Americans have some amount of pyrethroid in their blood (CDC, 2005). This widespread exposure is low-level and does not cause a health risk for most people. In fact, there are very few poisoning reports due to pyrethroid use around the home. However, misuse of the product can lead to excessive exposure and toxic effects, and children and those who are chemically sensitive may be particularly vulnerable. Of course, there is the ever-present danger of young children getting their hands on the spray can or liquid formulation and ingesting it.

> **MYTH:** The main exposure to pesticides in the home comes from inhaling the chemical when it's sprayed.
>
> **REALITY:** The exposure continues for days to weeks after the spraying is over, with more exposure actually occurring afterward. It's natural to assume that once you put the spray can away, you can let your kids back into the room. However, the pesticide actually vaporizes and enters the air you breathe, with some settling down on the floor or counter and merging with house dust. This portion won't go anywhere until the surfaces are cleaned. Contaminated house dust is a natural way for children to become exposed. They play at floor level and mouth their fingers and toys, which can be coated with contaminated house dust. The pesticide also soaks into plush toys; the levels in these toys continues to rise a week after spraying occurred (Hore et al., 2005).

Bottom line, use of an insecticide spray around the home leads to both direct and longer-term exposure via inhalation, ingestion, and skin absorption. This applies as well to "crack and crevice" treatments, wherein a pesticide is applied to specific spots. The reality is that many pesticides are fairly mobile in the indoor environment, and can result in exposures greater than what one may get from pesticide residues in foods, pesticide applications at school or work, or pesticide exposure from community spraying programs.

> **MYTH:** Neighborhood spraying programs to kill mosquitos and prevent the spread of West Nile virus are a major source of pesticide exposure.
>
> **REALITY:** Mosquito control programs in neighborhoods lead to less exposure than what many people get from using pesticides at home. They are typically not an important source of risk to the general public.

The sight of a tanker truck crawling through the neighborhood emitting a fine spray of pesticide can send chills up your spine. It looks like urban warfare against insects, with humans as innocent bystanders getting caught in the line of fire. The controversy surrounding such spraying is understandable given how bad it looks. Some people can still remember the 1950s anti-mosquito spray campaigns with DDT, which were stopped after it was discovered that DDT is toxic to wildlife and people. But millions had already been exposed. With that kind of history, it's no wonder people fear that a new spray program will prove to be risky as well.

It's important to remember that modern pesticides are more efficient than DDT, with very low levels needed to do the job. Furthermore, they break down relatively quickly outdoors (in less than a day). People are instructed to stay indoors with their windows closed and to bring in children's toys when the spraying occurs. These actions usually minimize the amount of exposure. In fact, studies in several states have shown that the baseline level of pesticide in people's bodies before spraying was the same as after spraying, showing that what we pick up from the spray truck is minor compared to what we receive indoors. As we discussed before, compared to outdoor spraying, pesticides used indoors lead to greater exposure because they are more persistent and because they are placed right where we spend the most time.

TREATING HEAD LICE

The scourge of elementary school, a head lice outbreak, can keep the school nurse occupied full-time and make parents throw up their hands in disgust. Who infected my child with this nasty condition? Really they should be asking, how do I keep the rest of my family from getting it? Head lice are very contagious, transferred from direct contact with infected hair or clothing. The treatment is painstaking and time consuming: inspecting the scalp, combing out the nits (eggs), killing off the adults and doing a lot of extra laundry and housecleaning. The reason we bring this up here is that the most common scalp treatment to kill lice contains a pyrethroid pesticide.

Direct application of pesticide-laden shampoo onto the heads of young children seems dubious from a public health perspective. However, the amount of exposure possible in a ten-minute application followed by a thorough rinse is not likely to be significant. The potential benefit of stopping a lice infestation in its tracks is a major benefit, so overall, there is more benefit than risk in using the pesticidal shampoo. That's with regard to the over-the-counter shampoos. There are prescription shampoos that are more potent and toxic, containing malathion or lindane—these should be avoided. On the other extreme, you can try one of the non-pesticidal lice shampoos that have recently been put on the market. They have enzymes that attack the exoskeleton, killing adult lice and their eggs.

THE RISK INDEX FOR HOUSEHOLD PESTICIDES

The combination of pesticidal products around the home, including killer sprays, crack and crevice treatments, insect bait stations, and flea products for your pet, can lead to long-term residues in air, dust, and toys, and excessive exposures to people. The current homeowner marketplace is dominated by the fairly low-toxicity pyrethroids. Risks for pyrethroid toxicity increase as you use more of more these pesticides, especially around children. Certain people may be sensitive to getting these pesticides on their skin or to inhaling them, which may trigger rashes or asthma.

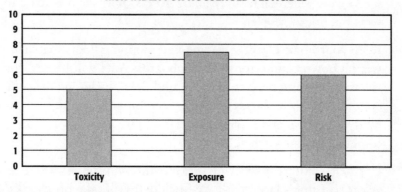

RISK INDEX FOR HOUSEHOLD PESTICIDES

DECREASING YOUR EXPOSURE TO HOUSEHOLD PESTICIDES

The guiding principle for reducing your pesticide exposure is to simply use less, or ideally no pesticide at all. Integrated pest management (IPM) techniques control insects with a minimum pesticide use. The first IPM point to consider is whether you need to do anything at all. A few ants in the springtime may just be scouts entering your home in search of food or water. They may not represent an infestation, but merely the usual springtime visitor who's gone in a week or two. Cockroaches and moths, on the other hand, may indicate that you have some live-in guests who have already colonized, and may call for more aggressive measures.

What follows are ways to fend off ant, cockroach, or moth infestations without using a lot of pesticides or calling in an exterminator.

These measures may not be effective if your infestation is too large, at which point you would be more likely to need pesticides. To eradicate other indoor pests, contact your local university agricultural extension agent.

Ant Control Measures

- Prevent access to your home. Follow the ant trail back out to where it enters the house. Ants often use foundation penetrances, pipes, or wiring to enter the house. Seal any entrance ways with caulking or filler material.

- Seal indoor cracks or crevices with filler material. Use boric acid powder (available at many pharmacies and hardware stores) in cracks where you believe ants are gaining access. Boric acid is toxic to insects but not to people.

- Keep your home clean, sweeping and mopping floors regularly and wiping down countertops and cupboards. Ants will be attracted to sugary surfaces wherever they can find them, including the containers of honey or molasses you may keep on your counter. Clean behind your stove and refrigerator. Don't give ants any reason to go foraging in your kitchen.

- Use bait stations instead of sprays. Ants will be attracted to the sweet bait that's laced with a pesticide; they'll take off chunks and bring them back to the colony, where it will poison everyone from the queen on down. Bait stations are an effective way to use a minimal amount of pesticide to get right at the colony, especially if you place them where you know the ants will travel. However, great care must be taken to keep them away from young children and pets, who may ingest the sweet bait and become poisoned.

Cockroach Control Measures

- Cockroaches can enter either as adults or as eggs in food you bring home from the store. This you can't prevent. However, when you suspect an infestation, search the pantry for evidence of a problem and throw out any foods that have insects growing in them.

- Cockroaches can chew through paper, cardboard, and thin plastic, so store foods in secure plastic containers and bins.

- Keep food waste separate from regular trash and discard it every day.

- Eliminate clutter. Cockroaches hide, mate, and lay eggs in tight, out-of-the-way places. Remove whatever hiding places you can. Caulking over cracks will also help in this regard.

- Put roach traps under counters and in cupboards where there is roach activity. These contain a sticky substance but no pesticide, and will only work for small infestations and if you have removed most other roach hideouts.

- Cut down on the availability of water. Don't leave standing water in the sink, dish drain, or dog dish. Cockroaches only need a drop a day to thrive, so even condensation on pipes can keep them going. Pipe insulation will help keep condensation to a minimum.

- Put dessicants in areas frequented by roaches. These powdery substances dry out a roach's body until it dies. No pesticide is needed if roaches come into contact with enough of these materials. The most common ones are diatomaceous earth and silica aerogel, which are both available commercially.

Grain Moth Control Measures

Like cockroaches, grain moths will usually enter your home through a contaminated food source. Your risk is greatest if you buy large quantities of grains and don't use them up quickly. Once in your house, the infestation can spread to other grain and non-grain products. Pesticide sprays are available but usually not called for if you catch the infestation early. Moth hatching is faster in warm weather, so you are more likely to experience the problem in summer.

- As soon as you see moths in the kitchen, start looking through all your foods, particularly grains and cereals, for webby, clingy formations. After hatching from eggs, the pupae living off the grain leave this spiderlike tracing. You may or may not see the pupae (small worms) themselves. In either case, immediately discard that bag of grain in the outdoor trash. Continue looking for more infested food supplies.

- Store bulk grains in sealed plastic or glass containers away from the kitchen, preferably in a cool, dry place. Only bring into the kitchen amounts you are likely to use quickly.

- Place moth traps in kitchen cupboards. The traps contain a pheromone to attract moths, and have sticky sides to trap them.

- Keep dog, cat, and bird food out of the house, storing it on a porch or in a shed. Pet foods are more likely to be contaminated than human foods, due to less quality control.

TOXIC FACT

MOTHBALLS CAN BE A SUBSTANTIAL SOURCE OF CHEMICAL EXPOSURE.

Moths are not only found in kitchen cupboards but also in bedroom closets, combing the racks looking for your nice wool clothing. You may not see them in action, because they avoid light. However, they leave behind their signature, circular holes that ruin your garments. The answer many people resort to is mothballs. These little white balls release a toxic gas that kills moths. They are made out of naphthalene or para-dichlorobenzene, two chemicals that can change directly from a solid to a gas (the technical term for the process is sublimation). It all seems so simple—just put your woolies into a sealed bag with a few mothballs for the summer, and the mothballs turn into a toxic gas that fumigates your clothes, killing any moths or eggs that happen to be there. Once fall comes, your clothes are as good as new. All you have to do is air them out before wearing them to get rid of the residual odor.

Unfortunately, it's not quite that simple, as mothballs are constantly emitting this toxic gas: when you bring them home from the market, when they are stored in your cupboard, and whenever you handle them. Opening the bag to take your clothing out exposes you to a big puff; improper use (sprinkling them around the bottom of your closet) causes even more exposure.

You don't have to worry about the gas being lethal—it won't even kill moths at the diluted levels you may experience around the house. However, naphthalene and para-dichlorobenzene are possible carcinogens that have toxic and reproductive risks. They are irritating to breathe and have a distinctive odor (that you may recognize from the men's room—para-dichlorobenzene is also in that white hockey puck deodorizer in urinals). The worst scenario is when a baby's blanket or clothing has been stored in mothballs and then not aired out before use. This situation has led to overexposure and toxicity in the exposed babies, including skin rash, jaundice, and anemia (RAIS, 1993).

In short, though we may think of mothballs as an old household friend, it's better to think of them as a gaseous pesticide that is best handled very carefully or not at all. Homes where mothballs are used have considerably higher levels of naphthalene or para-dichlorobenzene than homes without such use, indicating that it's easy for this pesticide to spread beyond where it's needed and permeate your house.

Moth Proofing Made Safe

Fortunately, there are non-pesticidal solutions to the clothing moth problem. Cleaning clothing prior to storage gets rid of perspiration and food stains, both of which attract moths. You can also try storing your cleaned clothing in a closet or chest with cedar chips, or better yet, in a cedar closet. Cedar emits an odor that is a natural, nontoxic moth repellent.

If you decide to stick with mothballs, minimize your exposure by storing the box in the garage. Bring your bagged-up clothing out to the garage for the addition of mothballs. In the fall, open the bag outside and thoroughly air out your clothes before rehanging them in your closet.

We almost forgot the most important safety tip: never leave mothballs where a toddler can find them (e.g., the bottom of your closet). They can look like nice round balls of candy, good for sucking or swallowing whole. A baby may not figure out that it doesn't taste so good until it's too late.

Safety Tips for When You Need to Spray

If the preventive measures described above do not work, contact your agricultural extension agent or your state pesticide office to find out whether you've exhausted all non-pesticide measures. If so, ask which pesticide product is best for your situation. They may recommend that you do the spraying yourself or, if the situation is too complicated, that you hire an exterminator.

Try to avoid building-wide spray programs that may be triggered by people in other units who have roach or ant problems. If you've managed to keep your unit under control, you shouldn't have it sprayed unnecessarily. However, insects may enter your unit as they flee your neighbor's sprayed unit—they will sense that yours is a safe haven. Therefore, it is critical to seal up any cracks and crevices between you and your neighbors, which is a good idea anyway to hold down general insect traffic.

If you do need to have your house or apartment sprayed by an exterminator, leave and do not come back for at least twelve hours after spraying is complete. Pack away as much clothing as possible to avoid it becoming contaminated. Make sure your children's toys are not left behind. When you move back in, air out the apartment and clean it thoroughly, including a shampoo of the carpets.

Cosmetics and Personal Care Products

Of all toxics issues, perhaps the one that's most overwhelming is chemicals in cosmetics and personal care products. It's easy to feel lost in a sea of toxics when you realize that the products we apply to our bodies on a daily basis to cleanse, coat, beautify, or make us fragrant contain hundreds of chemicals. Some of these products have been proven to be toxic to one degree or another, and many others haven't been adequately tested. A 2004 survey of 2,300 consumers found that on average, people use nine different personal care products a day, introducing 126 different chemicals onto their body (Campaign for Safe Cosmetics, 2004). Most people are surprised when they find out that these products are not subject to government safety reviews and receive only minimal evaluation, and that from an industry-led board.

The good news is that many of these chemicals are relatively simple alcohols, acetates, oils, polymers, surfactants (soaps), and preservatives. Though chemicals with names like methyl paraben, glycol stearate, or hydroxypropyl methylcellulose sound like they could be harmful, in fact they are fairly innocuous—skin irritation is the most common effect they cause. However, coating ourselves in a chemicalized marinade is bound to have some risks, and we can't ignore the fact that some chemicals have the potential to be carcinogenic or harm our reproductive systems if they get into our bodies. Recent efforts by consumer groups and certain governments, particularly in Europe, have shed more light on what has been a hidden source of exposure. While the needed research is just beginning to occur, it already appears that cosmetic formulations are in need of a makeover.

1,4-DIOXANE, FORMALDEHYDE, AND PHTHALATES

Of the myriad chemicals in cosmetic products, we're going to focus on three of the most worrisome, 1,4-dioxane, formaldehyde, and phthalates.

TOXIC FACT

1,4-DIOXANE IS A CARCINOGEN THAT IS PRESENT IN MANY BATH AND BODY PRODUCTS, INCLUDING THOSE USED BY CHILDREN.
The chemical we are describing here, 1,4-dioxane, sounds like dioxin, but in fact has nothing to do with it. It is chemically much simpler and will not persist in the environment or in our bodies. However, what's troubling about 1,4-dioxane is that, similar to dioxin, it is carcinogenic.

1,4-dioxane is a by-product of foaming agents of the ethoxylated surfactant class (e.g., propylene glycol). To put this into English, there are certain products such as shampoos and bubble baths that work best if they have lots of foam and suds. Chemical additives (ethoxylated surfactants) help this happen. In and of themselves, these surfactants are not much of a health risk. However, they bring along a contaminant, 1,4-dioxane, which is a health concern. 1,4-dioxane has been detected in a variety of personal care products; bubble baths, shampoo, laundry presoak, and soaps have been found to have levels in the 10–50 ppm range. Thus, there is potential for exposure on large areas of skin, and to young children in particular.

At high doses, 1,4-dioxane is carcinogenic and can promote the formation of tumors on the skin. We're still not sure if it's the kind of carcinogen that can produce cancer at very low doses, such as those we are likely to get from soaps and shampoos. This issue is currently under review by USEPA in an ongoing toxicology evaluation. While studies with monkeys suggest that 1,4-dioxane does not penetrate the skin very well, it may be a different situation when your skin is soaked with it while you're sitting in a high-temperature bath. The drinking water guidelines for 1,4-dioxane are in the 3–20 ppb range, which is more than 1,000 times lower than the levels found in personal care products. Of course, since we don't drink shampoo or bubble bath, this is an apples-to-oranges comparison. However, it indicates that a risky chemical that appears to be worth regulating down to low levels in drinking water is present at relatively high levels in our bath and body products; thus, it would be prudent to minimize exposure.

Easier said than done. Since 1,4-dioxane is a by-product and not an intentional additive, it will not appear on product labels. It is a hidden ingredient in products that list "foaming agents," "ethoxylated surfactants," or "polyethylene glycol" on their labels. We recommend that you be cautious with these products and consider switching to "greener" versions that lack those ingredients. An even more commonsense approach is to focus on protecting your children at bathtime, since it's children who are likely to receive the greatest exposures and risks. Look for shampoos and bubble baths that don't have the 1,4-dioxane-contaminated ingredients listed above. Bubble baths can be created from materials commonly found around the home (baking soda, hand soap, glycerin, Epsom salt), so you could even create your own homemade recipe (see box below).

RECIPE FOR HOMEMADE BUBBLE BATH

1 quart water
1 bar castille soap (4 oz)
½ cup glycerin
5–10 drops of an essential oil for fragrance (if desired)

Mix glycerin and water. Dissolve soap (heating the water/glycerin mixture or shaving the soap will help dissolve it). Then add the oil. Shake well when mixing and again just before use. Note: castille soap is very mild and made from olive oil. Glycerin is a natural, non-oily moisturizer. All ingredients are readily available at department stores, supermarkets, or on-line.

FORMALDEHYDE IS USED AS A PRESERVATIVE IN PERSONAL CARE PRODUCTS.

As you'll see in Chapter 8, formaldehyde is a contaminant of particleboard and veneer furniture, creating indoor air exposures that are irritating to some and potentially carcinogenic for everyone. If this weren't bad enough, formaldehyde is also widely used in cosmetics and personal care products. Its ability to mix well with water and kill germs on contact makes it an effective preservative for watery products like shampoos, conditioner, bubble baths, liquid hand soap, and shower gel; it is also present in many makeup formulations as part of a slow-release resin that prevents products from growing bacteria. The formaldehyde content of these products is relatively low (< 0.2%), but given that the chemical in question is going directly onto our faces and bodies, these products could be important sources of exposure. Unfortunately, the studies needed to determine just how much exposure have not been conducted. Europe has introduced at least a measure of control by banning formaldehyde from spray formulations, an attempt to keep a lid on how much gets inhaled.

Overall, the cancer risk from formaldehyde in soaps, shampoos, conditioner, and hand washes appears to be low. The main risk is skin irritation, especially in those who have sensitive skin or are allergic to formaldehyde in the air. As with 1,4-dioxane, exposing children to formaldehyde in bubble baths may be a serious concern. Check product labels to make sure the bubble bath products you bring home for your children do not use this preservative in any form.

PHTHALATES CAN AFFECT THE DEVELOPMENT OF YOUR FETUS.

TOXIC FACT

Most women make significant lifestyle changes during pregnancy to make sure they will have the healthiest baby possible. These changes often include stopping smoking and alcohol consumption, watching out for mercury in fish, avoiding prescription and even over-the-counter medicines, and following an overall healthier diet. However, one area that most women don't consider is cosmetics, primarily bath and body products, which often contain relatively high amounts of phthalates, chemicals that can alter a baby's development in utero. The specific concern is that exposure during pregnancy can affect the hormonal balance in the womb and tend to make baby boys less "male" (see Chapter 5). We already discussed the phthalate exposure that can come from food, but you should be aware that the greatest source of exposure for most people is likely from bath and body products.

Phthalates are multi-purpose additives that help nail polish maintain its integrity, give hair spray more hold, and make fragrances last longer. Unfortunately, phthalate testing is very limited. The most comprehensive study to date looked at seventy-two different brands covering five different categories: hair products, deodorant, nail polish, body lotions, and fragrance (Houlihan et al., 2002). Phthalates were found to be common in all of the products, with one type in particular (diethylphthalate, or DEP) being the most prevalent.

Even more frightening is the frequency with which DEP and other phthalates are found in people. Studies evaluating a wide array of phthalates in human urine detected nine different phthalates in most of the people studied (Swann et al., 2005; Duty et al., 2005). The fact that DEP is present at relatively high levels in both products and people suggests that the phthalates in bath and body products do penetrate the skin and are a key source of human exposure. If you are pregnant, they can be a risk to your baby's development. (It's noteworthy that the levels of phthalates in women and men are very similar. In the men's phthalate study, the amount of exposure increased as the number of bath and body products, including cologne, aftershave, hair gel, deodorant, and lotion, increased.)

Not all brands have phthalates, and in fact bath and body products would probably work just as well without them. Unfortunately, manufacturers do not have to label their products for phthalates, so you can't tell from the bottle. Some test results show brands that do and that do not contain phthalates (Houlihan et al., 2002); however, the testing has been very limited. Until the federal government fixes this testing and labeling problem, or removes phthalates outright, your basic approach should be "buyer beware." It would be prudent for pregnant women to avoid hair sprays, body lotion, deodorant, and perfume entirely during pregnancy, unless they can verify that the products are phthalate-free. (As with other issues, Europe is ahead of us on phthalates, with a 2003 ban removing two of the riskier phthalates from cosmetics.)

FRAGRANCES

Fragrances tend to evoke an all-or-nothing response: you either love them or hate them, with the anti side fueled by the issue of allergic or chemically sensitive individuals. Many of us have been asked to leave our scented products home when receiving invitations to attend a weekend workshop, in deference to those who don't do well with extra chemical exposures. Their susceptibility may be very real: fragrances are known to contain many chemicals, both from natural and synthetic sources, some of which are proven allergens. There have also been cases where a person's dislike or fear of a fragrance has led to a negative physiologic response.

There are approximately 5,000 different scents or ingredients in fragrance mixtures, which makes identifying all the allergens you might encounter in a fancy little bottle a daunting task. Certain fragrances are known to be more allergenic than others, with cinnimal, benzyl salicylate, and isoeugenol among the most common allergens in fragrance mixes (SCCNFP, 1999). However, it does little good for us to list allergens in fragrances for you because there are no labeling requirements—you won't be able to find these names on the bottle (a seemingly ridiculous loophole, given that one to two percent of all people have skin allergies to fragrance). People with allergies can simply try different fragrances until they find ones they are compatible with. The downside is, fragrances are usually blends of various ingredients, and it's common for a fragrance to have at least some amount of some allergen in the mix. That can make it difficult to find a scented product that you won't be allergic to if you are unlucky enough to have this kind of allergy.

And then there's the issue of being at risk because of other people wearing fragrances. Inhaling fragrances may cause allergic people respiratory distress, a situation over which they have little control if they go out in public. There has been some debate over whether fragrances can cause new cases of asthma. There is little data to concretely support or refute the possibility; however, what is known is that fragrances can help bring on an asthmatic attack in those who are especially sensitive to fragrances and already suffer from asthma. Fragrances can be a trigger that, along with other air pollutants, tighten airways and make breathing difficult.

Perfumes cause the greatest fragrance exposure, but it's worth noting that many products, from shaving cream to shower gel, from hair sprays to hand lotion, are often scented—even men's products like colognes, aftershave, hair gel, and deodorant. These products leave a scent on the skin that can affect other people, or possibly cause a rash on the wearer.

THE RISK INDEX FOR COSMETICS AND PERSONAL CARE PRODUCTS

The risks associated with these products are difficult to assess. On the one hand, we know there are some fairly toxic, allergenic, and carcinogenic ingredients in everyday cosmetic, bath, and body products. On the other hand, the levels of those ingredients in any one product are low. However, most people use numerous products in a day, and wear them around for many hours. Because the toxic potential of these chemicals is moderate and exposure appears to be common, we have given the four ingredients covered in this chapter (1,4-dioxane, phthalates, formaldehyde, and fragrances) a moderate overall composite risk ranking.

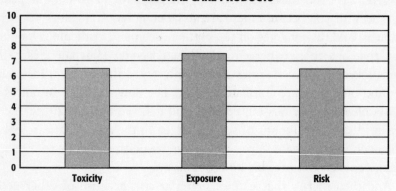

RISK INDEX FOR COSMETICS AND PERSONAL CARE PRODUCTS

AVOIDING CHEMICALS IN PERSONAL CARE PRODUCTS

Since labeling of personal care products for toxins such as 1,4-dioxane, formaldehyde, and phthalates is not required, an avid label-reader won't have much to go on. Instead you should:

- Select "green" products. Companies that sell these products will make claims about being free of toxic chemicals, but you may want to e-mail the company and ask to see their full ingredient list and test data. You can find out about green products at www.thegreenguide.com.

- If you stick with the traditional personal care products, cut back on their use before and during pregnancy. Transfer of the reproductive toxicants (phthalates) or carcinogens (especially 1,4-dioxane) to the developing fetus should be avoided.

- Only use bubble bath products that are free of 1,4-dioxane and formaldehyde, and also free of foaming agents of the ethoxylated surfactant variety.

- When using scents, be aware of the potential for skin irritation or breathing difficulties. If any arise, try to isolate the offending product by eliminating all personal care/cosmetics products and then adding one back at a time, noticing if you have a reaction with each new addition.

- If you or your family members are sensitive or asthmatic, avoid fragrances altogether by using "fragrance-free" or "perfume-free" products. Watch out for the word "unscented," as it does not guarantee the lack of fragrances—it typically refers to a lack of odor, which can be accomplished with masking agents that allow the fragrance to remain in the product.

The bottom line regarding fragrances is trial and error for the selection of your own personal care products. Use what gives you the least amount of irritation or respiratory distress, and be sensitive to those around you. You don't want to turn yourself into a walking asthma trigger.

CONSUMER PRODUCTS CHECKLIST

GENERAL PRINCIPLES FOR ALL PRODUCTS

❏ Keep all products with toxic chemicals away from small children. This is especially critical for harsh cleaning agents, coatings, adhesives, and pesticides.

❏ Follow label directions.

❏ Use only with adequate fresh air, usually the more ventilation the better.

❏ Stop using any product that is immediately irritating to your nose, skin, or throat.

❏ Choose low-VOC and "green" household products.

CLEANSERS

❏ Never mix ammonia and bleach.

❏ Avoid harsh cleansers, instead opting for milder disinfectants and soaps.

❏ Select carpet cleaners that are free of VOCs such as PERC.

❏ Use a pourable liquid rather than a spray cleaner, particularly for enclosed spaces.

COATINGS AND ADHESIVES

❏ For paints and wood treatments, use water-based rather than oil-based coatings.

❑   Keep children and other family members out of the work area until the coating or glue is dry and the odor has dissipated.

❑   Conduct the coating project in warm-weather months. Periods with low humidity are best for rapid curing.

PESTICIDES

❑   Carefully consider the need to use any pesticide at all.

❑   Use non-pesticide control measures for ants, cockroaches, moths, lice, etc.

❑   If you must use a pesticide, check with the local university extension agent to find out which one to use and whether it's safe for you to apply it.

❑   Avoid programs where your entire building will be sprayed, unless you have a heavy infestation.

COSMETICS AND PERSONAL CARE PRODUCTS

❑   Cut back on their use before and during pregnancy to decrease exposure to reproductive toxins (phthalates) and carcinogens (1,4-dioxane) in the products.

❑   Use bubble bath products that are free of 1,4-dioxane and formaldehyde. Consider opting for natural "green" products or homemade recipes.

❑   When using scents, be aware of the potential for skin irritation or breathing difficulties. If they occur, consider "fragrance-free" or "perfume-free" products.

SECTION 3

Toxics in the Air We Breathe

CHAPTER 8

Indoor Air Pollution

Normally, when we think of air pollution, our thoughts go to plumes of smoke exiting large industrial smokestacks or the tailpipe of diesel trucks, the brown haze of summer smog or the smell of the local landfill. Outdoor pollution, which is measured by state and environmental agencies across the country, has received the kind of high-level congressional attention that brought about the Clean Air Act of 1970, with major revisions since. But there's another form of air pollution that is less obvious, is not debated in Congress, and does not get measured very often, yet is more pervasive and can at times be a greater health risk: indoor air pollution (IAP).

You probably don't think of carpets, furniture, cleaning products, paints, and stoves as risks to your health. Unfortunately, many consumer products contain unwanted chemicals that can be released into your home's air. The situation has been made worse over the past twenty years because we've sealed our homes, offices, and schools to increase energy efficiency, unknowingly trapping pollutants in the places we spend the most time.

IAP is a complex topic that can fill an entire book. The amount in your home or office depends on what kind of furniture you have, what the furniture is made of, the size of the room in question, what cleaning products are used, and how much fresh air it gets. Over two hundred chemicals have been identified as "background" contaminants of indoor air, which means that they are present for no special reason. So, in an effort to narrow the IAP topic down to a manageable level, this chapter focuses on several commonly found and risky contaminants, although we point you to other chapters to learn about additional factors that can degrade indoor air quality (Radon, Chapter 2; Mold, Chapter 3; Asbestos, Chapter 4; Consumer Products, Chapter 7).

In this chapter, we will cover volatile organic compounds (VOCs) from wood and household furnishings and combustion products like carbon monoxide, particles, and nitrogen oxides.

Q *How concerned should we be about indoor air pollution?*

A *Very concerned.* IAP regularly ranks at the top of lists of important environmental problems. For example, in an environmental risk ranking by the USEPA, IAP came in as number three, while hazardous waste dumps ranked near the bottom (USEPA, 1987a). IAP ranks so high because of the large numbers of chemicals found indoors, and because we spend an estimated ninety percent of our time indoors.

Volatile Organic Compounds

What do carpeting and kitchen cabinets have in common with smokestacks at a chemical factory? They all expose us to volatile organic compounds, or VOCs. In fact, VOCs are the most ubiquitous indoor air contaminants. They are present in every home or office, and come in a bewildering array of chemical varieties.

The term "VOC" is very broad, referring to many different chemicals. They all have two characteristics in common: first, they are liquids that tend to evaporate into the air at normal room temperatures; second, they are organic, meaning they have carbon atoms in their structure. It's important to recognize that some but not all VOCs are toxic. Inhaling VOCs isn't necessarily a health risk, and even the more toxic VOCs can be tolerated if exposure level is low enough. This section will identify which VOCs and exposure scenarios you should pay particular attention to.

Thousands of VOCs are used in the manufacture of common household products and furnishings. VOCs themselves usually don't impart an important quality, but rather act as carriers to help other ingredients become embedded in a product (e.g., ingredients that provide stain resistance, resistance to wrinkling, or just hold things together such as glues).

As discussed in Chapter 7, when the VOC vaporizes from such products, during the process of curing or gelling, it escapes into the indoor environment. Pretty soon your air becomes a complex "soup" of VOCs. Although it's difficult to predict the dangers from inhaling this "soup" day in and day out over many years, most experts agree that it's prudent to limit exposure as much as possible. It's also possible that building-related illnesses such as Sick Building Syndrome (SBS) and Multiple Chemical Sensitivity (MCS) are triggered by indoor VOCs.

Consumer products and building materials that are sources of VOCs include:

- Carpets, drapes, and upholstery
- Fabricated wood products, such as particleboard and veneer surfaces
- Cleaning products and disinfectants (covered in Chapter 7)
- Paints (latex and oil-based—Chapter 7) and paint removers
- Gasoline, kerosene, and other fuels
- Dry-cleaned clothing (Chapter 7)
- Glues and sealants (Chapter 7)
- Air fresheners, candles, and aromatherapy products
- Caulking and drywall tape
- Vinyl flooring and wall coverings
- Insulation
- Furniture finishing products containing waxes and varnish (Chapter 7)

Of the several hundred chemicals typically found in indoor air, the following are the more common and toxic members of the club:

- Formaldehyde
- Methylene chloride
- Perchloroethylene (PERC)

- Benzene

- Toluene

- Xylene

- Trichloroethylene (TCE)

Up until the late 1980s, most people would have guessed these chemicals would have had much higher levels outside than inside, since they are often emitted in smokestacks and car exhaust. When actual measurements were made, scientists around the country muttered a collective, "Why didn't we see this coming?" In 1987, the USEPA conducted the groundbreaking Total Exposure Assessment Methodology (TEAM) study (USEPA, 1987b). They found important VOCs like benzene to be five times higher inside homes than in outdoor air, even in urban industrial areas in New Jersey. Investigators started looking more closely at consumer products and building materials, and finding VOCs on ingredients lists everywhere. They realized toxic VOCs are like a Trojan horse, welcomed into our homes in new consumer products, and once inside, slowly releasing vapors that create health risks.

TOXIC FILE

DON'T BE A VOC PACK RAT

Dave used to enjoy basement handiwork—doing light carpentry for family and neighbors, building birdhouses, dog kennels, basic furniture. He had a basement full of woodworking supplies. However, once his wife gave birth to twins, he didn't have time for those projects, and in fact hadn't been in his workshop in over a year. He wouldn't have given it a second thought, but on this particular day an environmental consultant was coming over to do some testing. Dave's neighbors had complained of a fuel odor in their basement, and studies had shown that the soil and groundwater in the area was contaminated with fuel leaking from a nearby gas station.

The consultant took some air tests in his basement and first floor and moved on to the next house. Since Dave did not detect any unusual odors in his basement, he thought no more about it. However, he took notice of the results when they came back several weeks later: twenty-one different VOCs were detected, and according to the lab sheet, seven were well above what could be expected indoors.

He checked on the Internet and found to his surprise that none of the elevated VOCs had anything to do with gasoline. Instead, they were chemicals like acrylates and solvents that you might find in glues and wood finishes. The environmental consultant told him what was already becoming obvious—that the basement readings were likely due to VOCs evaporating from his woodworking products.

What worried him most was the fact that some of the readings were also elevated upstairs. He felt terrible that he had let these chemicals spread throughout the house with the infants present. If he had discarded what he was no longer using, the basement and house air would have been much cleaner. He asked a doctor if there were any tests to determine his family's health risk, but was told there was nothing worth testing. The doctor assured him that it was unlikely the babies were harmed, but said it was important to remove any VOC-containing products from the basement, to throw out those he no longer intended to use, and to store the remainder away from the house.

Dave went through his workshop and the rest of his basement, reading labels and removing anything that had a chemical list of ingredients. He ventilated the basement and paid for a private testing company to come back in and see if his cleanup was successful. When this was shown to be the case, Dave and his wife could breathe easier, being very thankful that problems at a neighbor's house had alerted them to a different kind of problem of their own.

This Toxic File points out a common mistake: storing VOC-containing products that are no longer needed, leading to completely unnecessary exposure. Don't be a pack rat. Old cans of paint or varnish and tubes of sealants and adhesives don't seal tightly and allow volatile chemicals to escape. You need to treat these materials with the respect owed to chemical waste. In fact, you shouldn't even put them in your regular trash, but store them outside your house and bring them to the local hazardous waste collection day for disposal.

FORMALDEHYDE

Even before the TEAM study, formaldehyde raised the red flag on indoor air pollution. During the 1970s, many homes were insulated with urea-formaldehyde foam insulation, or UFFI. Home insulation became very popular during the energy crisis of that era, and UFFI became one of the major products on the market. However, some homeowners who had UFFI installed became ill, primarily with eye, nose, and throat irritation. Air testing showed that "UFFI homes" had elevated levels of formaldehyde. Around the same time, it was discovered that mobile homes made with large amounts of plywood or particleboard could also have high levels of indoor formaldehyde.

The UFFI and mobile home problems focused the public's attention on formaldehyde, showing how it's possible to contaminate our own homes with the materials we use to build them. Formaldehyde in general, and UFFI in particular, became a regulatory target, and some sources of formaldehyde were decreased or eliminated. (For example, UFFI has not been used to insulate homes since about 1980.) However, formaldehyde is still common in certain consumer products. It shows up in clothing and home fabrics, where it is designed to prevent wrinkling and discourage mold growth (e.g., in permanent press fabrics); as a binding agent in glues and resins; in smoke from your fireplace, cigarette, or other combustion sources; in paints as a preservative; and in pressed wood products.

Pressed wood products such as plywood and particleboard are the most important source of formaldehyde in homes today. Combined with other chemicals, like urea and phenol, formaldehyde forms resins that bind these processed wood sections together. Most of the formaldehyde in these products is locked up in the resin; however, some if it may be released if it did not totally react in forming the resin. Furthermore, water and humidity may cause resin to break down, resulting in formaldehyde release. In general, phenol-formaldehyde-based products release less formaldehyde than urea-formaldehyde-based products, and are also more resistant to water-initiated release of formaldehyde.

> **MYTH:** Homes insulated with urea-formaldehyde foam insulation (UFFI) are a health hazard and should be avoided.
>
> **REALITY:** UFFI homes do not, in general, pose a health risk; you need not worry about this risk when considering purchasing a home.

As we mentioned, when UFFI was first installed in the 1970s, it caused problems in thousands of homes. Pretty soon, UFFI inspection checkboxes started to show up on real estate buyer's contracts, which ensured that the question would at least come up in every home purchase; if the seller was fleeing a problem-UFFI house, the buyer had a shot of finding out about it. Within a few years, testing began to show that most UFFI homes no longer had formaldehyde levels that presented a hazard (Weintrub et al., 1989), a discovery confirmed by government tests. Apparently, UFFI had a limited amount of formaldehyde to begin with, and after several years inside the walls there wasn't enough left to be a health risk.

Today, you don't have to worry about UFFI homes—since almost all UFFI insulation is over twenty years old, there is little risk of elevated levels of formaldehyde. In fact, inspections or air testing of UFFI homes are no longer recommended by most government agencies. Still, some prospective homebuyers are concerned when they see the UFFI checkbox on a house disclosure form. Our recommendation is, don't worry if you are buying or live in a UFFI house. You don't need to inspect the house for UFFI. If you think you are having symptoms associated with formaldehyde, you might consider air testing, but usually that step is not needed, at least not right away.

Manufacturers have also made an effort to reduce the amount of formaldehyde emissions from pressed wood products. While formaldehyde levels are not zero, they are not in a range that would bother most people. The two exceptions are if you've brought numerous pressed wood articles of furniture into your home and if you are hypersensitive to formaldehyde. People can develop allergies to formaldehyde after a high-level exposure or after years of chronic low-level exposure (ATSDR, 1999) that can include rashes from direct contact and asthma attacks triggered by inhalation. For these sensitive individuals, even low to moderate formaldehyde exposure can be harmful. They should consider lowering the amount of formaldehyde in their homes by getting rid of pressed wood products and other consumer items likely to contain formaldehyde.

Q *I have asthma and know that formaldehyde makes it worse. However, I want to remodel my kitchen and have heard about formaldehyde coming from cabinets. How do I reduce the amount of formaldehyde that I bring into my home?*

A Start by buying products that are low in formaldehyde. Many cabinetry products are manufactured with at least some pressed wood products, and thus
formaldehyde. You can avoid pressed wood products by purchasing solid
wood cabinetry. When using solid wood products in general construction is
not practical, especially when installing sub-flooring, which is usually made
of plywood or particleboard, ask for "exterior grade" products that have lower
emission rates. You can also look for labels from the American National Standards Institute (ANSI). Particleboard should be labeled with ANSI codes of
PBU, D2, or D3 to assure lower formaldehyde levels. Medium-density fiber-
board, or MDF, also has ANSI criteria for lower formaldehyde emissions.

The federal Department of Housing and Urban Development (HUD)
has a standard requiring that materials used in manufacturing mobile
homes not create formaldehyde greater than .4 parts per million (ppm).
Look for pressed wood products such as cabinetry that have a HUD label,
indicating it meets their standards. The Greenguard Environmental Institute
also has a commercial certification program that helps identify low-VOC-
emitting products (including formaldehyde), and offers a fact sheet on
formaldehyde in pressed wood products (www.greenguard.org). Be aware
that the problem with pressed wood products is generally decreasing because manufacturers have voluntarily reduced formaldehyde emissions
from such products by up to ninety percent.

If you do bring formaldehyde-containing products into your home, it's
a good idea to ventilate the area during the first days to weeks after installation. Just keeping your windows open can help reduce emission levels, so
obviously save the remodeling project for warm weather if you can. However, keep humidity levels low by using a dehumidifier, since high moisture
levels can increase the breakdown of the resin into formaldehyde.

FORMALDEHYDE IS A HUMAN CARGINOGEN.

TOXIC FACT

The World Health Organization has concluded that formaldehyde is a human
carcinogen (IARC, 2004). It has been shown to cause nasal cancer in animals,
with evidence of the same in workers (e.g., embalmers) exposed to relatively
high levels. It has also been associated with leukemia and brain cancer.

It is unclear what these cancer findings in people subject to heavy exposures mean for the general population. We are all exposed to low levels
of formaldehyde, indoors and outdoors—in fact, our bodies produce
formaldehyde as part of our normal metabolism. Our natural defense

mechanisms convert formaldehyde to less toxic compounds, and these same defenses may protect most of us from our general low-level exposure to formaldehyde. Few, if any, studies document a link between cancer and formaldehyde in the general public.

In other words, although formaldehyde can be considered a human carcinogen, it does not appear to be a major cancer concern in a typical indoor environment. There are always uncertainties in such assessments, so it's prudent to reduce your exposure as much as possible. Just know that, given all the small sources of formaldehyde, it is impossible to get your exposure down to zero.

OTHER VOCS

It may surprise you to learn there are no standards for VOCs in indoor air for the general public—the amount you can safely breathe has never been formally defined or regulated. Which means that if you tested the air in your home and found it to have lots of VOCs, the government couldn't force the source of the pollution to stop (as opposed to VOC contamination of your tap water, which is regulated by strict standards; see Chapter 6). The problem with regulating VOCs in air is that there are so many sources. If you found a high level, you would need to conduct a study to prove where it was coming from and that might not prove anything. Standards only work when they are associated with enforceable actions that lower pollution to safer levels—it's hard to set them when the pollution sources are so numerous and varied.

Indoor VOC levels are generally low compared to workplace standards. There *are* actually workplace standards for VOCs. However, they are usually pretty high and not safe for the general public (e.g., pregnant women, very young children, the elderly). In fact, workplace standards are not a guarantee of safety, even for the workers they are meant to protect (see Chapter 9).

Instead of government standards, product makers have decreased VOCs in things like liquid paper, paints, magic markers, and glues. Ironically, this has been the result of attempts to control outdoor air pollution that comes from inside, not out of a concern about the levels of indoor toxics themselves (Chapter 7), a fact that shows the degree to which indoor air quality has been overlooked.

Another major source of VOCs is your car. Gasoline is a soup of VOCs, including benzene, toluene, ethylbenzene, and xylene, all just waiting for a chance to escape your gas tank. This becomes an IAP issue in houses with attached garages, because gas tanks are not airtight—VOCs escape into the garage and from there, into your house. New regulations in a number of states requires gas caps to fit better, a feature tested when cars go through annual inspections. While this measure cuts down on VOC emissions from cars, it does nothing about VOC emissions from lawn mowers or other gasoline-powered equipment stored in the garage.

Target indoor air concentrations have been determined by some states, as part of an effort to prevent VOCs from entering homes through contaminated groundwater (Chapter 6). But in this case, the source of the pollution is known, so state agencies have a means of requiring the proper cleanup. The target indoor air concentrations set for this purpose can be useful guidelines (not standards) for evaluating VOC measurements in homes and offices. Ask your state health department if it has established target indoor air concentrations, or find levels developed in other states as a point of comparison.

Another way to evaluate VOC levels is to consider the total VOC content (TVOC) of the air. When TVOCs are higher than five parts per million (ppm), some people may experience health symptoms such as tiredness, headaches, and general discomfort. In fact, you may notice levels as low as one ppm, sensing that there is something wrong with the air quality in the building. Hiring a consultant to measure TVOCs is very crude and nonspecific, but it can be a useful way to do a rapid screen of the air quality, and identify possible problem areas.

Q *Should I test my home or office for VOCs?*

A People react differently to the news that the air in their homes may be contaminated by the things they purchase to make it functional and beautiful, ranging from outrage and activism on the one hand to acceptance and apathy on the other. Some are determined to test their home's air, hoping to allay their fears, or if toxic chemicals are found, to figure out a way to remove the source. After all, you can successfully test indoor air for radon, and then determine a practical solution.

However, as we've made abundantly clear, the situation for VOCs is very different, because no standards have been established for air test results. Nothing is more frustrating than having a consultant conduct expensive tests, and getting a report that provides no real conclusions about the results. What's more, since there are so many sources of VOCs indoors, it is often difficult to decide what to fix or remove if the results are high. For those reasons, testing your house for VOCs is generally not a good first step. Instead, if you believe you have a VOC problem, look into what products, particularly new products like carpeting or furniture, might be emitting the contaminants into your air. Ventilate your house, remove suspect products, at least until they air out, and be careful not to buy any new products that will emit VOCs.

HEALTH RISKS OF VOCS

Sick Building Syndrome

Sick Building Syndrome (SBS) is a recognized phenomenon in which some occupants of a building feel ill only when in the building. The malaise most often occurs when workers move into a new building, or the old building is refurbished with carpeting and furniture, which might be giving off VOCs (though it's difficult to prove). The effects are usually mild and pass when the worker is moved to a different area. For more information, see Chapter 9.

Cancer and VOCs

We already know formaldehyde is a human carcinogen, but what about other VOCs? Some chemicals are known or suspected to be cancer-causing agents. Benzene is one such chemical: exposure to this proven human carcinogen, which causes leukemia in workers exposed to high levels, is widespread. As discussed, we breathe it wherever we go, indoors and out, due to cars and other equipment that run on gasoline. Background levels typically found in outdoor air and in homes are low and thus not a significant cancer risk; however, it is important to keep your exposures to a minimum. The main preventive measure you can take is to not store gasoline or other fuels in basements or attached garages. If you do have an attached garage, keep the door tightly closed and maintain weather-stripping along the door edges to prevent air leaking from the garage into the house.

MULTIPLE CHEMICAL SENSITIVITY (MCS)

Imagine living in constant fear of going places because of the risk of encountering a chemical that triggers breathing difficulty. This is the situation for thousands of people with multiple chemical sensitivity, or MCS. MCS is a syndrome experienced by people who have symptoms, frequently severe, when they are exposed to chemicals at low levels that ordinarily wouldn't cause problems for most of us. MCS sufferers often need to live in the barest of surroundings (either that, or wear a respirator).

The mechanism whereby people develop MCS is not well understood. Much controversy exists in the medical community as to whether or not MCS actually exists as a clinical entity—most professional medical organizations do not accept MCS as an established disease. The lack of medical consensus has resulted in distrust and anger among sufferers of MCS, and a dilemma for public health professionals seeking to provide effective advice to those sufferers.

Usually, MCS sufferers can identify a high-level chemical exposure at some point in their past that precipitated their problems. After that initial exposure, they find themselves uniquely susceptible to very low levels of the same chemical and often to other chemicals as well, which contradicts what is known about sensitization (where subsequent reactions occur only after exposure to the original chemical or allergic agent, such as mold or pollen). Currently, there is no accepted theory on how exposure to one chemical can trigger severe reactivity to many other, unrelated chemicals.

Despite these uncertainties, many physicians and other health professionals will diagnose and treat MCS. MCS symptoms can occur in different organ systems, but usually there is no physical damage and no change in objective measures of health (blood pressure, heart rate, etc.). Often symptoms appear in the nervous system, lungs, and gastrointestinal tract. These symptoms frequently include depression, fatigue, pain, memory problems, confusion, and breathing difficulty. Most MCS sufferers find little relief from standard medical treatments. Sufferers first have to identify the chemical exposures that may have triggered the symptoms. Then they have to carefully avoid those chemicals, often a difficult task in our modern environment, where industrial and consumer product chemicals are so commonplace. Some MCS sufferers lead limited lives, trapped at home or in other "safe" environments. In their attempts to avoid exposure, some people can take avoidance too far, developing an unrealistic "chemophobia" than can ruin their lives. Some sufferers may require psychological support in addition to normal medical care.

MCS is one of those tough subjects for which we don't have satisfactory answers. MCS patients *know* they are sick and know that the environment is the cause, but most doctors and scientists cannot substantiate their claims and can't even agree on a diagnosis. Research continues on MCS, so stay tuned for future developments.

THE RISK INDEX FOR VOCS IN INDOOR AIR

The following chart, which separates formaldehyde and other VOCs, shows risk levels that depend upon how much chemical is in the household product to start with, and how quickly it evaporates into the air. For formaldehyde, we have divided the chart into UFFI products and everything else. Because UFFI no longer gives off formaldehyde, we give it a very low overall risk. However, a variety of other products give off formaldehyde and combine to create a moderate health risk. Other VOCs (benzene, TCE, PERC, etc.) are widespread in consumer products and gasoline, but the levels that get into indoor air are moderate, so the overall risk is also only moderate.

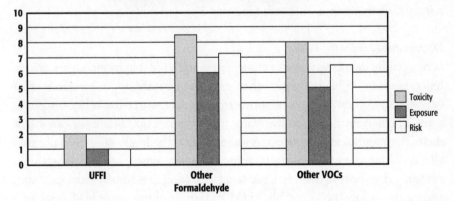

RISK INDEX FOR VOCs IN INDOOR AIR

DECREASING YOUR EXPOSURE TO INDOOR VOCS

VOCs in Carpets and Wood Products

Carpets, furniture, and other products containing VOCs should be "aired out" outside your home prior to installation. New carpets may give off VOCs for a long period, sometimes months, so it may be impractical to fully air out a carpet yourself. When you order it, you can request they roll it out at the warehouse and let it air out for some time before delivery. After the carpet is installed, put a fan in the room and draw the indoor air outside for a week or so until any noticeable odor dissipates.

Also, consider buying "greener," low-emitting products. The Carpet and Rug Institute has introduced a Green Label Plus testing program to identify carpets that meet the most stringent VOC emission standards. Green Seal is a non-profit organization that certifies products as environmentally friendly, using criteria set by the USEPA and other government agencies. The Green Seal website (www.greenseal.org) has fact sheets on some important indoor sources of VOCs, such as general-purpose cleaners and wood finishes, that also recommend products that are low in VOCs. The resources listing for this chapter shows how to get more information from these organizations.

As for VOCs in other consumer products, the best way to reduce your exposure is to not bring items containing VOCs inside to begin with. Become an educated consumer and choose products that have a lower VOC content whenever possible (see Chapter 7).

VOCs in Public Drinking Water

When public drinking water is chlorinated, unavoidable by-products are trihalomethanes (THMs) and other chlorine-containing compounds (See Chapter 6). When we take a shower or use hot water for other purposes, some THMs vaporize from the water to our indoor air, where we can inhale them. Although some exposure is unavoidable, the levels of THMs are usually too low to be a health concern. However, when combined with the amount of exposure we also get from drinking the water, risks can start adding up. While the allowable THM level in drinking water is 80 ppb, anything above 50 ppb is elevated above what is typically present and is more of a health concern. Your THM level should be reported in annual "consumer confidence" reports that water companies are required to send to their customers. If your THM level is on the high side (above 50 ppb), you should ventilate the bathroom with a ceiling fan to pull out any vapor coming from the water. A whole-house water filter is also an option; refer to the water filters advice provided in Chapter 6 for more information.

AIR FILTERS TO THE RESCUE?

If you still think you have a VOC problem after following the steps discussed above, you may ask, "Why not filter the air?" That's one of the most common questions posed about indoor air pollutants. The quick answer is that only charcoal-based air filters are effective for VOCs, and they are not recommended for long-term or large-scale problems. These filters need to be relatively large, even to filter the air in a single room, so if a charcoal filter is your solution of choice, it must be sized for the area in question. The filter can overload if VOC levels are high, in which case the charcoal will need to be replaced frequently.

In general, air filters are not a solution to IAP problems. They are really more like a Band-Aid, providing only partial and not very reliable help and not addressing the underlying problems (USEPA 1990; CARB 2001). They are often expensive and overadvertised, promising more than they can deliver. Different kinds of filters are needed for contaminants other than VOCs. You'll find a detailed discussion about other kinds of filters and how they may or may not be effective against allergens later in this chapter.

Combustion Products

Campfires are great to sit around as you tell stories and watch the flames consume the wood. However, all it takes is a shift in the wind direction to break your trance and send you scrambling out of the way of the smoke. Visible and highly irritating, smoke is a great warning sign that you are inhaling toxic gases, chemicals, and particles that are formed when fire burns any material. Inhaling these gases and chemicals can be hazardous, as each ingredient below has its own toxic properties:

- Carbon monoxide (CO)—acute poison, can cause death

- Particles—lung irritant, can make asthma worse, risk of death to elderly and infirm

- Nitrogen dioxide—lung irritant, decreases immune system

- Sulfur dioxide—lung irritant, can make asthma worse

- Aldehydes—nose and lung irritant, potential carcinogen

- Polyaromatic hydrocarbons (PAHs)—present in particles, carcinogenic

Wood stoves are more likely to produce particles, gas stoves produce more nitrogen dioxide, and furnaces are a major source of carbon monoxide. While carbon monoxide is the deadliest gas, as we'll discuss in the next section, it is important to minimize exposure to the entire list.

None of smoke's gases are more toxic than carbon monoxide. In the great outdoors, a campfire will not lead to toxic levels of carbon monoxide, but that same fire left burning in an indoor fireplace with the flue closed can be a formula for disaster as the gas builds up inside the house. Also, there are a variety of combustion appliances in the home that can release carbon monoxide. A combustion appliance is any device powered by the burning of fuel, whether it is oil, natural gas, kerosene, wood, or gasoline. Most combustion appliances are well known to us, and we usually feel safe having them in our home. However, if they are not operating properly, especially if they are not properly vented, they can become dangerous. These appliances don't usually give off smoke or other warning signs, and can cause a life-and-death situation if not properly vented to the outdoors.

Some common combustion appliances are:

- Furnaces (oil and gas)

- Gas stoves

- Wood stoves and fireplaces

- Water heaters

- Gas dryers

Other, less common combustion sources are only occasionally brought inside. These sources include:

- Portable electric generators

- Charcoal grills

- Portable heaters using propane or kerosene

- Gas-powered tools such as chain saws or cement saws

CARBON MONOXIDE

The CDC estimates that nearly 200 accidental deaths are caused annually in the United States by carbon monoxide. In addition, up to 10,000 people become ill due to carbon monoxide poisoning. The unfortunate case of tennis star Vitas Gerulaitis in 1995 put carbon monoxide poisoning on the map. He was visiting a friend's house and died from carbon monoxide poisoning while taking a nap; investigators discovered that carbon monoxide from a nearby hot water heater had been drawn into the room through the air conditioner. A more recent case is of an adult and three children who died while camping. They were found in a closed tent with a small propane stove still burning—they had apparently brought the stove in with them for heat.

Carbon monoxide is particularly dangerous because it is colorless and odorless. Victims often do not know they are being poisoned until it is too late; in many cases, they go to sleep and never wake up. Once inhaled, carbon monoxide has the extraordinary ability to replace oxygen in the blood, preventing it from being carried by red cells to the body's tissues. This leads to "chemical asphyxiation," as your cells are starved of oxygen.

Chemical asphyxiation has a number of health effects, depending upon how much carbon monoxide was inhaled. At high doses, it brings on confusion, loss of consciousness, and death. At lower levels, carbon monoxide poisoning is more insidious, causing symptoms that can be confused with the flu—headache, fatigue, and nausea. Some hints that you might be suffering from carbon monoxide poisoning are if the symptoms come on suddenly at home, and if all members of your household become sick at once. Because it can be mistaken for the flu, carbon monoxide exposure can go on for weeks without being diagnosed. Your symptoms may be the only sign that your house has a carbon monoxide problem. If the problem goes undiagnosed, you may go to sleep one night and not wake up.

Once elevated carbon monoxide levels are found, it is critical to remove all occupants from the house and fix the problem. If a carbon monoxide victim is promptly treated with the antidote, oxygen, most symptoms will fade quickly. Unfortunately, this may not be the case for those exposed to higher levels of the gas, or for longer periods of time. Chronic effects on mental ability may persist for years. Survivors of high-level carbon monoxide poisoning sometimes have difficulty with memory, and may experience behavioral changes.

SEVENTY-FIVE PERCENT OF ACCIDENTAL CARBON MONOXIDE POISONINGS INVOLVE HOME FURNACES.

Cold-weather months are generally the high-risk season for carbon monoxide poisoning. That's when the major combustion appliance in your house, the furnace, is working full-time. If the exhaust fumes from your furnace are not properly vented, they can back up into the basement. This accounts for seventy-five percent of all carbon monoxide in homes, and applies to gas and oil furnaces alike. Furnace fumes can back up into the house for a number of reasons. Sometimes material falling into the chimney or flue blocks the escape of carbon monoxide–bearing fumes; sometimes an animal nest built in the chimney causes a blockage; other times, the connections from the furnace to the chimney becomes loose or disconnected.

A less obvious cause of furnace fume backup is lack of adequate "makeup air." When a furnace burns any type of fuel, air must enter the furnace to feed the fire. That supply of makeup air is also needed to carry combustion gases up the chimney. If a furnace is enclosed in a small space, there may not be enough makeup air around it, resulting in a backup of carbon monoxide into the house. Also, the venting of other major appliances may interfere with air flow around the furnace and cause a carbon monoxide danger. These air-flow issues should be inspected by a furnace professional if a problem is suspected.

KILLER POWER OUTAGES

The highest-risk situation for carbon monoxide poisoning is a power outage. When ice or windstorms knock down wires causing blackouts, gen-

erators provide a backup supply of power for many people. These generators burn gasoline and produce carbon monoxide; therefore, they must be
located outside or be vented to the outdoors. But the fears and darkness
that come with a blackout often make people forget about basic safety.
They may decide to run the generator from their basement, attached
garage, or enclosed porch, all of which can be fatal mistakes. Power outages can lead to an epidemic of carbon monoxide poisoning. For example, a 1998 ice storm in Maine left in its wake 100 people with carbon
monoxide poisoning, although many more people may have been ill who
didn't seek medical attention. A study conducted by the Maine Bureau of
Health estimated that seventy-five percent of these poisonings were due to
improper locations of gasoline-powered electrical generators. Power outages can drive people to extreme behavior—some have even been known to
use gas ranges to heat their living spaces. While ranges are safe for the short
time they are normally used for cooking, they can produce harmful levels of
carbon monoxide when operated continuously over hours or even days at a
time. Some people use portable propane or kerosene heaters during
power outages as a supplemental heat source. Like furnaces, these heaters
generate carbon monoxide; however, unlike furnaces, they're not vented to
the outside. You guessed it—this can allow carbon monoxide and other
dangerous gases to build up in your house. While opening a window to let
in fresh air can cut down on your risk, we recommend you don't use these
types of heaters.

OTHER CARBON MONOXIDE SOURCES

You may be tempted to buy other appliances that give your house a warm,
cozy feel. Be aware that they may pose health risks due to carbon monoxide. Any appliance burning fuel that is not vented to the outside is a concern. For example, non-vented gas logs are marketed as safe to operate in
your fireplace with the flue *closed*, the idea being that keeping the flue
closed will trap more heat, making the living room feel warm and cozy.
You could never do this with a real (wood) fire because you would quickly
gag on the smoke that fills up your living room. While it's true that gas
appliances generate very little smoke, they do generate carbon monoxide
and other risky gases (nitrogen oxides). You might find yourself in an even
riskier situation because you won't be able to tell if these gases are building up. Despite manufacturers' claims, such products cannot be used

without some exposure to harmful emissions, and should only be used with the flue open.

During cold weather you may want to heat up your car before you take it on the road. Just don't do it in a closed garage! The car will be nice and warm, but your garage will have become a carbon monoxide chamber. The situation will be even worse if your garage is attached to the house, as other family members may be affected. Even idling with the garage door open will give you an unnecessary dose of carbon monoxide. Warming up the car when it is outdoors is safest.

CARBON MONOXIDE ALARMS

Homeowners and renters are equally likely to take their furnace for granted and end up in trouble. One of the best ways both groups of people can avoid carbon monoxide exposure is by installing a carbon monoxide detector. These detectors are like mini insurance policies—they'll ensure your safety even if something goes wrong during the long winter months, or if you simply have other carbon monoxide sources in the house.

Considering they're one of the most important security systems you can install, carbon monoxide detectors are easy to use, reliable, and inexpensive, usually costing between $40 and $75. Look for alarms that are labeled as meeting the standards set by the Underwriters' Laboratory (UL). Place your carbon monoxide alarms in locations as instructed by the manufacturers, usually in the hallway near bedrooms. Also think about putting a second alarm in another part of the house—an alarm placed in the basement can serve as an early warning system for furnace malfunctions. Locate your basement alarm in an area you use frequently so you can check it easily.

It's important to remember that every home has a small amount of carbon monoxide in the air—this background level is not a health risk. Carbon monoxide alarms will not go off from background levels. The alarm will sound if high carbon monoxide levels are detected over a short period of time, or if a lower level is present over a long period. Some brands do not show you what the actual level is but simply emit a loud beeping sound when safe levels are exceeded. The better brands have a digital readout that tells you the carbon monoxide level at all times. Any reading over 10 ppm is a sign that you have more carbon monoxide than is normally found in a home, and means that there is a source that needs to be investigated right away and fixed (though you don't immediately have to leave your home).

If a carbon monoxide alarm sounds, call the fire department *after* evacuating the house. If your digital carbon monoxide meter reads at or near 10 ppm, call your oil or gas service provider or the fire department to look for the problem before it gets to be life-threatening.

You can check the Underwriters Laboratory website to make sure your carbon monoxide alarm meets their specification. Also, the U.S. Consumer Protection Commission has a number of fact sheets and articles on carbon monoxide alarms that can be found at www.cpsc.gov.

THE ALARM THAT MAKES SURE YOU CAN GET UP IN THE MORNING

TOXIC FILE

Cathy had been feeling tired since the start of colder weather. She often was dizzy and had a headache, usually in the morning. She had seen a doctor, assuming it was a cold or flu, but he couldn't make a diagnosis. Around the same time, she saw a news story about a family that was tragically poisoned by carbon monoxide. They had been renting an apartment in which the furnace had not been properly maintained by the landlord. The reporter ended the story by saying they could still be alive if they had installed a carbon monoxide detector.

Cathy was also renting, and had no idea where her furnace was or whether it was ever checked. She couldn't get hold of the landlord but decided to buy a carbon monoxide detector just to be on the safe side, and installed it outside her bedroom according to manufacturer's instructions. She woke up extra early the next morning to the sound of the alarm's beeper. She called the fire department and was advised to leave the house immediately.

When the firefighters arrived, their measurements revealed moderately high carbon monoxide levels throughout the house. They found a loose connection between the furnace and the chimney flue. Cathy was taken to the hospital, where a blood test found elevated levels of carbon monoxide. The emergency room doctors explained the connection between her recent symptoms and the problem with her furnace. After her house was ventilated and the furnace repaired, Cathy returned home. She suffered no more symptoms.

CARBON MONOXIDE CHECKLIST

❏ Install at least one carbon monoxide detector in your home, preferably a digital readout detector. Remember, carbon monoxide is colorless and odorless—you need a sensor to detect it.

❏ If the carbon monoxide detector has a reading above 10 ppm, investigate possible carbon monoxide sources. Contact your local fire department and/or oil/gas company for on-the-scene help.

❏ If the carbon monoxide detector alarm goes off, LEAVE IMMEDIATELY and seek medical attention. Investigate the problem afterward.

❏ Have your furnace inspected and tuned up before the beginning of every heating season.

❏ Don't operate *electric* generators indoors or in any structure attached to the house or near an air conditioner on an outside window.

❏ Don't use gas stoves for heating.

❏ Don't use portable propane or kerosene heaters without ventilation.

❏ Don't use unvented gas logs.

❏ Don't run your car engine inside an attached garage.

❏ Don't cook on a charcoal or gas grill anywhere indoors, even in a garage with the doors open.

❏ *Medical Note: Pay attention to sudden onset of symptoms that mimic the flu, especially if more than one occupant of the house becomes sick during a short period of time.*

BOATING CARBON MONOXIDE ADVISORY

❏ Be careful when operating boats, especially if you are sleeping onboard. A surprising number of carbon monoxide deaths in recent years have occurred when fumes from boat engines were drawn into the cabin. Houseboats in particular have had problems with carbon monoxide sources such as power generators, stoves, and heaters in a relatively small, enclosed area.

NITROGEN DIOXIDE AND PARTICULATES

Carbon monoxide is by far the biggest concern as far as combustion sources around the home go. By following precautions to prevent carbon monoxide poisoning, you will generally reduce the dangers of other combustion pollutants. However, there are a few special contaminants that need to be considered, because their fate is different than carbon monoxide's.

NITROGEN DIOXIDE

Nitrogen dioxide (NO_2), is a common pollutant both in and out of doors. Outdoors, automobiles produce NO_2; USEPA regulations are in place to reduce pollution levels in that venue. Indoors, NO_2 is produced by any combustion source. Studies have found that unvented appliances that burn natural gas, such as gas ranges, can be a particular problem. Ranges with continuously burning pilot lights are associated with the highest levels of NO_2, though a ventilation hood or fan over the range can reduce these levels. Another solution is to keep the gas flames properly adjusted, which also reduces NO_2. If the flame's color has excessive yellow in it, call an appliance repair service to investigate. As we mentioned before, unvented gas logs and the operation of propane or kerosene heaters without ventilation are also sources of NO_2.

Nitrogen dioxide can cause breathing difficulties, especially in children and adults with preexisting respiratory diseases. Higher levels of nitrogen dioxide can quickly irritate breathing passages, causing shortness of breath, and asthma attacks in people who already have the condition. Such high levels of nitrogen dioxide are not usually found in homes, so you are not likely to see these acute symptoms. However, children who are exposed to nitrogen dioxide have a higher risk of respiratory infections, which may be due to nitrogen dioxide's ability to irritate deep within the lungs, making them less able to fend off pathogens. This serious effect is possible in homes with gas ranges (USEPA, 2006).

AIRBORNE PARTICLES

We know that soot accumulates in fireplaces and chimneys. But did you know it can also accumulate in your lungs? Wood stoves, fireplaces, and cigarette smoke release fine particles into the air, and these particles can have both acute and long-term health risks. For example, they can irritate the eyes, nose, and throat. The elderly and infirm with heart or lung conditions are especially susceptible to particles in the air. Studies of outdoor air pollution indicate that heart attacks are more likely when particle levels increase (Chapter 11). Particles can also trigger asthma attacks, and may contain cancer-causing chemicals, including a group of substances called polyaromatic hydrocarbons (PAHs). Cigarettes are the most infamous source of cancer-causing chemicals—they emit hundreds of carcinogens in every puff of smoke. Even non-smokers have an increased risk for lung cancer if they live around people who smoke.

The best way to reduce airborne particles in your home is to make sure fireplaces and wood stoves are adequately ventilated to the outside. Wood stoves should be sealed and operated with adequate air supply to create an updraft; it's also worth investing in good-quality, dry hardwood, which burns hotter and more completely than other woods, decreases the amount of smoke, and retards tar buildup in the chimney. (The USEPA certifies wood heating appliances and has fact sheets on the topic at www.epa.gov/woodstoves/.)

You can minimize particle pollution specifically from your fireplace by: making sure the damper is open before starting a fire; having your chimney cleaned regularly; and having a tight-fitting glass cover over the front of the fireplace to control air flow and keep smoke out of the room.

AIRBORNE PARTICLES AND CANDLES

Candles are another, much less dramatic or worrisome source of airborne particles. They are one likely cause of a strange phenomenon known as "dirt streaking," which is responsible for the dark streaks you may find on plastic items, walls near windows, and even on ice trays in your freezer. The streaks are due to particles and dirt (sometimes from candles) accumulating wherever air flows or where the air temperature fluctuates.

THE RISK INDEX FOR COMBUSTION GASES IN INDOOR AIR

As the following chart shows, you can't get much riskier than carbon monoxide. The risk levels for nitrogen oxide and particulate matter typically produced indoors are low to moderate.

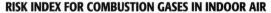

RISK INDEX FOR COMBUSTION GASES IN INDOOR AIR

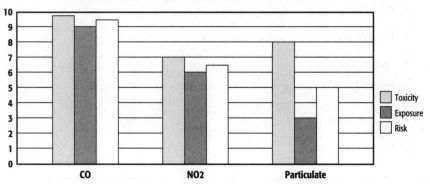

Other Indoor Air Pollutants

Some air pollutants are homegrown, a natural part of our indoor environment. We share our homes and offices with a variety of minute creatures, including insects, mold, and bacteria. These fellow occupants are usually harmless—in fact, some are a necessary part of our environment that have evolved with humans over the ages. However, our bodies are not totally happy with this arrangement. Some of these creatures contain substances that cause allergies, while others are pathogenic, causing infections such as Legionnaires' disease. Since the allergic contaminants are most common, that's what we'll focus on in this section.

As the name implies, allergens cause allergic reactions in sensitive people. We have already covered this concern with respect to mold, which is such a common problem that we dedicated an entire chapter to it (Chapter 3). However, there are a number of other agents that you should be aware of.

ALLERGENS

Allergens and allergies come in many forms. A common example is "hay fever," a condition many of us suffer from during pollen outbreaks in the spring or fall. Classic symptoms of hay fever, common to most of the indoor allergens, include:

- Irritated or watery eyes

- Runny nose

- Headache

- Sneezing

- Shortness of breath

- Skin rashes

- Sinus congestion

Most of us are allergic to something. We might even have become allergic after having an intense exposure to a particular allergen, thus becoming sensitized. After that point, even a small exposure can trigger a nasty allergic reaction.

Our immune system is to blame for this overreaction. As you know, our immune system recognizes and destroys foreign intruders, such as bacteria and viruses. A natural part of our immune response is inflammation, the body's way of sounding the alarm. In the case of allergies, the alarm is sounded way too loud, as either there is no real pathogen (e.g., pollen instead of a harmful bacteria) or the pathogen is not very dangerous. All the sneezing and secretions are our way of getting rid of the allergen, but we would much rather our bodies not put up such a fuss, since the inhaled material isn't actually dangerous.

Usually, allergic reactions are mild, with passing symptoms such as watery eyes and runny nose. However, in some people, allergies can be severe, even life-threatening. These people can have acute asthma attacks or even go into anaphalactic shock. One indoor air pollutant that can cause severe reactions is latex rubber. Latex particles from gloves, rubber bands, or balloons can become airborne, and those who are sensitive require latex-free homes and workplaces to breathe comfortably.

TOXIC FACT

ASTHMA RATES HAVE DOUBLED SINCE 1985.

For reasons that we can't quite fathom, the rate of childhood asthma has more than doubled over the past twenty years—in some communities, the rate is as high as fifteen percent. There are no firm explanations, though we can tell you the risk of becoming asthmatic is likely elevated by several factors: genetics, history of infections, and environmental exposures. As we discussed, indoor air pollutants, especially biological allergens, can also cause asthma or make it worse. The recent National Academy of Sciences report, "Clearing the Air: Asthma and Indoor Air Exposures," lists environmental pollutants that may instigate asthma (Nat'l. Inst. of Med., 2000).

Of the pollutants NAS examined, the only one confirmed to cause new cases of asthma is the dust mite. This tiny insect lives in most buildings but is too small to be seen with the naked eye, making it difficult to know if you have a dust mite problem. Their feeding habits appear to be scripted from a horror movie: they live by eating dead skin cells that regularly flake off our bodies. For that reason, they tend to live where we spend a lot of time—our bedding, carpets, furniture, and even stuffed toys. They grow best under wet or humid conditions. The dust mite's body parts and waste are highly allergenic agents that become airborne easily.

Many other indoor biological pollutants can trigger asthma attacks, and some may be able to cause new cases.

- Animal dander (flaked dead skin), saliva, and hair
- Mold
- Bacteria
- Pollen
- Cockroach body parts and waste
- Rodent urine
- Ordinary house dust and lint

KEEPING A LID ON BIOLOGICAL POLLUTANTS

Even a home that appears perfectly clean harbors biological pollutants. It's especially important to minimize biologic growth in homes with asthmatic children. Keep in mind, these organisms require food and water. Pay special attention to areas or items in the home that get damp or are prone to water damage, such as basements, bathrooms, air conditioners, and humidifiers. Thorough cleaning, preferably with a HEPA vacuum, can help control allergens. Removing or covering soft porous materials can also be effective. These measures are summarized in the following list:

ALLERGEN CONTROL CHECKLIST

❑ Keep humidity low and prevent moisture buildup.

❑ Cover pillows and mattresses with dust-proof covers.

❑ Vacuum regularly with a special HEPA-filtered vacuum cleaner. Damp-mop hard surfaces such as wood floors.

❑ Remove carpeting from bedrooms.

❑ Wash bed linens in hot water regularly. Wash stuffed toys whenever possible.

❑ Place a dehumidifier in the basement or other damp areas of the house.

❑ Vent crawl spaces.

❑ Use air conditioners during hot, humid weather.

❑ Don't place carpet on concrete floors, especially in the basement or other areas at risk for flooding or water seepage.

❑ Regularly maintain and clean dehumidifiers and air conditioners.

❑ Change filters regularly if you have an air handling system. Use high-efficient air HEPA filters whenever possible.

❑ Look for water damage in suspect places like doors, windows, porches, roofs, and basements.

❑ Make sure the exhaust fans in bathrooms and kitchens are working and venting outside.

AIRBORNE PARTICLES AND AIR FILTERS

Earlier in this chapter, we described how air purifiers have only limited value against VOCs. This is also true for allergens, which require yet another kind of filter, HEPA instead of carbon. The high-efficiency, or HEPA, filter can remove microscopic particles from the air, the kind that tend to be most worrisome. But although this filter can help, it's no magic bullet. It is generally not large enough to filter the air in an entire house and so is best used to filter the air in a single room where the asthmatic spends a lot of time. Air purifiers should never be used as the only approach to an indoor pollution problem. They can be a part of the solution, but the preventive measures described in this section are the most important.

Electronic purifiers, including ion generators and electrostatic precipitators, are advertised for clearing VOCs, allergens, and other particles from the air. Both work by producing charged ions that attach to particles in the air. In electrostatic precipitators, the charged particles pass through a pair of electric places that trap the particles. Ion generators do not have a trapping mechanism; instead the charged particles settle out on surfaces in the house. You should be wary of these devices because they may involve ozone, which when released into your home's air can present its own health risk. *Consumer Reports* recently reviewed a number of electronic filters and recommended only one. Many brands were found to be producing significant ozone levels, and performed poorly at removing particles from the air (*Consumer Reports*, 2005; *NY Times*, 2006). If you have an asthmatic in the house, electronic air cleaners should be avoided for that reason.

Believe it or not, there are other types of air filters that intentionally produce ozone, called "ozone generators." The ozone is supposed to react with a wide variety of pollutants, thereby reducing their levels and toxicity. However, ozone generators have not been proven effective in reducing pollutants, and in fact can actually create byproducts that may be more toxic than the original pollutants. In addition, ozone itself is a known irritant and asthma trigger. USEPA has sent out a notice alerting consumers to the possible health risks from ozone generators (USEPA, 2002).

Homes with forced hot air or central air-conditioning usually have a filter capable of blocking large particles. However, these whole-house filters are not very efficient at removing the types of particles that instigate allergy and asthma, and can now be upgraded to more efficient filters that approach HEPA standards. We don't recommend the use of electronic whole house filters (ion generators, precipitators, and ozone generators).

AIRBORNE MERCURY

Perhaps one of the more entertaining parts of high school chemistry class was mercury. This element could perform a number of tricks, starting with being the only metal that's actually a liquid at room temperature. On top of that, mercury could actually change and become a gas. Playing with it on the counter quickly revealed its most endearing property—it could easily fracture into small, perfectly smooth balls, gliding across the countertop like little marbles. Alas, the simple joys of yesteryear have been foiled by our new awareness of how toxic these gliding pearls can be.

As you'll recall from our food toxin chapter (Chapter 5), mercury in any form is a toxin that can damage the nervous system, affecting our ability to think and coordinate our movements; it can also damage the kidney at high doses. Liquid mercury is not that risky on its own. The problem starts when it vaporizes into a gas, which easily occurs at room temperature and even more so at higher temperatures. Mercury vapor is readily absorbed across the lungs, and can gain access to the brain and other vital organs.

While not quite as toxic as the form of mercury we eat in fish (organic mercury), mercury vapor is still a decided health risk. Unfortunately, it is still present in fever thermometers, blood pressure gauges, some thermostats, and even fluorescent light bulbs. The potential for human exposure is real whenever these devices break, releasing their mercury as silver beads that get lost in layers of carpet, settle in corners, or hide under radiators. From there it can slowly vaporize, spreading in the indoor air throughout your entire home.

Most cases of broken thermometers don't lead to a high level of exposure or toxicity, because people are generally good about searching for and discarding the spilled mercury. The brief exposure you may get while cleaning up the spill is not a health concern. However, longer-term exposure from mercury that you don't clean up *is* a health concern; so it's best to properly clean up a spill right away. In fact, the longer mercury remains on the loose in your house, the harder it will be to clean up—that's because more and more becomes a gas and enters the air over time.

CLEANING UP AFTER A MERCURY SPILL

Cleaning up spilled mercury is tricky because the beads are mobile, because they can easily break into smaller beads, and because there's the added pressure of needing to find and remove all of them. Therefore, if you have a mercury spill, it is important to do the following:

MERCURY CLEANUP CHECKLIST

❑   First, do not be alarmed. Mercury is not an acute toxin at the levels you may encounter from a typical spill. It's important to be calm and take your time to do the job correctly. You don't need to hire a cleanup contractor or environmental consultant for small spills.

❑   Isolate the spill area—one of the main threats is the spread of contamination. Keep people and pets out of the area. Walking on spilled mercury can contaminate shoes, leading to a trail of mercury thoughout the house. If someone has walked into the area, he or she should remove his or her shoes and leave them at the contaminated site. If mercury has been spilled on clothes, the clothes should also be removed and left on-site.

❑   Search for the beads of mercury. Make sure you have adequate lighting—as a silvery metal, mercury is shiny and so should be easy to spot. A flashlight may help you find mercury deposited in dark corners or shag rugs. In fact, after you have found the obvious beads, one strategy is to dim the lights and shine the flashlight around the floor; any remaining beads should reflect the light and stand out.

❑   Collect the beads of mercury. Avoid touching the metal to lessen the risk of spreading the contamination. Visible mercury can be picked up by an eyedropper or pushed up between two pieces of cardboard.

❑   Discard the mercury. Put the beads in a plastic bag and enclose within another plastic bag; seal tightly and discard in the outdoor garbage barrel.

❑   Dealing with mercury spills on carpets: porous surfaces such as carpeting or upholstered furniture may be difficult to clean. It's best to throw away these items if you know they have been contaminated with mercury because when you attempt to clean them, it's difficult to know that you got it all. If the item is valuable, have a professional environmental cleanup company do the procedure. They can also test the area to make sure the mercury is gone. **Never try to vacuum up the mercury—this will make it spread faster through the air.**

❑   Dealing with larger or more spread-out spills: the above steps will work for a situation where the mercury is contained within a single room, such as a broken fever thermometer. For larger amounts of mercury, like those that could be spilled from a broken blood pressure gauge, you should use the services of an environmental cleanup contractor from the start. The contractor can use a cleanup kit that has a powder that binds to mercury, making it easier to sweep up and discard. Additionally, you should notify your local health department.

❏   Seeking medical attention: this is not normally necessary unless you are in a mercury-contaminated environment for a week or more. Also, if you suspect that mercury was tracked through the house and contaminated clothing, bedding, etc., you may want to see a doctor. The doctor can check for symptoms of mercury toxicity and can test your blood and urine for mercury exposure.

❏   You should keep in mind that mercury spills can only occur if mercury is present in the house. New digital readout thermometers do not contain mercury. You can take your old thermometers to the town hazardous waste collection day for proper disposal. You should also check up on any other mercury-containing devices or products, and dispose of them properly. Removing these mercury sources from your house is the critical first step to becoming mercury-safe.

SUMMARY OF INDOOR AIR POLLUTANTS

CONTAMINANT OR ISSUE	LEVEL OF RISK	OPTIONS TO AVOID EXPOSURE
Volatile Organic Chemicals		
Formaldehyde	Low, but high for those who are sensitive	• Buy solid wood instead of pressed wood, particleboard, or veneer products • Look for products that are labeled as low in formaldehyde • Air out furnishings that may contain formaldehyde before putting them in occupied areas • Ventilate rooms in which these products are placed; keep humidity low
Urea-Formaldehyde Foam Insulation (UFFI)	Low	No actions needed. If UFFI is still present in a home, it can be left alone

CONTAMINANT OR ISSUE	LEVEL OF RISK	OPTIONS TO AVOID EXPOSURE
Other VOCs: benzene, perchloroethylene chloroform, trichloroethylene	Moderate, but high for those who are sensitive	• Don't park your car in attached garage • Seal off attached garages from your house • Store paints, glues, thinners, waxes in shed or unattached garage; discard unnecessary products on your town hazardous waste day • Choose low-emission carpeting and other products • Thoroughly ventilate rooms with new furnishings • Allow dry-cleaned clothes to air out before putting them into your closet • Run the bathroom vent fan during baths or showers • Consider the need for a water filtration system

Combustion Pollutants

Carbon Monoxide	High	• Tune up your furnace every fall • Don't use unventilated combustion appliances • Don't use an electric generator indoors • Use a carbon monoxide detector
Nitrogen Oxides	Low	• Ventilate gas stove with hood/fan • Tune the flame on your gas stove to be less yellow • Do not use unvented gas logs or similar combustion appliances
Particulates	Moderate	• Do not smoke in the house • Make sure your wood stove and fireplace are vented to the outside; have sufficient makeup air to create an updraft; keep the chimney and flue pipe free of blockages • Use a tight-fitting glass cover for the fireplace

Other IAPs

Biological Growth/Allergens	High for those who are asthmatic or allergic	• Keep your house clean, dry, well ventilated; use a dehumidifier in the basement or wherever necessary • Use a HEPA vacuum for carpet cleaning • Consider removing carpets from bedrooms • Fix water leaks and discard water-damaged materials • Don't rely on air filters as a primary solution
Mercury	Low	• Clean area soon after the spill • Follow cleanup guidelines • Hire an environmental cleanup crew for large spills

CHAPTER 9

Toxics in the Workplace

Modern workers usually don't have to deal with the subpar work conditions that were common fifty years ago. Today, employers pay attention to such basics as proper lighting and ventilation, and in some cases expand into things like stress reduction and fitness facilities. Our offices are more ergonomic than ever, and our factories have environmental controls that put a cap on how many chemicals we inhale. Occupational physicians, so-called Occ Docs, monitor workers to make sure they aren't getting the textbook work-related diseases and conditions of the past. Even the government has gotten into the act, creating agencies that regulate workplace safety, such as the Occupational Safety and Health Administration (OSHA) and the National Institute of Occupational Safety and Health (NIOSH).

While modern workers have the benefit of more protections, many of us are still working in inherently dangerous occupations involving chemical or physical hazards in factories, mines, power plants, and laboratories. Less hazardous but still of concern are service-industry businesses that routinely use chemicals, like dry cleaners, nail salons, printers, and photographers. These small Main Street businesses can harbor risky exposures that rival what takes place in chemical factories.

Finally, there are the jobs that appear to be totally safe: office workers, bank tellers, schoolteachers, etc. You might be surprised to know that some of these workers have experienced "Sick Building Syndrome," a modern phenomenon brought on by airtight buildings with windows that don't open, and centrally controlled ventilation systems (discussed in detail in Chapter 8). These systems usually work well, but when mold gets into the building or something goes wrong with the air supply, illness can ensue. Modern office equipment can compound the problem. In isolated cases, asbestos is a concern.

Bottom line, no matter what type of workplace we find ourselves in, we need to look out for potential hazards. Considering the amount of time we spend at work, there is ample opportunity for exposure. And let's not forget that, in some workplaces, the management might feel that strict compliance with health and safety standards is too costly, a hindrance to the bottom line. Ultimately, a safe workplace depends on ethical employers, governmental vigilance, and workers who keep themselves informed and hold their managers accountable for workplace safety.

This chapter is divided into two types of workplaces: those that handle toxic chemicals on a regular basis, and those where the dangers are more subtle (like office buildings).

Workplaces That Use Toxic Chemicals

MYTH: Workplace hazards are a relatively recent phenomenon that emerged after the Industrial Revolution.

REALITY: Historians have found evidence as far back as Greek and Roman times of hazardous working conditions. The worst conditions through the ages have been in occupations involving heavy metals, such as mercury and lead, as well as in mining for coal and asbestos. Toxic effects found in ancient workers demonstrated that chemicals can be hazardous and opened the door to toxicology as a discipline.

OCCUPATIONAL HEALTH

In spite of all of our advances in worker protection, there are still some pretty grim statistics. Although exact numbers are hard to come by, experts estimate that 5,000 Americans die each year from occupation-related illness, and 45,000 new cases of work-related disease are diagnosed annually (U.S. Dept of Labor, 2003). These numbers do not include the large number killed or injured by accidents.

A BRIEF HISTORY OF OCCUPATIONAL DISEASE

The Greeks first noted lead poisoning in slaves working in mines circa 300 to 400 B.C. In the first century A.D., Pliny, the Elder of Rome, described lead exposure in workers painting ships, reporting that they often wore loose bags over their heads to avoid breathing the noxious dust. Pliny devised a simple face mask made from animal bladders to provide more effective protection. One of the earliest recorded environmental cancers was noted by Percival Pott, an eighteenth-century doctor who found a high rate of scrotal cancer among chimney sweeps. He determined the cases were associated with soot in the scrotal area picked up from climbing around inside of chimneys. The fact that baths weren't that frequent caused exposure to be nearly continuous, compounding the health risk. That led to what might be the first worker health law, the Chimney-Sweeper Act of 1788. In the nineteenth century, toxics at work were made more visible when Alice came across the Mad Hatter during her adventures in Wonderland, an obvious reference to mercury-poisoned workers in the hat industry. (Mercury can damage the nervous system, and in these workers manifested as delusional and extreme behavior.)

In the twentieth century, a number of pioneers have documented occupational disease and pushed for government controls. Ironically, it was another Alice at the forefront, Alice Hamilton, the physician, who is credited with founding occupational medicine. Dr. Hamilton studied workers in the lead, rubber, and ammunition industries and was able to prove that chemical exposures were resulting in serious disease. She used this evidence to promote workers' compensation laws designed to keep employees financially solvent when disabled from workplace exposures. So-called workers' comp. laws became common by the middle of the twentieth century and laid the groundwork for later occupational health laws.

The most significant step forward in worker health was made in 1970, with the passage of the Occupational Safety and Health Act. This law is the basis for most worker safeguards, and founded the agency charged with enforcing the law, the Occupational Safety and Health Administration (OSHA). The 1983 Hazard Communication Standard Act ensures workers' rights to information about the hazardous materials they may encounter on the job.

The leading categories of work-related diseases include:

- Lung diseases, such as asbestosis, silicosis, black lung, and asthma
- Various cancers—lung, leukemia, liver, and bladder
- Cardiovascular problems—high blood pressure, heart attacks
- Reproductive effects—birth defects and infertility
- Nerve disorders—peripheral neuropathy and behavioral changes
- Skin diseases—contact dermatitis, acne, and skin cancer
- Kidney and liver damage

That's only a glimpse of what is possible in today's work environment. Given the fact that over 60,000 chemicals are used by industry (U.S. Office of Technology Assessment, 1995), almost any type of toxicity is possible from chemical overexposure. And these statistics apply to the U.S.—workers in the countries where we export our manufacturing jobs have fewer safeguards. One can only guess at the disease statistics in those countries. Nor do the above disease statistics include those caused by physical and biological hazards such as noise, extreme heat or cold, vibration, infection, and physical injuries. These are equally important concerns, but are not covered in this book because they do not involve toxic chemicals. However, you should be aware that OSHA has regulations covering physical hazards, and that your employer needs to comply with them as well.

Obviously, not all workplaces are created equal when it comes to chemical hazards. The worst exposures typically come via inhalation, so industries that put toxins into indoor air usually have the most risk. Some chemicals can be absorbed through the skin, so jobs that involve direct handling of toxins can also pose a hazard.

The following occupations involve major chemical risks:

- Chemical manufacturing—rubber, plastics, and other products
- Oil refining—benzene and other hydrocarbons
- Agriculture—pesticides and organic dust
- Fire fighting—carbon monoxide, cyanide, and other gases

- Painting—VOCs, lead from surface preparation

- Dry cleaning—PERC

- Nail salons—toluene, acrylates

- Hazardous waste cleanup—VOCs, metals, pesticides

- Metal working and machine shops—lead, chromium, chlorinated solvents

- Auto repair—cleaning solvents, asbestos brakes

- Welding and bridge repair or demolition—lead and metal fumes

- Boatbuilders—paints, adhesives, and solvents

- Art and printing—dust, solvents, and metals

- Mining—dust and radon

- Plumbing—asbestos, welding fumes

- Foundries—silicosis

- Medicine and dentistry—radiation, latex, acrylates, disinfectants, and mercury

- Road construction and roofing—asphalt, coal tar

- Textile industry—organic dust

- Toll collectors and tunnel workers—particulate matter and VOCs from auto exhaust

- Nuclear power industry—radiation

The list could go on. We only want to illustrate the types of jobs and exposures possible. If your job is not listed here, that doesn't mean it's free of toxics. For example, we don't usually think of farmers as being at risk from chemical exposure, but they can actually be at greater risk than a typical factory employee.

It is critical that workers learn about the chemicals used in their work environment, and the risks they pose. Learning about those risks will enable you to protect yourself and to ask the right questions of your employer. Government regulations help protect workers, but as described below, it's up to management and employees to make these regulations work.

THE BRIDGE WORKER

Dan was happy to land a job with a bridge repair company. He liked outdoor work, and the pay was good. The boss gave him some important responsibilities, one of which was operating the sandblasting machine, which shot sand at high force onto bridge surfaces to remove old paint, readying the surface for repainting. Dan was informed that most older bridges have lead paint and was told that he must wear a respirator to avoid breathing the lead dust generated by the sandblaster.

About a month after starting work, Dan's family noticed changes in his behavior. He became moody and irritable, was having trouble sleeping and sometimes woke with stomach pain. Another month went by and his symptoms became worse. His wife insisted that Dan go to his doctor, who could not find any obvious cause for his symptoms and suggested that they might be due to stress.

Back at work Dan talked with the other workers, some of whom had similar symptoms. He also learned that workers didn't last very long in this job, tending to quit after a few big projects. Maybe that's why the pay was good—they had trouble holding on to workers. His suspicions raised, Dan sought out another doctor, an Occ Doc at a nearby university hospital. The doctor found Dan to have the early stages of nerve damage. When he discovered what Dan did for a living, he immediately ordered a blood lead test. Sure enough, the level was more than double what is considered safe for workers (30 micrograms per deciliter). An industrial hygienist from the health clinic visited Dan's workplace and found a number of problems with their safety procedures. The respirators supplied to workers were not well maintained and did not fit tightly onto their faces. There was no shower or changing room on-site for workers to clean dust off after their shifts. The industrial hygienist advised Dan to have his wife and children tested for lead, since he might have brought home some dust on his skin and clothes. Dan's children tested within the normal range, but his wife had a slightly elevated level, probably from handling Dan's clothes.

The doctor informed Dan's employer that he should be removed from the sandblasting activity right away. He considered treating Dan with a "chelating agent" that would bind the lead in his blood, allowing it to be more quickly excreted from the body. But chelation has serious side effects, and Dan's lead levels were not high enough to risk the treatment. Within a few weeks of being removed from the job site, Dan's symptoms improved, although it took a few months for a full recovery. Regular blood tests showed a slow decrease in lead levels. Dan's wife was also monitored, and her lead levels dropped quickly once she stopped handling her husband's work clothes.

The federal Occupational Safety and Health Administration (OSHA) was notified by Dan's Occ Doc, and their investigation found a number of safety violations at his work site. OSHA ordered testing of all employees, and a majority came back with high lead levels in their blood. According to OSHA regulation, this testing should have been done on a regular basis by the employer. A total upgrade of the company's safety protocols and facilities, including the installment of showers and changing rooms, was ordered. New adjustable respirators were purchased, and all workers were properly fitted. A regular blood lead testing program was set up so that a problem in a particular worker could be identified before it became serious.

This Toxic File illustrates a classic case of workers being exposed unnecessarily due to negligent employers. Regulations and standards are in place to protect workers, but halfway adherence by employers can put them in harm's way. If workers are uninformed and inexperienced, they might not know what their options are if they're exposed. For example, Dan thought he knew how to avoid lead exposure, but he was provided with inadequate respirator equipment and did not receive the type of safety education required by the law.

TOXIC FACT

THERE ARE OVER 60,000 CHEMICALS USED IN OUR MODERN ENVIRONMENT. OSHA HAS WORKPLACE STANDARDS FOR ONLY 600 OF THEM!

One of OSHA's main functions is to set PELs (permissible exposure limits), enforceable limits on workplace air concentrations. The list of chemicals for which OSHA has developed PELs is old, stemming back to the priority list in existence when the administration was formed in 1970. Since then, they've developed new standards for only a few chemicals, which means the PELs that are in existence are badly out of date and certainly don't reflect the advances in toxicology in the latter part of the twentieth century (Nighswonger, 2000).

OSHA is not totally to blame, as industry has effectively blocked the agency's attempts to update the PELs, by tying up the process in the courts. Other bodies, such as NIOSH and an independent body called the American Council of Governmental and Industrial Hygienists (ACGIH), have developed more updated workplace air standards. Their lists cover approximately 100 more chemicals than the OSHA PELs. But unfortunately, these values are not enforceable. Furthermore, not all of them are that much of an improvement over the OSHA PELs.

MYTH: The NIOSH and ACGIH limits protect workers from the toxic effects of workplace chemicals.

REALITY: Even though the NIOSH and ACGIH limits are updated and improved relative to OSHA PELs, they are not fully health-protective. Typically, they are set precariously close to the levels known to elicit mild toxicity or irritation. They don't factor in a safety or uncertainty margin, or consider the long-term risks for things like cancer. Therefore, some workers may develop health symptoms and disease from exposure at the NIOSH or ACGIH limits, or at the OSHA PELs.

It's important to note that there are other types of OSHA requirements that provide important safeguards, including:

- Medical monitoring of workers
- Mechanical controls to reduce levels of airborne chemicals
- Protocols for air sampling and analysis
- Requirements for respirator programs
- Training of employees regarding workplace hazards
- Posting of warning signs

ENFORCING OCCUPATIONAL REGULATIONS

As you might have guessed, OSHA has a lot to do besides setting workplace standards—they also have to enforce them, which is a very large task. There are over five million workplaces under OSHA's jurisdiction. Although the number of OSHA inspectors fluctuates from year to year, on average only 1,200 inspectors are on duty nationwide, which adds up to almost 5,000 workplaces for each inspector!

Obviously, it is impossible for OSHA to inspect every workplace on a regular basis. The highest priority goes to sites where there have already been accidents, illnesses, violations, or written complaints from workers. Employees have a right to file a complaint and request an inspection by submitting a signed letter; "whistle-blower" laws protect employees from retaliation by their employer. Without those brave people, flagrant violations and unsafe practices might never come to OSHA's attention.

Since most workplaces won't see an OSHA inspector anytime soon, there must be other ways to ensure safety. By law, employers must be aware of OSHA standards and regulations, and they must set up programs to guarantee compliance. Many larger companies accomplish that goal with occupational health programs involving industrial hygienists and occupational physicians.

One of the most important workplace regulations was adopted by OSHA in 1983, the "Hazard Communication Standard," more commonly known as the "Worker Right to Know Act." This standard requires employers to inform their workers of the harmful effects of chemicals in use at the workplace, which employers accomplish by making available the Material Safety Data Sheet (MSDS), a compilation of information on the toxic properties of a particular chemical or of all the chemicals in a product. Amazingly, before this standard was adopted, workers could spend their entire career working with chemicals they didn't know anything about, not even the name. Having this information is a key step to understanding your health risks on the job. If you call OSHA or the health department to discuss chemicals in your workplace, the first thing they will ask is whether you have the MSDS. That document will tell them all the types of chemical hazards present in your workplace.

If you can't obtain the MSDS, you can usually get some information from the label on the containers you work with. The Right to Know standard requires manufacturers and importers to place a label on all containers, identifying the chemicals inside, and listing a health hazard statement and contact information for the manufacturer or importer. As we said before, OSHA also requires employers to train workers about the hazardous chemicals found in their workplace. MSDSs are normally a key part of this training, along with protocols for handling spills and other emergencies, and the use of personal protective equipment like respirators, gloves, and eye protection.

Q *What happens if I do get sick at work?*

A If you do become ill on the job, there are a few things you can do. First, stop working in the area that made you sick. See a physician to explore where the illness came from. Your regular doctor may not have the expertise to determine if there is a connection between your symptoms and work, so consultation with an Occ Doc may be necessary. The Association of Occupational and Environmental Clinics has a list of occupational health clinics (www.aoec.org). Your company may employ an in-house physician with expertise in occupational health issues, whom you could also consult.

Whether your illness is temporary or has lasting effects, you will probably want to be paid for the missed work days. This requires filing a claim with your state's workers' compensation agency. You will need documentation from a physician that your illness is work-related. Employers carry workers' compensation insurance to cover disability and medical costs—a kind of no-fault insurance where workers do not have to sue their employers for compensation. However, employers may contest your claim in an effort to keep a lid on their insurance premiums.

Workers' compensation was originally designed with physical injuries in mind. In these cases, it's clear that you are missing work due to something that happened on the job. It is more difficult to make the connection with chemical-induced illnesses, because other factors may have contributed to the problem. For example, if you get skin rashes from being around workplace chemicals, an employer may claim that rashes are simply commonplace, and that yours could be due to dry skin or some bath and body product you use (see Chapter 7).

If you are trying to get workers' compensation because you fell ill with cancer, you may have a difficult case. Many different factors can contribute to cancer, and thanks to the disease's long latency, the exposure may be years removed from the effect. The same is true for heart and lung diseases. Some states have limits on the types of diseases for which workers' compensation can be claimed. Since you may have trouble getting your compensation claim approved, you should document your working conditions and how they have affected your health, getting medical documentation and legal advice, if needed, early in the process.

WAYS YOUR EMPLOYER CAN MAKE YOUR JOB SAFER

- Reduce toxins! The easiest way to reduce chemical risks in the workplace is to substitute toxic chemicals with safer products. More and more manufacturers are finding less toxic alternatives that can do the same job. For example, many carcinogenic solvents such as benzene and TCE have been phased out of manufacturing processes, and replaced with less toxic substances such as toluene.

- Local ventilation. A tried-and-true method to reduce exposures is to have exhaust fans in areas where chemicals are used to remove airborne toxics before they can be breathed by workers. Similar to the exhaust hood in your kitchen, these ventilation systems draw air up and out of the building.

- Isolation or segregation. Another easy way to reduce exposure is to have hazardous operations in rooms or buildings separate from where most workers are located. A good example are spray paint booths, closed rooms in which manufactured products like cars get a final coating of paint.

- Personal protective equipment (PPE). PPE is the last line of defense. Employers should try to reduce exposures with one or more of the options listed above, but if they fail to reduce toxics to a safe level, respirators and other PPE will be necessary. PPEs must be fitted carefully to the individual worker and well maintained. Using this equipment may be inconvenient, but it is essential to protecting your health.

- Education. It is the employer's responsibility to provide health and safety training in workplaces where chemical exposure is possible, including the health effects of the chemicals involved, the use of PPE, and what to do if there is an accident or spill.

- Housekeeping. Keeping a clean and safe workplace depends on mundane but critical housekeeping tasks such as:
  - Cleaning small spills promptly

- Keeping chemicals safely stored
- Proper labeling of hazardous materials

- Medical and industrial hygiene surveillance: if your job involves working with one of the more toxic chemicals, such as lead or pesticides, your employer should have a medical monitoring program, which would have measured your health status when you started working and at regular intervals thereafter. The company should also conduct regular air testing and workplace inspections by an industrial hygienist.

Q *This job is toxic: who can I call?*

A Don't wait for someone else to speak up—if you think your workplace contains chemical hazards, go first to your supervisor. The company may not know about the problem and may be willing to follow up. Government help is also available. Many state occupational health agencies offer a consultation service through which an employer can request a "consultation inspection." The results of this consultation will not get the company in trouble with state or federal agencies; the inspector will simply make recommendations on how to reduce exposure and risk.

If your company is not cooperative, you can file a complaint with OSHA. Most private sector workers should file the complaint with the local federal OSHA office, which is listed in the blue pages of your telephone book and online (www.osha.gov/html/ramap.html). Also contact your state's occupational health unit to find out where you can get help. Remember, complaints can be filed anonymously. You are protected by OSHA whistleblower laws against retaliation by your employer.

THE RISK INDEX FOR WORKPLACES THAT USE TOXIC CHEMICALS

While the chemicals, exposure levels, and risks can vary widely in different workplaces, we have to rate the overall potential for toxic effects to be high. This is based upon the relatively large number of workers who have to discontinue work due to chemical exposures, either accidental or because they are a normal part of the job. Workplace exposures can be much higher than what is experienced by the general public. Governmental oversight is generally not strict enough to prevent all workers from being affected.

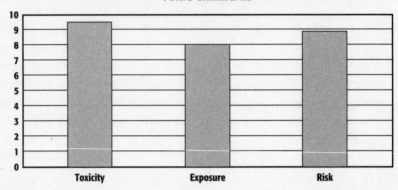

**RISK INDEX FOR WORKPLACES THAT USE
TOXIC CHEMICALS**

CHECKLIST FOR A SAFER WORKPLACE

You are your own best inspector when it comes to making your workplace safer—that is, if you are an educated worker. Due to cutbacks, you cannot depend on OSHA to conduct regular inspections. Most employers try to do the right thing, but financial considerations can take priority, compromising health and safety.

GET EDUCATED

❑   Get a complete listing of the toxic chemicals in your workplace.

❑   Find out about the hazardous properties of these chemicals from the MSDSs that should be available from your employer.

❑   Ask about any OSHA violations or occupational illness at your plant.

❑   Know the emergency plan in case of a spill. Participate in drills and training sessions whenever they happen.

❑   Obtain the NIOSH *Pocket Guide to Hazardous Chemicals.* This is the bible for many workers in the field, listing recommended exposure limits that are often more protective than OSHA standards. It also recommends respirators and other personal protection equipment as needed. Visit the NIOSH website to order the guide: www.cdc.gov/niosh/npg/default.html.

REDUCE YOUR EXPOSURE TO TOXIC CHEMICALS

❏ If there are volatile chemicals (that enter the air from a liquid or solid state) or agents that fume, make sure you are getting ample fresh air or that you have an adequate respirator.

❏ If there are chemicals that can damage the eyes or skin, make sure you have safety equipment such as gloves and goggles. Some chemicals can penetrate right through a protective glove, and you may need something more resistant. Make sure your equipment is suitable to the task.

❏ If there are flammable or explosive chemicals, keep them away from any flame, sparks, or other reactive chemicals. There will likely be special storage and handling precautions you will need to follow for safety's sake.

❏ Do not eat, drink, or smoke in the workplace, except in break rooms or other clean areas.

❏ Wash your hands and face thoroughly before going on break and at the end of the day.

❏ Leave work clothes at work. Your employer should provide changing and locker room facilities.

❏ Follow your nose—find out the source of what you smell and how toxic it is.

COMMUNICATE YOUR CONCERNS

❏ Contact your union, if you are in one. Ask them to help you improve safety conditions.

❏ Contact your workplace Health and Safety Committee.

❏ Contact OSHA if you have questions or a formal complaint against your workplace. Don't wait for OSHA to come to you.

❏ Get a medical checkup before starting a potentially risky job. See an occupational physician if you think your current job is making you sick.

Office Buildings

Far from the manufacturing floor, office workers busily peck away at key-boards, looking forward to their next coffee break. Sneaking into this tranquil work environment is the chronically congested nose, the frequent headache, irritated eyes and throat, and in some cases, asthmatic attacks. Why? Because some buildings harbor biological agents, mold and bacteria, that can lead to a variety of respiratory symptoms. Others have poor air quality due to ventilation systems that don't work right, allowing for a buildup of VOCs, carbon dioxide, and health symptoms. The office building array of indoor air quality issues is epitomized by the phenomenon labeled "Sick Building Syndrome," which we've already discussed in Chapter 8.

MYTH: Sick Building Syndrome (SBS) is a well-documented medical condition with known environmental causes.

REALITY: Sick Building Syndrome is a term often used by the media and general public as a catch-all phrase to describe any set of symptoms that people experience in a building. Often, the environmental causes are uncertain. SBS doesn't mean the building is sick, just that, for one reason or another, a group of workers feels ill when in the building. The typical symptoms include headache, eye, nose, and throat irritation, nausea, lack of concentration, and fatigue. SBS has been associated with high levels of volatile organic compounds coming from building materials in new or recently renovated buildings, or buildings with a lack of ventilation or fresh air. Mold can also cause Sick Building symptoms.

Few studies have definitively tied SBS health problems to VOCs or any other contaminants in the building. The most common situation is that a small number of workers in a specific part of the building become ill. However, there have been cases where an entire office building had to be shut down because so many workers were affected. Ironically, one classic example is the USEPA headquarters in Washington, D.C. The USEPA was housed in a refurbished mall for many years, and in the 1990s, a number of USEPA employees became ill. A series of investigations were conducted, but despite having top experts at their disposal, they were unable to identify the source of the problem. Parts of the building were evacuated while investigation and remediation occurred. In the end, the chemical 4-phenyl cyclohexene, used in the backing of new carpets in the building, was postulated as the cause of the problem, but never proven. Lots of carpets were removed and replaced. Eventually the USEPA moved into different offices and the space in the mall was not used again (USEPA, 1991).

Controlling the air quality for a large building containing hundreds to thousands of employees is an engineering challenge. There are many checkpoints in the system to maintain, and even more things that can go wrong. But in contrast to the industrial workplace, air quality hazards in the modern office building are less obvious. There are no MSDSs to warn of particular chemicals, and no protective gear. Office personnel are wise to learn how their ventilation system works, and how to recognize when it's not functioning properly.

OFFICE BUILDING INDOOR AIR QUALITY

Evidence has mounted over the past twenty years that indoor air quality (IAQ) problems in office buildings can cause respiratory symptoms and lost work days. Though these effects may be primarily caused by chemical and biological contaminants, people's reaction to them is often influenced by physical factors such as temperature, lighting, and social factors. For example, workers often tolerate tainted indoor air if there is open communication between labor and management and proactive steps are being taken to fix the problem. But the situation can become intolerable when the employee feels ignored and powerless.

TOXIC FACT

MANY INDOOR AIR PROBLEMS ARE CAUSED BY POOR VENTILATION.

Modern office buildings can almost be thought of as spaceships with critical life support systems needed to supply fresh air. These buildings are often designed with windows that do not open, or at least aren't the primary source of fresh air, instead opting for mechanical ventilation systems called HVAC (heating, ventilation, and air-conditioning) systems.

HVAC systems take in fresh air from the outdoors, heat or cool the air, and mix it with air already circulating through the building. Thus, HVACs do not provide one hundred percent fresh air, but rather recycle about eighty percent of the air with every pass through the system. This blended indoor and outdoor air is then distributed via ducts to all sections of the building.

HVACs also contain a return system, which partially exhausts the indoor air out of the building. Bringing in twenty percent fresh air is usually sufficient to get fresh-air delivery rates up to the recommended level of 15 cubic feet per minute per person. This ventilation rate is designed to provide enough fresh air to keep a lid on the transmission of airborne germs from person to person, as well as provide enough oxygen and remove enough carbon dioxide for your brain to function normally. Less fresh air would cause the room to feel stuffy, people to get uncomfortable, feel tired, and perhaps think less clearly.

During the energy crisis of the 1970s, many building managers reduced or even eliminated fresh air intakes in order to save energy, which led to an increase of indoor air pollution and was one of the factors leading to emergence of Sick Building Syndrome in the 1980s. Today's building manager balances energy costs with the need for fresh air to keep workers healthy.

While there is no government regulation of indoor air quality, the guidelines for fresh air delivery developed by the American Society of Heating, Refrigeration, and Air-Conditioning Engineers (ASHRAE) set the standard for building managers to match; however, building managers are not required to maintain their system at that standard. This is perhaps the single biggest factor leading to IAQ problems. HVACs may be neglected, preventing them from functioning as well as they should. Inspectors often find broken belts or clogged filters inside HVACs. It's also common for engineers and maintenance staff to make alterations to the ventilation system in the hope of fixing a problem, when in fact the measures they take make the situation worse.

To determine if a building is getting enough fresh air, inspectors measure the level of carbon dioxide. Yes, the same carbon dioxide that is at the center of heated debates about global warming is present in our indoor air. That's because it also comes from us—the more of us exhaling into a work space, the more carbon dioxide is present. If carbon dioxide levels are over 1,000 parts per million, it's likely that not enough fresh air is coming in to the workplace. (Don't worry, carbon dioxide by itself has no toxic effects at these levels; it is just a simple barometer of IAQ.) If carbon dioxide is elevated, it is likely that chemical and biological pollutants are also elevated, since, like carbon dioxide, they are not being vented from the building.

In fact, ventilation systems themselves can become a source of contaminants. If not properly maintained, air filters that take particles out of the air may become overloaded and actually add particles back to the air stream, or simply block the movement of air through the system. For that reason, air filters need to be changed regularly. Another key maintenance area is air conditioner drip pans. Air conditioners take the moisture out of the air, which collects in a drip pan until emptied. This collection of water can grow mold or bacteria, so drip pans must be inspected and cleaned regularly.

Contaminant Sources: Mold and Chemicals

Pollutants do not magically appear indoors—they must either be brought in by people, come in through windows from outdoor air pollution, or be created in the building. The first rule of indoor air investigation is to look for the source(s) of air contamination. Most biological contaminants, including mold, are caused by water entering the building. If materials get wet and stay damp, mold will grow! When investigating mold problems, look for places that are damp or where water has intruded in the past. (See Chapter 3 for more details.)

One of the most common types of building contaminants are volatile organic compounds, or VOCs. As in homes (see Chapter 8), buildings with

DUCT WORK: TO CLEAN OR NOT TO CLEAN

The pros and cons of cleaning ventilation system duct work are hotly debated—what seems like a logical precaution may actually make matters worse. A single vacuuming or wiping will remove most of the dust that has accumulated inside the ducts. However, if the cleaning process is not done carefully, it can also dislodge some of the dust and send it into occupied rooms. Since most of the dust was probably firmly attached to the duct walls, some indoor air experts question the benefit of disturbing duct dust at all. The USEPA does not recommend routine cleaning of duct work, saying instead that it should be done only when truly necessary (USEPA, 1997).

One thing that has become clear is that chemical cleaning agents should not be used in duct work. Cleaning companies may want to use disinfectants and sealants to discourage bacterial and mold growth, but it's actually an unnecessary step that puts chemicals into the ductwork that later enter the airstream and get inside of people. The USEPA has put out a warning about the use of sanitizers and disinfectants in ductwork as a potential health risk (USEPA, 1997; USEPA, 2002).

new furnishings or carpeting can have excessive levels of VOCs that can be irritating to the nose, eyes, and throat. Having inadequate fresh air compounds the problem. So does office equipment—copiers and printers give off fewer emissions than in the past, but the ink and heat do create vapors that should be ventilated. Large copiers in particular should have dedicated air exhausts to vent the VOCs that come off the machine. Another unexpected source of VOCs is floor cleaners and waxes. These products can contain VOCs (see Chapter 7) that continue to evaporate from the floor and into the air for hours after their use.

Even our own bodies are sources of indoor air pollution. Early attempts to set ventilation standards were actually directed at controlling body odor!

TOXIC OFFICE NEIGHBORS

Betty had worked for years at a travel agency, and was tired of answering to a boss. She had plenty of her own clients and so decided to open her own agency. She was lucky enough to find an inexpensive office to rent on the second floor of a small commercial plaza. The office was roomy, with plenty of light for her plants.

Betty settled in and business began picking up. But all was not smooth and trouble free—within a month of moving in, she began feeling tired and headachy at work, not every day but often enough to make her worried. She had noticed odors from time to time, which vaguely reminded her of being in traffic, something like driving behind a bus or truck. She got used to the odors and was preoccupied by her new business, but couldn't shake her symptoms. In fact, they got worse. Realizing that she felt better at night and on the weekend, she became determined to find out why her workplace was making her sick.

She began by knocking on doors, going down the hallway to her second-floor neighbors. No one had the kind of symptoms or odors she reported. On her way out that night, she bumped into a maintenance man for the complex. She told him her problem, and asked whether there was anything in the building that might cause that type of odor.

The workman didn't hesitate. "Have you ever gone around back? There's a dirt road that leads under the building to a garage where some guys work on cars. Most people don't know it's there because there's no sign of it in the front. Come to think of it, it's just about right under your office." While it wasn't absolute proof, Betty felt much better about her sanity.

But now what could she do? She knew she wouldn't get very far asking the garage guys to stop working for a few days so she could see if their shop was the problem.

Instead she called the plaza management company, from whom she rented her office. They were polite, but told her that no one had ever complained about the auto mechanic in the past and that they had just as much right to rent a space in the building as she did. Betty's next call was to the local health department. The sanitarian said he'd be able to come out later in the week and look around. Betty was thrilled that the health department would come out and inspect the premises.

That week was particularly chilly for mid-October, and Betty had closed the windows and door to her office. She was thankful for the heat that was coming up in the baseboard grill. However, the closed windows made the smell and her headache particularly bad—she even felt nauseous and dizzy, and went home early on Wednesday. Feeling better the next morning, she went back in and managed to reach the health department. The sanitarian promised to come out that day.

By the time he got there, Betty was feeling bad again. He immediately noticed the smell and recognized it as car exhaust. Hearing her symptoms and seeing how close the car repair shop was to Betty's office, the sanitarian told her: "I think you should go home now, since the office may not be safe. In fact, I'm going to call in the fire department to test for carbon monoxide, since it's one of the most toxic ingredients in car exhaust."

While waiting for the fire department to arrive, the sanitarian paid a visit to the repair shop. He found that there was no venting system. The fumes were going right up into the ceiling, Betty's floor, especially in this cold weather with the garage doors closed. The fire department's carbon monoxide test found a level of 55 ppm, far above what it should be and into the health risk range.

The local health department called Betty and told her to work from home because it was too dangerous to go back to the office. Next, they called the management company and explained that there was a hazardous situation in the building, and that having a shop that generates air pollution beneath other occupants is unsafe. The management company promised to talk with the building owner and get back to the health department. Weeks and months went by. Betty had long since stopped paying rent and moved out. Finally, after the health department had issued a violation and fine, the owner hired an engineer to install a venting system for the car mechanic shop.

This Toxic File points out the hazards of mixed-use buildings. It is not unusual for light manufacturing, chemical storage, dry cleaners, nail salons, and even car mechanics to be housed in the same building as office workers. If businesses that use chemicals are not properly vented, the neighboring offices can be affected. Workers in such offices should be aware of what businesses surround them, especially if they feel that their indoor air quality is compromised.

THE RISK INDEX FOR OFFICE BUILDINGS

Most office buildings do not harbor indoor air hazards—their health issues usually involve ventilation problems or mold, not highly toxic chemicals. The following chart indicates a low level of risk for office buildings in general, although in particular cases (e.g., mixed-use buildings) the risks can be higher.

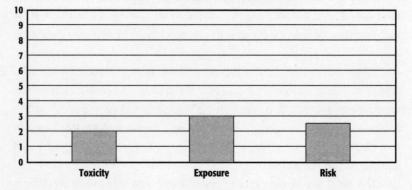

RISK INDEX FOR OFFICE BUILDINGS

OFFICE BUILDING CHECKLIST

❑   Notify your employer if you believe the indoor air quality to be inadequate, or if there are water problems, mold, unusual odors, or large office equipment that is not vented to the outside. You may also call OSHA, but their regulations are not really intended for these kinds of office IAQ issues.

❑   Make sure your employer performs routine maintenance on the ventilation system and troubleshoots problems as they arise. Ask how much fresh air is brought into the building with each cycle of air movement (should be approximately twenty percent).

❑   Do not cover over exhaust and ventilation ports in the ceiling. Some workers feel they have too much air blowing on them and will manually block the vent. This can send the HVAC out of balance and create local hotspots of poor air quality.

❑   In small office environments, find out about your neighboring businesses. Look further into any that work with toxic chemicals, especially if there is a chance they could get into your office.

CHAPTER 10

Toxics in School

You were fastidious during your pregnancy. No alcohol, not even a glass of wine. You avoided taking drugs, including over-the-counter medications. You took all your pre-natal vitamins and paid attention to which fish had mercury and PCBs. You read to your burgeoning belly, and were sure the being inside was attentively listening. You did your all to keep your child safe and help him or her learn from conception forward. However, when your child enrolls in kindergarten, both his safety and his formal education are out of your hands. There are certain aspects of schools that can impair not only your child's ability to learn, but also his health, most importantly the school's indoor air quality. And it's not just students who may be affected. Teachers, who spend more time at school, both in terms of hours per week and years per lifetime, may also be at risk.

School Indoor Air Quality

The USEPA estimates that up to fifty percent of all schools, old and modern alike, have indoor air quality (IAQ) issues, ranging from simply not having enough fresh air, to the more complex world of mold and chemicals encountered in art and shop classrooms. Health symptoms can vary widely from child to child, some reporting worsening of asthma, others headache and tiredness, and others cold or flu-like symptoms. Some kids may just feel better at home than at school. And if parents pull their child from the school, they typically do so against the backdrop of anger, blame, and denial, with school administrators and teachers caught in the middle. What's often sacrificed is learning, as the health questions and controversy can take months to years to figure out.

A 2004 report by the U.S. Department of Education concluded that indoor pollutants such as nitrogen dioxide correlate with school absenteeism, and that dampness and mold are associated with poor school performance (U.S. Department of Education, 2004). Children in schools with serious IAQ concerns may need to be transferred to a different school (or makeshift facility) until the problem is fixed. In fact, it's not uncommon for a town to abandon the old school altogether and hastily craft a totally new school—great for future students, but not great for the kids who actually have to deal with all the upheaval.

Listed below are problems schools frequently encounter, some of which you may recognize from the previous chapter on workplaces. The main issues tend to be inadequate ventilation, chemical-containing products, student mischief, and the one that's the biggest showstopper of all: mold.

COMMON IAQ ISSUES IN SCHOOLS

Inadequate Ventilation

Causes: Overemphasis on saving energy leads administrators to keep air recirculating, instead of bringing in fresh air; it can also be caused by blockages or imbalances in the HVAC (heating, ventilation, air-conditioning) system.

Effects: Poor ventilation causes increased levels of carbon dioxide and other air contaminants; temperature extremes and localized areas of poor air quality are possible (e.g., old wing versus new wing differences); health effects can range from feeling tired, to the inability to concentrate, to the greater chance for the spread of infection because germs are not swept away from students.

Outdoor Pollution Brought into School

Causes: Improper location of air intake for school; if the system is too close to the ground, it can suck car and idling bus exhaust into classrooms.

Effects: Elevated levels of particulates, carbon monoxide, and irritating gases; health effects include headache, irritation, increase in asthma symptoms.

Chemical Usage
Causes: Art room and vocational/technical/shop classroom use of products that contain chemicals that can get into the air; exposures can also occur in chemistry labs.

Effects: Increased levels of volatile organic chemicals and dusts in the air; health effects can include headache, dizziness, tiredness, irritated eyes and throat, respiratory difficulty.

Student Mischief
Causes: Students decide to pull a prank and close school for the day by releasing a stink bomb or playing with liquid mercury.

Effects: Panic and hysteria; toxic exposures possible if mercury exposure is extensive.

Mold
Causes: As in other buildings, leaky roofs, broken pipes, damp basements, and wet carpets lead to mold growth that can close down the school.

Effects: Can include respiratory symptoms similar to allergy or infection.

TOXIC FILE

A MYSTERIOUS RASH AT SCHOOL

After a long, hot summer, custodians at Springfield High found a few classrooms on the ground floor that had areas of fuzz growing on top of the carpeting. Since the school had not been used over the summer, the ventilation system had been shut off, which allowed the heat and humidity to build up, creating the conditions for mold growth. The maintenance staff were not particularly phased, and applied some carpet shampoo. They removed what had been visible, and didn't give it much thought beyond that.

During the first week of classes, a few students and teachers in the rooms where mold had been detected complained of allergic reactions whenever they were in those rooms. A consultant was called in and he found mold lingering under the carpet. He recommended that those rooms be sealed off and the carpeting replaced. It came out that the mold had originally been found during the summer, and some parents and teachers were more than a little angry that they had not been informed sooner. Students had to be transferred to other parts of the school, some classes had to double up, and the general state of confusion of early-semester high school was magnified to chaos.

Finally, when new carpets had been installed and students moved back in, a new and bigger problem arose. A student from a classroom that did not have mold reported to the school nurse with a severe rash on her hands and neck. Her rash improved once she went home but returned when she came back the next day, literally as soon as she stepped into the classroom.

At a loss, the principal closed that classroom, but by the next day, over twenty students from all over the school were gathered outside the nurse's office, complaining of itching. Some had visible flushing on their necks. A bunch of students went home at lunch, and by 1 P.M., TV trucks had arrived outside the school, asking students what was happening and projecting their rashes into thousands of homes across the area.

The principal sent all students home early and planned to keep the school building closed. The local health department was called in to investigate, along with the indoor air consultant who had come in previously. They spent most of the night and the next day going over the school in minute detail. The original moldy carpet problem appeared to have been solved—there was no evidence of water damage or mold anywhere else, and no obvious source of chemicals could be found. The new carpeting may have been releasing some chemicals, but the students weren't spending a lot of time on that floor. It was unlikely that was the source of the rash outbreak. For the want of a recommendation, they suggested that the school be professionally cleaned with special HEPA vacuums. (HEPA vacuums don't let any dust particles back into the air; even the tiniest particles are trapped in the machine.) In trying to undo their earlier communication failures, the school drafted a Rash Investigation Factsheet and held a public meeting to respond to questions. On the following Monday, the school reopened with a dermatologist on hand to take a closer look at any new cases.

Sure enough, a few more students complained of rashes, but the dermatologist could find no clinical evidence of real problems. She thought that some of the students might have gotten overexcited with all the fuss. Some parents wanted to close the school again, but others were just as upset with the possibility of their children missing more school days. After consulting *with the dermatologist and health officials, the superintendent decided to keep the school open. On ensuing days the number of complaints dropped to just one or two each day. In the end, two students could not remain in the building and were transferred across town. The crisis slowly subsided and the school administration breathed a collective sigh of relief.*

This Toxic File illustrates some technical and some very non-technical issues that can arise from an IAQ problem. The school's initial reaction to do a quick cleanup without informing parents backfired from both a communication and an environmental perspective. People lost trust in the school administration for not coming forward right away once the mold problem was found, and the quick cleanup during the first week of school only worsened perceptions of how the school handled the mold problem.

The subsequent outbreak of rashes probably had nothing to do with mold or other environmental factors at the school. The first student may have developed a real rash due to sensitivity to something she encountered in a science lab or art class; she may have had a latex allergy and been around balloons in the school auditorium. But because of the heightened distrust from the earlier incident, students assumed that the mold problem had not been resolved. The power of suggestion led other students to develop rashes, which can be brought on by emotional responses as well as allergic agents.

The outbreak of symptoms among a group of people, even when there is no obvious biological cause, has a medical name: mass psychogenic illness. A June 2002 *New York Times* article, "Hysteria-Hysteria," reported an epidemic of rashes in schools across the United States. In case after case, no medical or environmental factor could be found. These psychogenic outbreaks can be kept to a minimum by proactive communication that addresses fears and discusses the actual risks at hand.

TOXIC FACT

AIR SAMPLING IS USUALLY NOT NEEDED TO INVESTIGATE AND IDENTIFY INDOOR AIR PROBLEMS IN SCHOOLS.
When confronted by an indoor air issue, school administrators often respond with the knee-jerk reaction of hiring a consultant to test the air. Testing gives the appearance of being responsive to concerned employees and parents, and it seems like a logical step to take, but in fact, air data often do

not provide useful information and sometimes raise more questions than answers. All indoor spaces contain low levels of chemicals and mold. Testing will always find these background contaminants, but at the same time won't necessarily locate the source of complaints. The best IAQ investigation method starts with a thorough visual inspection, consisting of a walk-through done by IAQ experts. After the visual inspection, the expert may decide to follow up with some limited air testing to confirm an initial conclusion. It's important to note that, in many cases, the most important step in an investigation does not even require the services of an environmental professional. An evaluation of the HVAC system and its fresh air delivery apparatus by building maintenance staff can reveal problems that can be fixed right away (see Chapter 9).

The final step in an indoor air investigation is to identify possible solutions. Almost every school can benefit from better housekeeping and upkeep of the ventilation system. In specific cases, more drastic measures, such as removal of ceiling tiles and carpeting due to mold growth, may be warranted. Improved ventilation in areas of the school where chemicals are used or stored can also be a part of the solution. Of course, the ideal solution is to prevent problems before they arise by following the program outlined in the next section.

"TOOLS FOR SCHOOLS" TO THE RESCUE

A highly effective way for schools to safeguard IAQ is to implement the USEPA's "Tools for Schools" (TFS) program. In partnership with the states, the USEPA has made TFS a success, sending kits to most schools around the country with instructions on how to implement the program. Many states also offer TFS training.

TFS kits contain a series of checklists that allow the school to do a self-examination and establish an IAQ plan. The most crucial component of the TFS program is establishing a team of people to get the plan going— essentially, an IAQ swat team that actively manages the school's air quality issues. The team typically consists of a teacher, a parent, the school nurse, a custodian, and a school administrator. The school nurse is usually a key member, often functioning as the IAQ coordinator.

The IAQ team conducts a series of inspections, using the following TFS checklist:

- Complete a walk-through inspection, noting the level of cleanliness, evidence of moisture and mold problems, as well as the condition of the roof.

- Document the condition of office equipment and ventilation system; take steps to ensure the system is properly maintained.

- (Custodian) Keep track of cleaning supplies, noting the occurrence of spills.

- (Nurse) Maintain health records and a complaint log.

- Document pest management and pesticide use.

- Keep track of renovations: Are construction projects or painting spreading contamination into areas occupied by staff and students?

- Track waste management, including waste containers, science chemicals, rubbish removal.

The TFS checklist provides an IAQ management plan, which includes solutions for problems found by the team, as well as recommendations for ongoing prevention and maintenance. The goal is to find "low-hanging fruit" first—in other words, simple, low-cost items that won't wreck the current school year budget. Long-term or high-cost items, such as new roofs or ventilation systems, can be placed on a priority list to be addressed in future budgets. In some cases, funding from the state government might be immediately available for these bigger items.

The Tools for Schools program is not a one-shot deal. IAQ issues at a school usually don't entirely go away, and new ones arise frequently. The TFS team should meet at the start of each new school year and plan necessary activities, such as a new round of inspections, revisiting unresolved items from last year, and updating the IAQ plan.

BUILDING OR REMODELING A SCHOOL

Parents need to make sure that their tax dollars are going to a building project that will actually create an upgraded new school, compared to the old one. There are certainly new school disaster stories, where bad design led to ventilation or moisture/mold problems all over again. There are several programs to help parents make sure their child's new school is energy efficient and has state-of-the-art air quality. Encourage your school system to follow one of these programs:

- **Design-Tools for Schools:** This program is an offshoot of TFS. The USEPA provides guidance on how to construct a school that prevents problems by selecting low-emitting (low-VOC-content) building materials and furnishings, and gives suggestions for moisture-resistant construction materials and an energy-efficient ventilation system that provides plenty of fresh air and comfortable temperatures indoors.

- **Leadership in Energy and Environmental Design (LEED):** This program was created by the U.S. Green Building Council. If your school system enrolls in the program and follows the LEED design and construction approach, after the completed building gets inspected, you end up with a certified "green" building that is healthy and energy efficient.

ART CLASSROOMS, SCIENCE LABS, AND VOCATIONAL CLASSES

Art class, science lab, photography, woodworking, ceramics, auto mechanics, and other vocational/technical programs are all part of a well-rounded curriculum. The problem is that these activities can expose students and staff to toxic substances if precautions are not followed. The first step, of course, is for teachers to reduce the amount of toxic chemicals used, and to limit exposure as much as possible when chemical use can't be avoided. But there's some specific advice we can give you for art classrooms, science labs, and vocational classrooms.

Art Classrooms

Art supplies are usually not treated with the level of caution and respect their toxic ingredients deserve. This goes for artists and art teachers alike, and, in the latter case, can lead students to chemical exposures. Until the 1970s, the toxicity of art materials was virtually unregulated. Potent toxicants were often present, containing carcinogens such as asbestos and benzene and neurotoxins like lead and hexane. Today, there is better regulation of toxics in art supplies, requiring labels to list harmful substances; some of the worst offenders have been phased out. Nevertheless, toxics in art materials are not controlled as tightly as they should be, so we need to pay attention to the risks.

Many art materials can contain toxics. Some of the more common ones include:

- **Paints:** Acrylic paints may be particularly problematic, because volatile solvents like mineral spirits can get into the air and be inhaled by children. In general, oil-based paints should not be used in the classroom, and young children (under 12) should not use paints made from powder, which may become airborne and inhaled as a dust. Be wary of white pigments because some still contain lead (look for it on the label). Other pigments can contain heavy metals and other toxics, so read carefully! Spray paint should also be avoided in the classroom.

- **Glues:** Any glues that are solvent-based, such as rubber cement, should not be used by children. When the glue dries, toxic compounds like xylene and heptane evaporate into the air (thankfully, the more toxic solvent, hexane, was taken out of rubber cement several years back). If teachers or parents do use rubber cement, make sure the old bottles containing hexane are no longer in use. Also, epoxy glues can be very irritating on the skin and release toxic chemicals into the air (see Chapter 7). In general, children should only use water-based glues like library paste or glue sticks.

- **Spray-on Adhesives and Fixatives:** These art supplies are used for matting a framed picture or coating a piece of artwork to make it "smudge proof." However, they contain solvents that, once released into the air, can cause headache and other neurologic effects. These should not be used by students, and only by parents or teachers with proper ventilation (e.g., outdoors or with exhaust fan indoors).

- **Crayons:** Most are now considered to be nontoxic, but it's still a good idea to keep kids from eating them.

- **Pottery:** Firing ceramic pottery in kilns can release airborne toxics, including the metals contained in glazes. In general, young children should not work with glazes, and the kiln should be well-ventilated during operation, preferably with a dedicated exhaust hood. Do not use glazes with lead. Also, be aware that working with clay leaves a dust residue that can get into the air and your children's lungs. Good housekeeping is especially important to hold down dust in the ceramics room.

- **Print Making, Silk Screening, and Lithography:** The pigments and solvents used in printing can release air toxics, including lead, cadmium, chromium, and solvents. Children should not be directly involved with these processes. Use water-based inks whenever possible, and keep the area well-ventilated with a local exhaust system.

- **Photography:** Developing chemicals can be very toxic and need to be handled with utmost care. Children should not be directly involved in the developing process. Acetic acid, which is used in photographic processes, can be corrosive on the skin or if splashed into the eyes. You should use protective equipment, including eye goggles and gloves, and should be sure you have adequate ventilation.

- **Woodworking:** Dusts created by sawing and sanding can be very irritating; and some woods like cedar can be particularly problematic because they contain natural oils that are allergenic if inhaled. Use more common hardwoods and softwoods, and prevent dust exposure with good housekeeping and adequate ventilation. (Note that common dust masks you can buy at the hardware store are not very effective.) Wood finishes such as polyurethane and varnish contain VOCs and should be used in well-ventilated spaces. Water-based coatings are a safer choice than solvent-based, but even water-based coatings contain some VOCs (see Chapter 7).

MYTH: Lead has been completely taken out of glazes and other art materials.

REALITY: Lead can still be found in some paint pigments, especially in oil-based paints. Usually these pigments are white. "Flake White" is one pigment in particular that is known for containing lead. Some ceramic glazes still contain lead, but can be food-safe if they are fired in a kiln at very high temperatures. Our advice is to avoid these glazes unless you are very experienced, and always read labels, as lead must by law be listed.

It's a lot to keep track of. We don't mean to suggest that these materials can't ever be used safely—you just need to be sure you proceed with caution. Here are some simple precautions that teachers (and parents) can take to reduce risks and keep arts and crafts fun and safe.

- **Storage:** Keep all art supplies stored out of the reach of children, especially any that contain toxic ingredients.

- **Ventilation:** Art rooms should be well ventilated, and teachers should use exhaust fans in windows whenever products that release dusts or solvents are in use. Ceramic kilns and printing operations should have a dedicated local exhaust fan.

- **Glueing, Matting, Fixative Projects:** Children should not use rubber cement or spray-on fixatives. Those parts of a project should be done by adults, either outside or next to an exhaust fan that vents to an open window.

- **Communication:** Inform the students about hazards they may encounter. Post signs and keep warning labels nearby.

- **Eating or drinking:** No one should eat or drink in the art room.

- **Washing:** Wash hands after every art class. Wear smocks to protect clothing.

- **Purchasing:** Buy products labeled as nontoxic, especially for younger children. Water-based products are safer than solvent based. Some states like California list safe products you can buy. (See next section for more details.)

- **Cleaning:** Keep the art project area dust-free, and keep clutter to a minimum.

- **Mixing:** Pre-mix dry materials before students arrive.

Q *How can we be sure our school is buying nontoxic art supplies?*

A Read labels! Fortunately, a federal law passed in 1990 requires art materials to contain labels that list toxic ingredients and provide warnings where needed. The Art and Creative Materials Institute (ACMI) is the main organization that reviews the safety of art products. This nonprofit organization has evaluated the toxicity of approximately 60,000 art and craft materials. ACMI certifies a product as "nontoxic" when they find that it will cause no harm, even to a small child (look for labels with the approved product or "AP" symbol on them), and requires warning labels when they cannot guarantee that a product is nontoxic; these products bear the "CL" designation meaning "certified as properly labeled." Take note, this does not mean the product is safe for children! In fact, you should keep "CL"-labeled products away from children, since we can't expect them to read labels or follow a teacher's safety instructions. You should also check the California artguide website: (www.oehha.ca.gov/education/art/artguide .html). It lists art supplies that have been banned from classroom use in California.

Science Labs

It should come as no surprise that school science labs are a likely place to find chemicals. Many dangerous chemicals, including benzene, mercury, hydrochloric acid, and, most notably, formaldehyde, can be found in high school chemistry labs, as well as a few in biology labs. Strong acids and bases are a special hazard because they are corrosive and can injure the skin and eyes on contact. Students must always wear goggles, gloves, and a lab coat to protect them against accidental exposure. But really, the key to chemistry lab safety is the exhaust hood. The exhaust hood is a section of lab bench that is enclosed or "hooded" with an exhaust fan at the top, ensuring that the vapors go up and out of the building. For example, opening a bottle of ether, a highly volatile and flammable liquid, out in the open near a lit Bunsen burner can create a trail of flames from the burner right back to the open bottle—the vapor hanging in the air will ignite. But opening that bottle of ether in the hood would prevent the accident from happening.

The following compounds should only be handled under an exhaust hood:

- Reactive compounds like phosphorous (red or white) or concentrated acids

- Other irritant gases such as ammonia, chlorine, bromine, and hydrogen sulfide

- Flammable chemicals such as ethers, hydrogen gas, and pentane

Some carcinogenic chemicals may still be in the lab and should be identified and removed as much as possible. These include:

- Acrylamide
- Benzene
- Beryllium
- Cadmium
- Carbon tetrachloride

- Chromium 6
- Formaldehyde
- Nickel
- Arsenic salts
- Asbestos

Every school with a chemical laboratory should designate a "chemical hazard officer," who develops a plan for safe handling of chemicals, from purchase to disposal. The chemical plan should include guidelines for:

- **Purchasing:** Only obtain chemicals that are absolutely needed and from an approved safety list.

- **Storage and labeling:** Keep chemicals safely locked when not in use. Ensure proper labeling and have Material Safety Data Sheets posted.

- **Spill response:** Have a spill response plan posted and train teachers for its use. Make sure they know where first aid kits and showers are available.

- **Personal protection equipment:** Make sure goggles and gloves are available.

- **Ventilation:** All exhaust hoods should be in good working order. They should have an air velocity of 100 linear feet per minute.

- **Students:** Inform students of hazards at the beginning of each experiment, and teach them general safety precautions. Students should always be supervised when handling chemicals.

- **Disposal:** Have a written plan for removing chemicals, including a shelf-life limit. Extremely dangerous, explosive, and/or unused chemicals like mercury should be disposed of immediately. Companies that properly dispose of hazardous materials should be hired to take care of the waste chemicals off-site. Do not flush chemicals down the drain.

- **Record keeping:** Maintain a current inventory of all chemicals, including designated disposal dates

Obviously, lab chemicals get us into a complex and potentially dangerous area. Much of the day-to-day responsibility for safety belongs to the chemistry faculty, but the school administration must support lab safety by providing students and laboratories with proper safety equipment. Parents should find out about chemicals used in the lab environment, and what safety measures are being taken. High school students should be encouraged to ask questions if any aspect of chemical use or safety is unclear.

SCIENCE LABS—STILL A SOURCE OF MERCURY

Most schools have taken mercury out of the classroom. However, because some schools have failed to dispose of that jar of mercury at the back of the storage closet, problems still occur. These errant stores of mercury somehow get into the hands of curious students. In such situations, mercury is inevitably spilled and tracked around school on students' shoes. This can trigger an emergency response where professionals in haz-mat suits chase beads of mercury and school may be shut down for a day or two. Students have to change into uncontaminated clothing before they are allowed to go home. Schools should search high and low and remove any mercury still on the premises, including mercury thermometers, barometers, and blood-pressure gauges (Chapter 8).

Vocational Classes
High schools with vocational training curriculums also need to be concerned about toxic hazards.

The following types of classes are of chemical concern:

- Engine repair—gasoline, lubricants, oils
- Woodworking—varnishes, solvents, wood dust
- Agriculture—pesticides
- Auto body—paints, epoxy

- Cosmetology—hair dyes, chemicals in nail salons

- Health technology—latex, disinfectants

- Metalworking—welding fumes, solvents

- Plumbing—welding fumes

- Graphic arts—solvents, heavy metals

Each of these classes involves hands-on training that can expose students to a variety of chemicals. Most of the precautions for art and science classes apply to these vocational work areas. The primary focus should be on safety training, reading labels, toxic use reduction, and exposure prevention with adequate ventilation. Material safety data sheets for all chemicals used should be on hand. We need to teach our students how to properly dispose of waste chemicals. The school environment is a perfect place to teach chemical safety to our future scientists, mechanics, carpenters, and beauticians.

THE RISK INDEX FOR SCHOOLS

Many schools have improved air quality by implementing Tools for Schools and spending money to fix things like leaky roofs and broken ventilation systems. However, the problems are still widespread and need ongoing attention. The risk index chart is divided into problems that plague the building itself (mold, ventilation) vs. problems that come from how the building is used (art, shop, vocational classes). Mold and ventilation are not associated with particularly toxic agents, although the exposures are common and potentially allergenic, leading to a moderate degree of risk. In contrast, art, shop, and vocational classes can involve products containing high-toxicity chemicals (e.g., lead, VOCs) or can generate high levels of dust. Therefore, the toxicity ranking is high while the exposure is considered to be low because students typically spend only a small part of the day in these classes. This leads to a moderate risk, but the risk can be higher for students that spend more time in such classes or for teachers. The risks for both the mold/ventilation problems and specialized classroom exposures are high enough to warrant active participation of parents, teachers, and school administration to decrease exposures and risk.

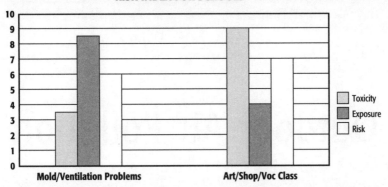

RISK INDEX FOR SCHOOLS

SCHOOL IAQ CHECKLIST

Much of the advice in this chapter is for school administrators, teachers, and custodians. But you as a parent have an active role to play, even if you are not on the Tools for Schools committee. You should be on the lookout for unsafe practices and materials in your child's classroom, and bring them to the attention of the teacher. Also bring up issues with the Tools for Schools committee, and if one doesn't exist at your school, talk to the principal about getting one started. The following checklist is a to-do list for parents and school staff alike.

❑ Encourage your school to adopt the Tools for Schools program.

❑ See that the school is clean and well maintained.

❑ Report any water leaks or moisture problems at once, and make sure something is done to stop the leak and prevent mold from growing.

❑ Make sure that renovations and construction projects around the school are done after school hours; if this is not possible, such projects should be isolated from the rest of the school with closed doors or plastic sheeting.

❑ Encourage your town to build new schools with IAQ in mind. Follow the USEPA's "Design—Tools for Schools" and/or U.S. Green Building Council's "Leadership in Energy and Environmental Design" (LEED).

❑ For art and science classes, purchase less toxic products whenever possible and make sure materials are stored and used safely.

❑ Have communication on IAQ issues occur early and often; parents and teachers should be informed of all problems and programs to improve IAQ.

CHAPTER 11

Outdoor Air Pollution

We are surrounded by an atmosphere that bathes us in life-giving oxygen, sunlight, and water vapor—but that also serves as a disposal site for many man-made wastes. Think of a goldfish in a bowl of water. The fish's existence depends upon the finite amount of water in its enclosed environment, water that fills up with pollutants that the fish excretes. Without a fresh supply of water, the fish will succumb to the toxics in its environment.

Our fish bowl is vastly bigger but still finite, and we have to remember there's a limit to how much waste material it can absorb and still support life and health. Like the fish's gills, our lungs take up whatever is in our living medium, the air we breathe. We've been sending our waste products airborne for hundreds of years, creating environmental nightmares such as acid rain, greenhouse warming, smog, and clouds of choking particulate pollution. But unlike other types of contamination (food, water, indoor air), we don't have much choice in the outdoor air we breathe, especially if our job and lifestyle demand that we live in suburban or urban areas. In fact, of all environmental hazards discussed in this book, the one you have the *least* control over is outdoor air pollution. We depend upon our local and federal governments to prevent pollution sources, which are often spread across an entire state, degrading air quality and harming public health. But government protection isn't always foolproof, and you need to understand where and when the risks are the greatest and learn how to avoid toxic air pollution.

The air we breathe is a mixture of natural gases, including oxygen, nitrogen, carbon dioxide, and water vapor. Natural processes put additional gases into the air: well before man created industrial pollutants, natural events were releasing toxics into the air from forest fires (smoke, particles, gases), volcanic eruptions (sulfur dioxide, silica, mercury), and lightning (ozone). Of course, humans have done more than our share to pollute the skies, beginning with the discovery of fire for cooking and heating. Fire represented a leap forward for mankind, and a giant step backward for the environment. This has been magnified over the centuries by the ever-expanding combustion of fossil fuels to run our cities and factories and power our cars. Fossil fuel combustion remains the main source of man-made air pollution, but we have increasingly used incineration to burn whatever we don't want, from municipal garbage to old tires to toxic waste. When you add the fact that factories send over a billion pounds of industrial chemicals into the air every year (USEPA, 2003), you're left with an unappetizing mixture of airborne toxics.

Fortunately, as we said before, there are government regulations to curb air pollution. The USEPA established air standards for six "criteria pollutants" beginning in the 1970s. These pollutants were prioritized because they had bad track records, and were obviously in need of regulation due to the death, disease, or environmental degradation they caused. These six criteria pollutants are:

- Ozone: toxic and irritating to lungs, can worsen asthma; formed in the atmosphere when car exhaust and other emissions mix with sunlight.

- Particles: toxic to lungs; causes premature death in elderly and infirm; released from all combustion sources, with particularly high levels from diesel trucks.

- Carbon monoxide: harms the body's ability to use oxygen, but today is mostly an indoor air concern (Chapter 8).

- Sulfur oxides: toxic and irritating to lungs; can worsen asthma and enhance toxicity of particles; also cause environmental degradation via acid rain; a major source is combustion of sulfur-containing coal and oil for power plants.

- Nitrogen oxides: irritating to lungs; decrease immune function; a likely asthma trigger; present in car exhaust and other combustion emissions.

- Lead: toxic to nervous system; lead fallout near factories (e.g., smelters, battery manufacturing) and roadways has caused excessive lead in soil and risks to children.

Criteria pollutant standards are updated by the USEPA every five to ten years. The standards for particles and ozone have been made more strict in recent years, amidst evidence that people can be affected by levels at or even below the former standard. Given how toxic these pollutants are, there is pressure from the public health community to lower the standards even further. But even with environmental regulation and air quality improvements, large amounts of criteria pollutants are still released into the air. For example, approximately 1.2 billion tons of particles are emitted annually in the United States (EWG, 1997). The public usually focuses on industrial smokestacks because they are obvious and an eyesore. However, we as individuals also have a big hand in polluting the air. The majority of air pollution comes from cars, and even though cars burn cleaner today than ever before, we drive more miles than ever before. Under the current framework, air quality seems destined to fight a losing battle against the automobile.

Lest all the attention given to these six pollutants makes you think there is little else to worry about, there are in fact many additional chemicals that our cars, combustors, and factories send into the air. The potential list of hazardous air pollutants (HAPs) is practically endless. In any one location, air quality may be impacted by general background sources (e.g., cars, buses, and trucks); layered on top of that are the emissions from local industries, landfills, or small businesses. Factories that make chemicals (e.g., pharmaceuticals, pesticides, industrial chemicals) or products that require chemicals (e.g., plastics, rubber, chrome plating, other synthetics) usually have an airborne waste stream. Gas stations, dry cleaners, nail salons, and farms that spray pesticides also produce airborne toxins. Both large and small sources of pollution can degrade air quality and lead to health risks.

Are there federal regulations to address HAPs? Fortunately, yes. These are separate from the regulations governing criteria pollutants. Industries can't just put HAPs into the air to their heart's and pocketbook's content. However, the system is far from perfect, and HAPs are an ongoing public health concern.

THE DAWNING OF AIR POLLUTION AWARENESS

TOXIC FILE

On Thursday, October 28, 1948, an unusually heavy layer of air pollution settled over the small industrial town of Donora, Pennsylvania. Townspeople were used to air pollution from a local steel plant and other factories, but this was different. A peculiar weather pattern had created an inversion that trapped pollution at ground level.

By the next day, the smog was so thick that fans at a local high school football game could not see the players on the field. Soon, the day became nearly as dark as night, and normal activities became impossible.

At midday Saturday, people began to get sick from the effects of the smog. They developed sore throats, coughs, and watery eyes, which progressed to more severe conditions. Some people were rushed to the hospital or died at home. Fortunately, a rainstorm and change in weather pattern cleared the air, but the damage had been done. Thousands were hospitalized, overwhelming local medical facilities, and at least twenty people died. Many more died in the following weeks due to lingering effects from the pollution.

The tragedy in Donora woke America up to the hazards presented by out-of-control air pollution. It demonstrated that when there are enough pollution sources in one area, all it takes for people to start dying is an unfortunate weather pattern to trap the pollutants and fill up the fish bowl. Donora became a rallying cry for early environmentalists who were beginning the clean air fight. Also, in 1952, a severe air pollution episode in London called the Killer Fog claimed scores of lives. Detailed studies showed how hospitalizations and death from respiratory conditions correlated closely to periods of high air pollution in London (Brown, 1994). The "smoking gun" evidence from Donora and London led to congressional action, and the passage of the Clear Air Act in 1970.

The key culprits in these cases were probably particulate matter and sulfur oxides. However, over the years additional pollutants have emerged as dangerous to public health. We focus on ozone, particulate matter, and HAPs in this chapter, because they are today's leading air pollution concerns.

> **MYTH:** If you don't see air pollution, there's not enough there to harm you.
>
> **REALITY:** Our eyes are not a good measure of air pollutant levels. Numerous toxics are invisible gases—in fact, the most toxic type of particulate matter is actually invisible, because only the very tiny particles reach the deep lung, where they can stir up an inflammatory reaction. Ozone isn't visible at street level, either. Only when you look up into the summer sky and notice that the natural blue has been replaced by a yellow-brown haze do you have a visual hint that ozone (also known as smog) has you in its grip. Emissions from gas stations, landfills, and many industries are gaseous and thus invisible. It's also important to note that the opposite is true for the plumes emitted from smokestacks, which may look much worse than they actually are. The emission may be mostly steam, which in the wintertime rapidly condenses to form thick, dark clouds of water vapor but little else.

OZONE

Ozone is probably the number-one air pollution risk for those living in cities and suburbs, especially for those with airways that tighten up when confronted with irritants. The effects on the respiratory tract are both immediate (in the form of increased chance for an asthma attack) and chronic (in the form of long-term lung damage). Fortunately, there are ways you can lower your exposure to this primarily summertime pollutant.

OZONE AND OUTDOOR EXERCISE

Lucy liked to go running in her suburban Connecticut town, located just over the border from Westchester County, New York. After years of running early in the morning, a change in her schedule forced Lucy to begin running during her lunch hour, which was fine until summer came. The warm weather brought shortness of breath, and she found she couldn't run as far or as fast. She was surprised at how easily she became winded. She eventually developed a slight wheeze and resorted to using an over-the-counter inhaler to control it.

One day, after a run in particularly hot weather, Lucy had her first full-blown asthma attack since she was a child. The emergency room doctor told her that he had seen a number of patients that day with asthma and

other respiratory problems. He went on to say it was no coincidence that an
air pollution alert had been issued due to high levels of ozone. Lucy was ad-
vised not to run during the heat of the day when ozone levels are the worst.

Lucy did some research on her own, discovering that ozone is a known
trigger for asthma attacks, and that her region in Connecticut did not meet
federal ozone standards during summer months. A respiratory specialist
told her to keep an eye on the "Air Quality Index" (AQI), issued daily by the
USEPA. He said Lucy should not run when the AQI was above "moderate"
for ozone. On those days, she was told to try to rearrange her schedule and
run first thing in the morning, because ozone wasn't usually a problem
when the sun was still low in the sky. Another option would be to join a
health club, as ozone levels were much lower indoors than out.

This Toxic File teaches us a number of lessons about ozone. First, it's
a warm-weather pollutant, requiring sunlight and high temperatures to
reach high levels. That's because ozone is not emitted directly into the air,
but rather is formed when two other common pollutants combine with
the help of energy from the sun. Nitrogen oxides (from cars and power
plants) join with volatile organic compounds (from evaporation of gasoline and other consumer products) to create ground-level ozone. The common term to describe this mix of summertime pollutants is "smog."

Ozone is chemically very simple, a close cousin of oxygen. Gaseous
(O_2) oxygen has two atoms in its natural state. Ozone has an extra oxygen atom (O_3), making it very unstable, reactive, and damaging to everything it comes in contact with. It can damage forests, agricultural crops,
and manufactured products like plastic. Ozone also acts like bleach in humans, oxidizing the cells lining our respiratory tract, causing inflammation and permanent damage. The main symptoms of ozone exposure are
shortness of breath, coughing, and asthma attacks, which can lead to hospitalization and death. Long-term exposure can cause increased susceptibility to infections and accelerated aging of the lungs.

Don't confuse ground-level ozone with "good" ozone, which occurs
naturally at the highest levels of the atmosphere known as the strato-
sphere. This form of ozone is beneficial, forming a layer that shields us
from ultraviolet rays coming from the sun. The hole in the ozone layer
created by chlorofluorocarbons (propellants that were once used in spray
cans and refrigeration units) has led to an increased risk of UV overdose
and skin cancer in certain parts of the globe. Which means, ironically,

there is too much ozone down at ground level, and not enough in the upper atmosphere.

Some people are much more sensitive to ozone than others. Asthmatics are especially sensitive to irritants in general, and ozone in particular. Children are more sensitive, because they spend more time outside and take in more air per body weight than adults. As our Toxic File makes clear, adults who engage in vigorous exercise at midday are also at risk, because their high breathing rate delivers ozone deeper into the lungs.

Ozone levels are generally highest in cities and adjacent suburbs. Since cars are the main culprits, regions such as Los Angeles and the northeast corridor tend to have high levels (USEPA, 1999); other major cities can also have ozone excesses. Ozone can travel substantial distances and be high even in rural areas downwind of the cities. For example, Acadia National Park in Maine, hundreds of miles north of the nearest big city, found it necessary to have an air pollution warning system that alerts hikers to avoid heavy exertion on high-ozone days.

Again, ozone levels are greatest on any given summer day between 11 A.M. and 4 P.M. Because ozone is so reactive, the levels fall off quite rapidly with the setting of the sun, so nighttime and early morning levels are low.

Steering Clear of Ozone

Ozone is what we call an air-shed issue. In the summer, ozone alerts often cover a whole county or even a whole state. Therefore, it's usually difficult to get out of the alert area. You can't simply buy a house on the other side of town to decrease your exposure—it engulfs an entire region. So, since fleeing isn't an option, here are some behavioral changes you should consider:

- Be on the lookout for air pollution alerts in the summer months. The alerts will typically be on the news, and may be a highlighted feature of the weather broadcast.

- Avoid vigorous exercise between the hours of 11 A.M. and 4 P.M. on alert days.

- If possible, spend most of your time indoors during peak ozone hours, especially if you have asthma.

- Consider spending summer months away from high-ozone areas if you're sensitive to ozone.

Air Pollution Alerts and the AQI

If anyone doubted that air pollution is a serious health threat, all they need do is mull over the air pollution alert system. Normally, the basic strategy in government is to not alarm the public, because people tend to overreact—their stress and anxiety may turn out to be worse than the actual risk. In this "don't rock the boat" mindset, a health risk must be pressing and immediate for regulators to send out warnings. And what warnings they are—for example, that the air outside is so unhealthy, you can't exercise, and really should stay in and close the windows. Sometimes it's hard not to feel like a prisoner in your own home, a captive to ozone and other air pollutants. But we should be thankful that the USEPA has been bold enough to alert the public.

Air pollution alerts come in the form of the Air Quality Index, or AQI. Produced by the USEPA and made available through a number of media outlets, it forecasts the air quality for the next twenty-four to forty-eight hours (www.airnow.gov). The AQI provides color-coded warning levels, each with its own advice to reduce exposure and risk. Much like a weather forecast, AQI forecasts can help you plan for the day ahead—when to mow the lawn or take a hike, and when to do the indoor chores or reading. It's important to watch out for the high to severe (orange to purple) alerts, especially if you have asthma or other respiratory conditions.

Q *Where are ozone levels lower?*

A The American Lung Association has a website that shows the number of air pollution violations by location (www.stateoftheair.org). Ozone violation records should also be available from your state environmental agency, so check their website. Regions that don't meet USEPA standards for a given pollutant are said to be in "non-attainment." If you are looking to relocate to a low-ozone region, find those with the best ozone attainment record.

AIR QUALITY INDEX: A WARNING SYSTEM
TO PROTECT YOUR LUNGS
(FOR MORE INFORMATION, GO TO WWW.AIRNOW.GOV)

AQI	COLOR	HEALTH CONCERN	SIGNIFICANCE	RECOMMENDATION (FOR OZONE)
0–50	Green	Good	Poses no risk	No limitations
51–100	Yellow	Moderate	Acceptable for most, but a few sensitive people may have moderate concerns	Unusually sensitive people should consider limiting prolonged outdoor exertion
101–150	Orange	Unhealthy for sensitive groups	Members of sensitive groups may have health problems	Active* children and adults and people with respiratory disease such as asthma should *limit* prolonged outdoor exertion
151–200	Red	Unhealthy	Anyone may be affected and sensitive groups may have serious problems	Active* children and adults and people with respiratory disease should *avoid* prolonged outdoor exertion. Everyone else, especially children, should *limit* prolonged outdoor exertion
201–300	Purple	Very unhealthy	Triggers "health alert." Anyone can have serious health problems	Sensitive groups should *avoid* all outdoor exertion. Anyone else should *limit* prolonged outdoor exertion

* "Active" means regular aerobic exercise or other activities during which individuals are breathing deeply.

Q *Are ozone levels improving?*

A Our outdoor air is cleaner today than it was in 1970, when the Clean Air Act was passed. Our cars burn cleaner fuel, and most of our factories and power plants have some level of pollution control. However, more cars are on our roadways and we are each driving more miles. As a result, ozone levels have not improved as much as is needed to protect public health. The National Academy of Sciences has stated that regulatory efforts to reduce ozone have "largely failed" (NAS, 1991). Over forty U.S. cities are currently in violation of the ozone standard to one degree or another, which is especially worrisome because that standard may already be too high to protect public health. Government agencies have been pushing industries to create low-VOC consumer products to cut down on our individual emissions of ozone-forming gases. However, the main culprit is still our cars.

To reduce ozone, we need to either drive cleaner automobiles that get better gas mileage (or don't use gas at all), or drive less. Greater use of mass transit is a big piece of the puzzle. We can also try to minimize our use of VOC-containing products such as lighter fluid, paints, paint thinner, floor coatings, and furniture waxes, all of which contribute to ozone production. Unfortunately, these personal steps are important, but don't add up to much unless tens of thousands in your area do the same. That's why we need government intervention to make what we drive and buy friendlier to the skies and our lungs. The USEPA has voluntary initiatives under the heading of "smart growth" to cut back on suburban sprawl to help fight traffic-related air pollution. However, many clean air advocates argue that Congress and the USEPA have not done enough to force automakers to make fuel-efficient cars or make mass transit more available. The fight will continue for years into the future.

PARTICULATE MATTER

Some particles that are blowing in the wind are large, like the kind that come from weathered soil and resuspended street dust. And some particles are quite small, microscopic in fact, like the kind that come from our tailpipes and smokestacks. Herein lies the key distinction: larger inhaled particles get stuck in our nose and upper airways, never making it to the deep lung. We get rid of these particles when we cough or blow our nose. It's only the tiny particles that get past our natural filtering mechanisms and accumulate in our lungs. The critical size cutoff is ten microns, only 0.0005 inches or one-seventh the thickness of a human hair. Any bigger, and the particle is pretty much harmless. In this special case, the smaller it is, the more dangerous the particle becomes.

The USEPA's standards take size into account, specifically targeting particles less than 2.5 microns in diameter (PM2.5). While there is little debate over that focus, many public health advocates and lung experts would like the USEPA to tighten the current standard to better protect at-risk groups. That's because since 1996, more than 800 studies have confirmed that particulate matter is associated with respiratory disease and death. In some studies, these effects were seen at levels lower than our current standards. In fact, researchers have been unable to find a consistent threshold level below which particles are safe (Samet et al., 2000). At very low levels, few people are affected, but for those who are, the effect can be severe.

Most particulate matter–related deaths are caused by a strain on the heart and lungs. The risk of heart attack spikes sharply during and immediately after particulate pollution episodes for the elderly and the infirm. Affected individuals can experience chest pain, heart beat irregularities, breathing problems, and abnormal fatigue as immediate effects.

TOXIC FACT

PARTICULATE AIR POLLUTION KILLS THOUSANDS OF AMERICANS EACH YEAR.

Fifty thousand deaths may sound like a World War II statistic, but in fact it's the number of deaths attributed to airborne particles (fine soot) each year in the United States. That huge number of casualties makes "particulate matter" (PM) one of our leading environmental risks. Unlike some chemicals whose risk is mostly theoretical, the public health impacts of particulate matter are proven (Samet et al., 2000)—the Donora, Pennsylvania, and London episodes have made that all too clear. Many follow-up studies have demonstrated that much lower levels are still a health risk, able to worsen respiratory disease, increase hospital admissions, and cause premature death. Particulate matter levels found in many U.S. cities can still get into a risky zone even after twenty years of federal regulation.

As you can imagine, a contaminant with such serious consequences is the subject of important federal regulations and political debate. But there are a lot of obstacles. PM is ubiquitous, with many sources in need of control. Regulating its emissions can have economic impacts on many industries. New studies that keep lowering the safe level of particulate matter have made striking a balance difficult. Also troubling is the fact that we still don't know exactly what makes particulate matter so toxic.

Reducing Your Exposure to Particulate Matter

Particulate matter is a little different than ozone. It's nearly impossible to decrease your exposure to ozone by traveling from one part of town to another. By contrast, with particulate matter we can identify a concrete source to avoid—highways and busy surface roads. Although fine particles can travel long distances, there is a difference between particulate matter levels near roads and farther away: those dwelling within 300 feet of roadways experience elevated exposures to particulate matter and a number of other pollutants (USDOT). They have a greater risk for asthma, infections, and cancer (Janssen et al., 2003). This shouldn't come as a surprise, as cars and especially diesel trucks are the largest sources of particulate matter.

Given that traffic is a major source of particulate matter, an obvious strategy to lower exposure is to not live, work, play, or go to school right next to a highway or major surface artery that carries trucks and buses. Of course, we realize you might not have much of a choice in the matter. However, if you have any leeway in choosing which house to buy, which senior housing facility to place a loved one in, which school to send your child to, which park to play in, take into account how close they are to heavy traffic. This is especially true when considering where the elderly, infirm, and young children in your life will be spending most of their time.

Watch out for alerts on particulate matter. The AQI system is responsive to high particulate matter conditions, and will issue an array of mild to severe warnings about the need to avoid exercise and stay indoors on high particulate matter days. Particulate matter does not have as marked a daily or seasonal cycle as ozone; it could be as high at night as during the day, and as high in winter as in summer. Particulate matter does tend to be highest when the air is stagnant and trapped at the surface by temperature inversions, which can happen any time of the year.

Another significant source of particulate matter in our local air comes from burning trash in your backyard, or wood in your fireplace. Your fireplace may bring enjoyment and warmth, but the burning wood puts lots of particulate matter into your personal smokestack and out into the neighborhood—it's a totally uncontrolled release of particulate matter pollution. And if you don't have the flue open with a proper updraft, the pollution may come right into your living room. Wood stoves are considerably better, especially the newer ones that have control equipment like catalytic converters. However, even newly designed, USEPA-certified wood stoves produce many times more particulate pollution than oil or gas furnaces (USEPA,

2006). In more rural parts of the country, smoke from wood stoves is the major source of particulate matter. In fact, some towns have "no burn" days, if forecasts indicate stagnant weather that will keep particulate matter hanging around.

If you must burn wood, make sure you get a newer, clean-burning wood stove. Always burn dry, seasoned wood that produces less smoke. Never burn wood that has been varnished or painted.

Wood-Burning Backyard Furnaces: The Ultimate Source of Particulate Matter Pollution

Traffic and fireplaces are minor sources of particulate matter pollution in comparison to a relatively new product, wood-burning backyard furnaces. These furnaces have become a popular alternative for home heating and hot water. They are stand-alone structures about the size of a small tool shed. Wood is burned inside the shed and water is circulated around its exterior; the heated water is then piped into the adjoining home.

Wood-burning furnaces produce large amounts of smoke and particles, which are released into the air at a low height, impacting nearby homes. USEPA studies have demonstrated that they produce much more smoke than a wood-burning stove, and since the smoke is emitted at ground level, they can immediately impact your air quality. And even though they are located outside, they can be an important source of both outdoor and indoor air pollution (NYS, 2005).

Some towns in the Northeast have banned these furnaces, but there are no federal and few state restrictions on their use. We can only hope that their design and pollution controls improve in the future. Until then, it is best to steer clear.

Federal and State Programs to Address Particulate Pollution

Aside from the measures we've talked about, particulate matter pollution is largely out of the hands of the individual. Most urban/suburban dwellers are forced to be passive, in some cases unknowing recipients of particulate matter–laden air. The major pollution sources, cars, trucks, heavy equipment, and industry, need to be controlled by federal and state agencies. There have been improvements over the past two decades—particulate levels are approximately thirty percent lower than they were in 1978. Quite an accomplishment, considering how many more gallons of fuel we burn to run our cars, power plants, and industries. Further reductions are needed to ensure the health of everyone.

The recent focus on diesel buses, trucks, and construction equipment as a source of pollution is appropriate, as these sources contribute high amounts of fine particulate matter. Communities are converting their school and commuter buses to low sulfur fuel, and retrofitting them with filters that trap particles. The USEPA has a "National Clean Diesel Campaign" to support such efforts with grant money and technical support. Getting diesel particles out of school buses and children's lungs is a very good thing for public health. While most of what needs to be done is at the regulatory level, you can help in your own way by driving less, carpooling more, and lobbying your town to sign up for the clean diesel and anti-idling campaigns. (Idling school and city buses make a significant contribution to local particulate matter levels.) See if your town can join the growing movement to end this wasteful and unhealthy practice.

HAZARDOUS AIR POLLUTANTS (HAPS)

Just because a chemical is not one of the high-profile six criteria pollutants doesn't mean that it's not a health risk. It does mean that it's regulated differently, typically with less monitoring and fewer controls.

The USEPA lists 188 hazardous air pollutants, or HAPs, which is really the catch-all category of air toxics. Regulating HAPs is more complicated than regulating criteria pollutants, because there are so many of them and because they come from diverse sources. In addition to the 188 that are prioritized for federal action, there are hundreds of other HAPs that may merit special attention in certain communities. Therefore, federal and state regulators have their hands full with a laundry list of pollutants.

Some of the more important chemicals on the HAP list are:

AIR TOXIC	SOURCE
Acrolein	Car/truck exhaust, industry
Benzene	Cars, trucks, gas stations
1,3-Butadiene	Car/truck exhaust
Chromium	Metal plating shops
Formaldehyde	Car/truck exhaust, industry
Perchloroethylene	Dry cleaners

MYTH: Most hazardous air pollution comes from industrial smokestacks.

REALITY: While this used to be true, it's far from true today. Like particulate matter, mobile sources (cars and trucks) are the main source of HAPs. This shift has a large impact on how you might prevent exposure: you can't simply live as far away as possible from local industry to get away from air pollution.

Thirty years ago, the main source of HAPs was industries such as power plants, oil refineries, chemical and steel factories, cement and glass manufacturers, coke ovens, and many other stationary sources. The large amounts emitted were sometimes a health threat to the local community. Initial attempts to address the problem involved raising stack height, sending pollutants higher and farther into the atmosphere, where they could more readily be diluted. However, this measure didn't prevent pollution—it just spread it around, leading to long-distance problems like acid rain. Eventually, controls were established that required industries to use scrubbers to capture the bulk of the pollutants before they left the stack. That measure, combined with other approaches (e.g., using cleaner fuels to run power plants and industries), has helped cut back on emissions. Unfortunately, we've all but cancelled out this positive trend by driving more, and shifting the main producer of HAPs to mobile sources (e.g., traffic). In addition, smaller businesses that use chemicals, like dry clearners and nail salons, add to the air pollution load.

Take note: while industrial smokestacks are no longer the major source of HAPs in general, they still can be a major risk if you live near one, and the wind is blowing in your direction. It's difficult to document the effects of industries on the immediate community because weather conditions and emitted levels are so variable. Also, the location of greatest impact may not be right at the fence line, but on the nearest hill where the plume actually hits ground level. But all the variables and uncertainties mean is that it's prudent to find out what your local industries are putting into the air, and to live as far away as possible from major pollution sources.

HAZARDOUS AIR POLLUTION CAN INCREASE YOUR CANCER RISK.

TOXIC FACT

One of the main concerns with HAPs is cancer, as many toxics on the list of 188 are carcinogenic—and not just to the lungs, but to other sites as well. For example, benzene causes leukemia; formaldehyde, nasal cancer; chromium, lung cancer; and perchloroethylene, kidney cancer. Some HAPs are also associated with birth defects, damage to the nervous system, and lung disease. These effects have been definitively documented in animal studies, and in some cases, in workers exposed at high levels; it's more difficult to document effects in people living near industrial emissions. Some studies in urban populations suggest elevated cancer risk in city dwellers (Hemminki et al., 1994). We can speculate that this is due to greater levels of HAPs in cities than in small towns, but we can't ignore the many lifestyle, dietary, and economic differences that may contribute to the cancer risk findings. In any case, the less we inhale of carcinogenic HAPs, the better (which is why they've been especially targeted by USEPA regulations).

Thus, the link between HAPs and human cancer risk is hypothetical, but troubling nonetheless. In fact, the USEPA's estimates are that cancer risks due to HAPs are fifty times higher than the target for maximal protection of public health (USEPA, National Air Toxics Assessment, or NATA). The lion's share of this cancer risk comes from vehicle exhaust and small businesses, with only eleven percent coming from factories.

You can look up the USEPA's cancer risk estimate for your area by visiting the USEPA NATA website (http://www.epa.gov/ttn/atw/nata/). Note that the site will not tell you about cancer risks from specific industries. You can get information on individual factories from websites that report Toxic Release Inventory (TRI) data. TRI is an annual accounting of the amount of chemicals released into air or water from large emitters. However, though it will give you a rough estimate of the total pounds of chemicals released, TRI information won't indicate how much cancer risk those chemicals cause. If there are large emitters in your neighborhood, you may want to talk to local and state health officials about what the chemicals mean to you, and what

the industries are doing to lower emissions. TRI is a good community em-
powerment tool for those who want to influence regulations of chemical
emissions. Check out the USEPA's TRI website (www.epa.gov/tri/).

Q *What is the government doing about HAPs?*

A The USEPA does not regulate HAPs as closely as it regulates criteria pollutants such as ozone—it has not established air standards or emission limits
that industries must meet. Instead, the USEPA's approach is to require industry to use the latest and best control technology. It's an "as good as you
can get" approach that generally does improve emissions from what they
otherwise would be. However, it doesn't guarantee protection of public
health. In addition, many industries aren't prioritized for review, and so slip
through the cracks. That's why it's so important for community residents to
learn about the major air toxics sources in their area, and ask state officials
what assurances there are that emissions are being controlled to protect
public health.

Reducing Your Exposure to HAPs

As with most outdoor air pollution, there isn't that much you can do
directly. We rely on government programs to control major pollution
sources and decrease the general background level in communities, as well
as ensuring that people living closest to industrial emissions aren't highly
exposed. However, these programs are not perfect, and need constant updating to ensure that the latest pollution issues are being addressed and
modern controls are in place.

One option some people can afford is to live where there is no industry
and less traffic. Of course, we understand most of us can't relocate that easily. If you do live in an industrialized area, you can find out what chemicals
are produced and how much pollution is emitted by looking up the TRI
data, as discussed in the previous section. You can also talk to local and
state officials to make sure the facility near your home is being inspected
and properly run.

Some states have air quality complaint hotlines where the public can report odors or smoke plumes coming from farms, industries, landfills, sewage treatment plants, construction projects, etc. Ask your state official to investigate any source that is noticeably affecting your air quality. Remember that you, the public, are the eyes, ears, and nose for government agencies. They rely on you to tell them where control programs are not working in the community. So don't be shy—let your state and local health officials know your concerns.

MYTH: If the air smells bad, it must be toxic.

REALITY: Odor does not equal risk. A detectable odor does not necessarily mean that toxic levels of chemicals are present. It simply means that something is reaching your nose that isn't ordinarily in the air. If the odor is unpleasant enough, it can make life miserable, increase stress, and lead to health symptoms. The classic example is hydrogen sulfide, the rotten eggs odorant that can be detected by our nose at levels a hundred times lower than what is actually toxic. The unpleasant odor can cause health symptoms, even at low sulfide levels. On the flip side, some more dangerous chemicals do not have much odor, so you can be exposed to toxic levels without knowing it. That is actually the more risky situation.

LANDFILL GASES

Tom lived in a nice section of town where there was little industry or traffic. He was surprised when he and his wife noticed a foul odor in their yard one summer morning. It was there early in the day, but didn't last long, so they thought little of it. However, the next morning was different—a powerful rotten eggs odor woke them up and drove them outside. Lights were on in their neighbors' homes. Apparently, this 5 A.M. wakeup call was affecting others as well. Tom went back inside to find his four-year-old son complaining of a stomachache and nausea.

Something was radically wrong. He had heard that the inside of a sewage treatment plant can smell pretty awful and wondered if the town plant had sprung a leak. But the plant was several miles away; the scenario just didn't make sense. That's when it hit him—the town landfill was about a half-mile away by car. He couldn't see it from his house, but he knew it took up a lot of land. Maybe it was closer than he thought. Looking at a town map proved his suspicion correct. As the crow flies, the landfill was within one-quarter mile of his neighborhood. At sunup, he drove over to the main gate of the landfill and walked onto the grounds. The smell was noticeable but not as strong as at his house.

Tom didn't go to work that morning. When the town offices opened, he called to register a complaint, finding that many of his neighbors had beaten him to it. Although the odor had once again dissipated in the morning breeze, he waited around town hall to see the health director, the town engineer, and finally the first selectman.

The town officials had themselves been meeting to formulate a response to the many complaints they'd received from Tom's neighborhood. They were able to give Tom some measure of good news: the source of the odor was pretty clear. Tom's suspicion about the landfill was correct. A fire had started deep within the dump several weeks ago, so workers opened large areas on top in order to fight the fire. The water they poured in subdued the fire but fed the bacteria that produce odorous gases inside the landfill. Apparently, the latest warm spell plus all that moisture caused the landfill to crank out some heavy odors. The hastily formulated plan was to reseal the landfill over the next few days, putting a lid on the odors.

Tom felt that the town had listened and was on his side. The next few days were rough, but he knew that the problem was being worked on. The odor wasn't constant; in fact, some days when there was a strong wind, he barely even noticed an odor, even in the early morning. But the problem did not go away, and some mornings were just as bad as that first bad one. His son was ill when it was bad; his mild asthma case had worsened overall. Tom and some neighbors went back to town hall a week after his first visit to get a progress report. They complained of insomnia, headache, breathing difficulties, and unexplained rashes. The town informed them they had finished putting a soil cover back over the entire landfill, in fact twice as deep as the original cover. They acknowledged the problem might still occur from time to time and that they were hiring a consultant to help them figure out what to do next.

It wasn't exactly good news for Tom and his neighbors—the ones who were actually living with the odor. The citizens contacted an environmental lawyer and the media, demanding immediate action, relocation expenses for those who had become ill, and a health study in the affected area. The town met some of the demands, speeding up the process and clearing a budget to spend on fixing the landfill. However, the most optimistic estimates were that the full repair would take six months. The town was unwilling to do a health study, afraid that it would be biased and could be used in a lawsuit against the town. Instead, it brought in the state environmental agency, who took outdoor samples during times when the odor was bad.

The testing found low levels of hydrogen sulfide, which could easily explain the awful odors. The state officials admitted that the odors could cause reactions such as headache, fatigue, and nausea, and could even trigger an asthma attack. However, the testing did not find any other chemicals at levels of concern. Given that the hydrogen sulfide results were below toxic levels, it seemed reasonable for town officials to tell Tom and his neighbors not to worry, that things would gradually improve. But that response was completely inadequate for many people, including those trying to sell their house at that time. Who would buy a house in a neighborhood with an odor more reminiscent of an outhouse than a nice house in the suburbs?

It took six months of study, engineering, and bulldozing to finally suppress the landfill odors. A new, permanent "cap" was placed on the landfill and a gas collection system was installed to trap the noxious odors and burn them for energy production. In the meantime, Tom's wife and son had moved into a hotel across town at their own expense. Tom felt ill from time to time, but not too ill to visit town hall weekly and keep the pressure on.

Once the landfill started burning its gases, the odor was much improved. Houses started selling again and people's lives went back to normal. However, every so often Tom would wonder whether the landfill would rise back up to take over their neighborhood.

This Toxic File points out how dedicated citizens can make the government sit up and take notice. Tom got the town to do the right thing, but it took a long time and a lot of work. Sometimes the resources of town governments are too limited to pay attention to a localized pollution source affecting only a few houses. Citizens need to form an action group, contact elected officials, work with local health departments, and, if necessary, go to the media to make sure their health concerns are aired. When this happens, the town often shifts its focus to protecting public health.

CHEMICALS AND TERRORISM

Factories that store large amounts of hazardous chemicals or radioactivity may be targets for terrorist activity. A bomb or fire started in such a facility may have particularly serious consequences for the surrounding neighborhood. The accidental release of forty tons of a hazardous gas, methyl isocyanate, in Bhopal, India, killed or severely injured thousands—this 1984 accident was a wake-up call for large industrial facilities to install preventative measures.

However, every year, accidental releases of toxic gases, most commonly chlorine gas, from chemical plants or rail cars, leads to health effects, death, and evacuation in the surrounding community. While our post–9/11 society has beefed up security measures at potentially vulnerable sites, those living nearby should be aware of the potential risks and have family evacuation plans in place.

To find out if you live near such a site, you can contact your Local Emergency Planning Committee (LEPC). Local industries must report the amounts of stored chemicals to the LEPC so that firefighters will know what they are confronting if things go wrong, and must file emergency response plans with LEPCs that include plans for community notification, warning, and evacuation.

NIMBY Industries

HAPs can come from a wide variety of facilities that can impact the quality of life and property values in a neighborhood. Very often, citizens try to fight the location and operation of these facilities in their town. Not in My BackYard (NIMBY) is the phrase that's been coined to describe citizens who protest the siting of new industry or municipal facilities in their area. The protected sites can run the gamut from pollution sources such as power plants to recreational facilities like bike trails and picnic areas.

We've already mentioned a couple of facilities that rank high on the NIMBY list: chemical plants and landfills. But there are some other important ones that you should know about.

ASPHALT PLANTS

We all recognize that tarry asphalt odor from driving past road crews resurfacing a stretch of highway. Hot asphalt gives off fumes that not only have a strong odor, but also contain toxics ranging from volatile organics to aldehydes to PAHs and particulate matter. The construction of new asphalt plants can be a frequent occurrence, because often the plants are portable, moving around a state to be close to road projects where the new asphalt is needed. That means plenty of opportunity for communities and regulators to butt heads over where they get built.

Fortunately, states typically require asphalt plants to operate control equipment that scrubs the emissions of dangerous pollutants, and catches almost all of them. These standards also limit asphalt production rates to levels that hold down emissions. Local ordinances often require a setback or buffer zone of 500 to 1,000 feet to keep asphalt plants from being built right on top of homes, schools, or businesses. Overall, monitoring of these asphalt plants has found very little air toxics getting out to the community.

So, though asphalt plants may be an eyesore, involve extra truck traffic, and can have an odor up close, they typically have limits placed on them by state and local regulators that make them safe neighbors. If one is proposed for your area, make sure it implements the controls that have come to be state of the art for this industry. Also inquire about the buffer zone. If you already live near a plant and sense emissions coming into your yard, report the problem to local or state officials. They can usually pressure the plant to improve their controls and prevent these exposures.

CREMATORIUMS

Some people object to crematoriums near them because of the dead bodies; others don't want the additional truck traffic, potential odors, and pollution. The main toxic in question is mercury from dental amalgams—when teeth filled with mercury amalgams are incinerated, the metal is liberated and gets out into the atmosphere. However, there is too little mercury in people's mouths to create a significant problem, and the mercury that is released forms a gas that typically travels away from the source. Therefore, living close to a crematorium is not particularly risky in terms of exposure to mercury; in fact, other mercury sources in our environment far outweigh what crematoriums release. In general, crematoriums are not worth battling about from an air toxics perspective, although it's a good idea to have a reasonable buffer zone (500 feet or more) between you and the building.

NUCLEAR POWER PLANTS

Memories of the Three Mile Island nuclear plant meltdown and even more so, the disastrous Chernobyl meltdown of 1986, paint a frightening picture for many people. And they're right—the fact that there are tons of high-level radioactivity under one roof is pretty scary.

However, there is little evidence that living near a typical nuclear plant poses any health risk. Cancer studies in these areas have shown almost no occurrence of disease associated with radiation or other theoretical risks (NCI, 1991). The Nuclear Regulatory Commission (NRC) requires exposure monitoring near nuclear plants, and ensures they meet limits that are lower than our exposure to radiation from natural sources. Overall, you shouldn't worry about an increased risk from the normal day-to-day operations of a nuclear facility.

The more serious concern with nuclear plants is the potential for accidents and the release of large amounts of radioactive gas into the community, a concern also addressed by controls and inspections placed on the industry by the NRC. Between those controls and industry standards for safe operation, the more than one hundred U.S. reactors have accumulated a track record of decades of safe operation. Many reactors have had NRC violations of one form or another, in some cases serious enough to shut a plant down until the deficiencies were corrected. However, there have been very few accidental releases big enough to raise a health concern.

The other important thing to know is, living near a nuclear plant means living ready to evacuate in the event of a major accident or terrorist incident. All nuclear plants have annual drills, when they practice notifying nearby communities up to ten miles away. In some states, preparedness also involves giving everyone living within a ten-mile zone potassium iodide (KI) pills, which protect the thyroid from radioactive iodine should a nuclear accident occur. The pills are a stopgap measure to protect people until they can be evacuated, and only protect one bodily organ from one form of radiation. Since the Chernobyl accident increased thyroid cancer twenty-fold in parts of the Ukraine, it's prudent to have these pills handy (Lomat et al., 1997). However, the best form of protection in a nuclear incident is rapid evacuation.

Not many new nuclear plants have been built in recent years, so this issue is much lower down the NIMBY list than in earlier times. That said, societal concerns over safety and unresolved issues with radioactive waste continue to plague the industry. If you're considering moving into a neighborhood that is close to a nuclear plant, you should seriously consider the safety issues, especially in this era where terrorism in the United States continues to be a concern.

MUNICIPAL WASTE COMBUSTORS

Given how hard it is to find new sites to dump our trash, and the problems that have cropped up in existing landfills, many communities have opted for trash incineration. This is a high-tech version of an ancient practice—rather than everyone burning their trash in their backyards and creating a lot of ground-level pollution, we send it to one central location, where it's burned under controlled conditions at high temperature with lots of scrubbers to intercept pollutants on the way out of the stack. Because the emissions are tested and regulated by government agencies, waste combustors usually have little impact on local air pollution.

Communities are often particularly concerned with dioxin, since this potent carcinogen forms when burning organics in the presence of chlorine, two ingredients in garbage. It's true that, in years past, waste combustors were one of the main sources of dioxin released into the environment. However, federal regulations implemented in 1995 and 2003 improved dioxin controls that lowered combustor emissions a hundred-fold below 1990 emission levels. While zero dioxin emission is a laudable goal, it's currently unrealistic and perhaps unreasonable, given that there are natural (e.g., forest fires) and societal (backyard trash–burning) sources of dioxin. The dioxin exposure for people living close to combustors will be greater from the food they buy at the store than from any fallout from the facility.

Another issue is the truck traffic that hauls garbage to the incinerators, which poses a greater local pollution issue than emissions from the incinerator itself. Contact your community board to make sure truck routes are planned to minimize particulate pollution in residential areas.

SEWAGE TREATMENT PLANTS

Most of us are all too familiar with the odors caused by municipal sewage treatment plants, caused by sulfur and ammonia compounds that are produced from decaying waste materials. As with landfills, the sulfur compounds, especially hydrogen sulfide, have very low odor thresholds, so even a small amount can be highly objectionable. However, studies around such treatment plants have not found high enough levels of any chemicals to cause toxic effects, despite the nasty smells.

Many newer plants are installing control processes and equipment that can significantly reduce odors; many older plants have been retrofitted and are controlling odors much better than they used to. If you live near a plant that has objectionable odors, find out what controls have been installed. Consult with your state environmental agency to see what regulations they can enforce to improve the plant.

THE RISK INDEX FOR OUTDOOR AIR POLLUTION

Decades of air pollution regulation have improved overall air quality. Yet the risks are still high, especially to vulnerable members of the population: children, the elderly, and the infirm. The major risks are highlighted in the chart below. All three pollutant types, ozone (smog), particulate matter (PM), and hazardous air pollutants (HAPs) produce a high overall level of risk. Ozone poses a risk to the lungs, with the key concern being an increased potential for asthma; for particulate matter, the major risk is increased illness and even death in the elderly and infirm due to the stress particulate matter pollution places on the heart and lungs. While HAPs can produce a wide variety of effects, the main concern at levels commonly experienced in urban, suburban, and even rural areas is an increased cancer risk.

RISK INDEX FOR OUTDOOR AIR POLLUTANTS

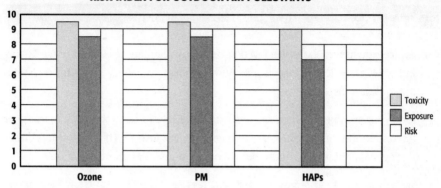

Remember, the main source of ozone, PM, and HAPs is the tailpipe emissions from our cars, trucks, and buses, much more than power plants or industries. Although an industrial smokestack may look like a behemoth polluter, it's often a better neighbor than it appears. It's our cars that are killing us. However, local industries merit some background checking and a watchful eye.

AIR POLLUTION CHECKLIST

❑ Avoid exposure to excessive PM and ozone by regularly checking the Air Quality Index (AQI). Follow the advisories and warnings, especially if you have respiratory or heart disease.

❑ Plan your summer exercise or yard work schedule to be in the early morning or late afternoon, times when ozone levels are the lowest. That's most important during stagnant weather periods when ozone pollution (smog) is worst.

❑ Try to live, work, and play at least 300 feet (a football field) from the nearest highway or busy street.

❑ Find out what pollutants are emitted by factories in your neighborhood by examining the TRI data. Contact local and state officials to make sure these plants are inspected and adequately controlled.

❑ Call local and state officials if you notice any odor or visible smoke plumes coming from local factories, landfills, etc.

❑ To decrease your part of the problem, drive less and buy cars that get better gas mileage. Use wood as a fuel sparingly or not at all. Do not use outdoor wood furnaces.

❑ Lobby your local officials and congress to require more fuel-efficient and lower-polluting cars, trucks, and buses. Ask them to support initiatives that make mass transit more available and attractive.

SECTION 4

Toxics in Your Yard and Neighborhood

CHAPTER 12

Toxics in Your Yard and Garden

As we learned in Chapter 11, NIMBY issues can be a major catalyst for local activism. But while people are quick to defend their neighborhood against a new housing development or industry, they may be overlooking important toxics issues literally in their own backyard. NIMBY needs to be transformed into WHIMBY: *What's* in my backyard? You may not have realized that backyards have chemicals hidden in soil or structures like playscapes, decks, sheds, or even outdated heating oil tanks. And then there are the not-so-hidden chemicals you or your lawn company apply to keep insects, fungi, and weeds under control. If you want to protect not only your investment but also your family's health, you need to move beyond NIMBY to WHIMBY and begin turning over the toxic rocks in your own yard and garden.

As with all toxic risks we describe, not every house will have all backyard contaminant issues. A clear dividing line kicks in at 1978 for one of the yard contaminants, paint—that's the year lead was finally taken out of paint. The dividing line for another key contaminant, chlordane, is 1988, because that's when this persistent pesticide stopped being used to kill termites. Thus, if you have a house built after 1988, you don't have to worry about either of those yard toxics. On the other hand, the arsenic-based pesticide in pressure-treated wood was not phased out until the end of 2004, so most of us with a wood structure in the backyard have that to worry about.

Yard and garden toxics were phased out of the home environment for a good reason—they were proven to be too hazardous in yard and garden materials to be safe for adults, for pets, and particularly for young children. However, just because they were removed from the stores doesn't mean that they were magically cleared from your yard. In fact, many of them are persistent chemicals that hang around in soil for decades and can be an ongoing source of exposure if you don't take matters into your own hands. A number of banned persistent pesticides may also be present as part of the legacy of converted farmland: When the farmer sold out to the developer, pesticide-contaminated soil was often an unrecognized part of the transaction. This contamination was passed along to you, the home buyer, and could still be lurking in your yard. Pesticide contamination continues today with homeowner application of modern pesticides, which, while less toxic and persistent, can still confer a degree of risk. Your yard may be plagued with another relic of the past, a buried heating oil tank. Even if your house switched to natural gas long ago, a heating oil tank may still be hiding in the ground, or even worse, leaking oil.

So, if you bought a house built after 1988, on land never used as farmland, and are sure there's no old tank in your yard, you're safe from pollution, right? Wrong. (See chart below.)

SOURCES OF YARD AND GARDEN TOXICANTS

Source	Not a Risk if Home Built After:
Leaded paint	1978
Lead from car exhaust	Date home built does not matter
Chlordane (ant and termite treatment)	1988
Arsenic in pressure-treated wood	January 2005
Persistent farm pesticides	Date home built does not matter
Modern pesticides	Date home built does not matter
Buried heating oil tank	More likely a problem in older homes (pre–1995), although new tanks can still be buried

THE GREATEST AMOUNT OF TOXIC CHEMICALS IN YOUR YARD IS PROBABLY RIGHT NEXT TO YOUR HOUSE, AND COMES FROM SOURCES YOU MIGHT NOT THINK TO CHECK.
Yard contamination doesn't spread around evenly—it's typically concentrated in hot spots. These hot spots are more likely to occur right next to your house. Why? Three main reasons: paint, pressure-treated wood, and a persistent pesticide. All three were used directly on or next to the house, so that's where soil contamination is the worst.

Lead in Outdoor Paint

We've already dedicated an entire chapter to lead in paint. Why do we bring it up again? Because most people think of lead as an indoor rather than an outdoor problem. And it's true, it doesn't get much worse than lead paint chipping onto floors where infants crawl. However, lead paint on outside shingles and trim is still an important, if often overlooked exposure source. Weather attacks paint and turns it into flakes and chips that land in your yard; there it remains, with new chips falling all the time, causing lead levels in soil to build up. Lead may have been accumulating in your yard's soil for years, even if your indoor environment is completely lead safe.

Paint chips usually land close to the house, within zero to five feet, so the narrow strip right next to the foundation is where the hot zone is likely to be. This may not seem like a big area to worry about, but it may be a sunny spot where you'd like to grow tomatoes, or the spot where the dog always digs, or your children play. You need to proceed with caution, especially if your house was built before 1978.

As a refresher, lead is toxic to the brain, especially early in life; it can decrease a child's ability to learn, and cause behavioral changes. Overall, it's one of the most toxic elements in our lives, causing damage to many vital systems (heart, blood elements, nervous system), even in adults. As mentioned in Chapter 1, a single paint chip has enough lead to send a child's blood level into the danger zone. Fortunately, once recognized, outdoor exposure to lead can be prevented, if you're careful about following lead-safe practices. For example: paint removal. The slow accumulation of lead in soil from exterior house paint can be greatly accelerated by a sloppy scrape and paint job (Jacobs et al., 2003). Whether you are a do-it-yourself homeowner or you hire a painter, it's essential that you follow the lead-safe practices outlined in Chapter 1. Be aware that your average painter from the classifieds may not be familiar with these practices—it's up to you to make sure he or she learns.

So far we've focused on lead paint near the house, but any old, painted structure in the yard, including old fences, sheds, swingsets, and play houses, should raise a red flag. All of these structures can create hot spots of lead contamination in your yard. Take note, you may well have moved the structures around your yard, so the location of hot spots won't always be obvious. Therefore, it's important to conduct soil testing for lead at different spots around the yard, especially if you live near a busy road or highway. That's because lead fallout from car exhaust may have contaminated your entire yard, regardless of the age of your house.

CHILDREN EAT ENOUGH DIRT TO PUT THEM AT RISK FOR LEAD POISONING.

TOXIC FACT

The main way children get lead into their body is by ingesting contaminated soil or house dust. In fact, children under the age of six eat a relatively large amount of dirt. Some toddlers will actually stick an occasional handful into their mouth. Even if they spit it out, a lot of lead gets left behind and swallowed. Now, you may be saying: "My child doesn't eat dirt, so I don't have to worry." The fact is, even normal activity brings dirty little fingers or play objects into the mouth. In risk assessment, we assume young children ingest 200 milligrams of soil a day, about the amount of soil in a fine coating on a teaspoon. Not a lot, yet enough to introduce toxic amounts into children if their yard is contaminated by lead, or other toxins such as arsenic. Bottom line, if you have an older house (pre-1978) and young children, you need to be especially vigilant for lead paint.

LEAD CAN GET INTO GARDEN PRODUCE.

TOXIC FACT

Gardening is another hazard of lead-contaminated soil. The first risky exposure is to the gardener who gets dirty and inadvertently ingests lead from contaminated lips, hands, and clothing. However, it doesn't stop there—lead in garden soil can be taken up into plants. Leafy vegetables like lettuce and spinach, and root crops like potatoes and carrots, tend to have the greatest uptake (Peryea, 1999).

Community gardens in inner cities are a wonderful concept, but may have several lead-contamination issues. Located in high-traffic areas, they are at greater risk for lead fallout from automobile traffic. In some cases, where the land has been reclaimed from an old building that was demolished, the soil can be contaminated from lead in the building's paint.

Whether you're working in a backyard or community garden plot, it's important that you test your soil before you plant, not only for lead, but also for soil pH (i.e., acid-base balance) and phosphates. Lead is much more mobile in acid soils and in soils lacking phosphate, an important nutrient that binds lead. Properly adjusting these factors and enriching your soil with organic matter can keep lead out of your produce, even if it's in your garden. Also, creating a raised bed where you bring in fresh topsoil can dilute out lead to insignificant levels. It's always important to thoroughly wash produce, and to peel root crops, since lead concentrates in the skin of root vegetables.

PETS: A VECTOR OF CONTAMINATION

Rover digging in the yard can be a nuisance, if he is ripping up nice lawn or disturbing your bulbs. However, it becomes more than a nuisance if the soil is contaminated. Pets pick up dirt on their paws and fur and track it right into the house, exposing children to lead-contaminated dirt on floors and carpets, and of course, on the dogs themselves. People are similar vectors, tracking contamination into the house on shoes and gardening clothes. (It's always a good idea to leave your shoes by the door when entering your house, but especially if your soil is contaminated.) The best solution is to control the contamination problem at its source, in your yard.

THE RISK INDEX FOR LEAD IN THE BACKYARD

The following chart reflects the fact that lead is a highly toxic chemical. However, the exposure side of the backyard lead equation is highly variable. It's generally low, because most lead contamination is contained within a narrow strip close to the house, but it can be high if that's where your toddler likes to play, or if it's where you've put your garden. Your exposure can also be high if your house is near a busy road due to lead fallout from car traffic. Overall, the lead exposure index is low to moderate, which combined with a high toxicity level, leads to a moderate risk ranking for lead in outdoor soil. Which means you should definitely control or remove any areas of lead contamination in your yard.

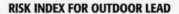

RISK INDEX FOR OUTDOOR LEAD

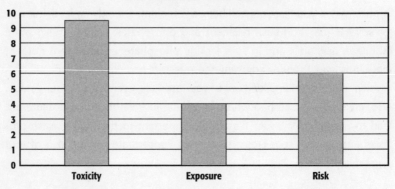

Preventing Lead Exposure from Soil Contamination

If you live in a house built before 1978, the basic precautions are testing, encapsulation, good ground cover, and proper attention to hygiene (summarized below). Review the resources listed at the end of the book for more details on how to be lead safe.

- *Soil Testing:* Make sure you test around the foundation of your home, and in other areas of the yard. Focus sampling in areas where children play, on the garden, and near any yard structures that may be pre-1978. Also, take samples in a few random locations to check for hidden sources of lead (removed structures, fallout from roadways). Find a lab that can analyze the samples for what you need: lead, soil pH, and perhaps also arsenic and chlordane (see the rest of this chapter). The lab should instruct you on how to collect the sample, and where to send it. The state college agricultural extension office may provide some of this testing for a low cost or tell you where it's available. You can find a contact for your state's agricultural experiment station on the web. For example, the listing for the western states can be found at http://www. colostate.edu/Orgs/WAAESD/AESGenInfo.html.

■ *Interpreting Your Test Result:* Naturally occurring lead in soil is less than 200 mg/kg; levels over 400 mg/kg represent a potential health hazard for young children. You should follow up on any result over 400 mg/kg by determining: 1) If the results are uniformly spread across the yard, or seem to occur in hot spots; 2) What structures the hot spots are near that might have put lead in your soil.

■ *Encapsulating or Removing the Source:* If lead paint is still present on your house or elsewhere in the yard, you can use lead encapsulants to seal it in place (see Chapter 1). When repainting or encapsulating, control the amount of dust generated by using wet scraping methods, and put down tarps to collect fallen chips.

■ *Soil Remediation:* Lead usually remains in the uppermost layer of soil (topsoil), making it very accessible to young children but also easier to clean up. Soil remediation is best done by an environmental contractor who can confirm that lead levels are less than 400 ppm when the job is done.

■ *Cover Contaminated Zones:* In lieu of soil removal, you can put a healthy layer of sod or grass over the hot spot to keep the contaminants below the surface and out of reach of young children. You must prevent dogs from digging into or otherwise disturbing the grass layer. If children's play areas are contaminated, you should consider bringing in sand or a fresh layer of soil to cover the contamination.

■ *Follow Precautions for Growing Produce in Lead-Contaminated Soils:* The most important things you can do are to neutralize the contaminated soil if it has an acidic pH, add organic material and phosphate, and wash vegetables, especially root crops.

■ *Personal Hygiene:* If you have lead-contaminated soil, remove clothing that has gotten dirty while doing yardwork or gardening and put immediately into a hamper. Leave your shoes at the door.

Wash your hands and other areas that may have become dirty. Wash children's hands and change their clothing after playing in the yard.

PRESSURE-TREATED WOOD

Backyard decks have become very common in the past twenty years, providing millions of homes with a natural-looking outdoor entertainment area. But the majority of those decks came loaded with a hidden toxic intruder: the age-old poison turned pesticide, arsenic. Along with chromium and copper, arsenic was part of a pesticide formulation known as CCA that made the wood resistant to mildew and decay, allowing decks to last twenty to thirty years. That arsenic-based pesticide was injected into the wood under pressure, thus coining the name "pressure-treated wood."

> **MYTH:** The arsenic in pressure-treated wood is locked into the wood and never comes out.
>
> **REALITY:** This has been the mantra of the wood industry for thirty-five years. However, it is false. Yes, the vast majority of arsenic stays bound to wood over its life span; however, a small percentage does leach out, a percentage sufficient to create a risky situation. The truth started emerging in the early to mid-1990s with careful studies done on decks in California and Connecticut, which demonstrated that arsenic leaches from the wood to contaminate the surface of the deck and yard below (Stillwell, 1997). What was an honest attempt to make outdoor structures safer and more durable turned out to be a short-sighted introduction of arsenic into the home environment.

Arsenic was the poisoning agent of choice for much of the Middle Ages and on into the twentieth century. However, the main concern with today's environmental exposures to arsenic is not acute poisoning, but rather cancer. We know this because large numbers of Taiwanese drinking arsenic-contaminated water got cancer, earning arsenic the label of a clear-cut human carcinogen (ATSDR, 2005). Arsenic leaching starts when rainwater penetrates into the wood and then puddles on top of it. This pulls arsenic out of the wood, bringing it up to the surface. From there it can drip down to the soil below or remain on your deck. When the weather clears and the water evaporates, you're left with a fine coating of arsenic dust on the wood boards and handrails that's easily picked up by clothing and hands. It's insidious, because you would never know that you were carrying around pesticide dust on your hands. Even worse, young children are at a high risk for swallowing the dust when they put their hands and toys into their mouths.

The amount of arsenic used to preserve wood topped thirty million pounds per year by the end of the 1990s. The wood was shipped off to lumberyards, where homeowners and contractors used it to build new decks, playscapes, treehouses, stairways, handrails, garden beds, and compost bins. The USEPA had approved the use of CCA, banking on the pesticides binding tightly to the wood and not leaching; however, facing mounting evidence that leaching did occur, industry and government agreed to start phasing out CCA and switch to safer wood preservatives. Be aware that if the deck in your yard was built before 2005, it may well have arsenic leaching from it.

TOXIC FILE · BABY-PROOFING YOUR DECK

Baby Bonnie was bright-eyed and curious like all toddlers, but at the age of fifteen months she had her parents worried. She hadn't spoken her first word, and now was approximately three months behind the toddler-talking world. Amanda brought Bonnie into the pediatrician, who was not alarmed but did share her concern. "Some children are just naturally late bloomers," he told her. "However, to be sure, let's check some things out." The pediatrician found that Bonnie's hearing was fine and reflexes normal, and felt the next step was to make an appointment with a speech pathologist.

After examining Bonnie, the pathologist said to Amanda, "Your daughter has no clinical condition that we can recognize at this time, but It's worth doing a blood test for heavy metals. Lead and mercury can cause your baby to learn and develop more slowly." Amanda didn't think her house was a source of either metal, but she agreed to have the blood test done on Bonnie.

Two weeks later, Amanda got a call to come back in to discuss the results. "The good news is, Bonnie's lead and mercury results were normal. However, we found surprisingly high levels of arsenic, more than double what we would expect in children." Another two weeks later, a test of Bonnie's urine also showed high arsenic. By now Amanda was meeting with the medical toxicologist at the children's hospital. "Mrs. Jones, arsenic is not known to cause speech or learning delays in children, so this finding may have nothing to do with Bonnie's delayed speech. But to be honest, it really hasn't been studied well. High doses of arsenic in adults do affect the nervous system."

The toxicologist then asked Amanda about possible sources of arsenic around the house. "Does Bonnie eat any shellfish? You see, shellfish contains a lot of arsenic, but it's in a nontoxic form that's not a health risk." Amanda explained the family didn't eat shellfish. Ruling out that option, the next question was about drinking water. "There are high levels of arsenic in groundwater in certain parts of the state. Where do you get your water from?" Amanda told the toxicologist that her water comes from a public reservoir on the outskirts of town. Not likely a source of arsenic. "What about soil contamination? Orchards used to use arsenical pesticides on fruit trees until that practice was banned. The arsenic could still be in the soil." As far as Amanda knew, her house was built on woodland, not an old orchard, but the soil had never been tested.

Finally the toxicologist asked about the backyard. "You don't have a deck or playscape where Bonnie likes to play, do you?" The question hit Amanda like a ton of bricks. "That's exactly where Bonnie plays, on the back deck. We made it Bonnie-proof with a baby gate, and she's happy being outdoors for much of the day." The toxicologist established that the deck was probably about five years old, and hadn't been coated with a sealant in years, maybe never.

The toxicologist told Amanda: "You did as good a job as you could in baby-proofing your deck. It's the health department that didn't do such a good job. They have a fact sheet that warns the public about arsenic leaching from decks made of pressure-treated wood like yours. However, you never got the information."

Amanda learned that arsenic used to be used in outdoor wood until 2005. Since her deck was built before that, she would have to deal with arsenic for as long as the deck was still standing. Angrily, she vowed to take the deck apart one board at a time and burn it. When she cooled down, she learned that there really wasn't anything she could do for Bonnie but keep her away from the arsenic-laden deck. In the meantime, the deck was off-limits to everyone in the family including the dog. They had the soil in the yard tested and found high levels of arsenic right under the

deck; they barricaded the area so the dog couldn't go under there and be-
come contaminated.

Two weeks later Amanda and Bonnie were dropping another urine
test off at the doctor's to see if Bonnie's arsenic level had come down. On
the drive over, Amanda heard Bonnie's babblings from the back seat start
to sound recognizable, almost like a word forming. Suddenly the word
came out. It wasn't the "mommy" or "car" you might expect, but a word
spoken almost nonstop for the past month by her parents: "r-snic." Bonnie
was being a little parrot, probably the first child in history to utter a heavy
metal as her first spoken word. The mix of thrills and chills left Amanda cry-
ing at the side of the road.

Over the next few weeks the words came tumbling out of Bonnie's
mouth, quite a vocabulary, too: "doctor" and "toxic" mixed in with the ex-
pected words. Her urine tests came back much lower as well. It was proba-
bly more coincidence than cause and effect, but no one could be sure. Later
that summer, the family got rid of the deck and cleaned up the soil beneath
it. They wanted no part of something with all that arsenic in it, even if they
could coat it every year to make it safe. As much as Amanda would've liked
a bonfire in the backyard, she found out how toxic it is to burn pressure-
treated wood, and agreed to see it sent off in a truck to the dump.

Amanda and Bonnie's story points out the potential hazard of setting
up a child's play area on a pressure-treated deck that has not been sealed.
In fact, the number-one rule of deck safety is to keep kids away from them
until they have been properly sealed (more on sealing at the end of this
section). The under-deck area is another concern—you should assume it's
contaminated with arsenic if your deck has gone more than a year without being resealed. The same is true of playscapes, treehouses, stairs, and
any other pressure-treated structures.

Although Bonnie's arsenic levels dropped quickly after her exposure
ended, that doesn't mean her risk for cancer or other toxicity disappeared.
The risk from early-life exposure to carcinogens stays with you for a lifetime. We don't mean to suggest that you screen your children for arsenic.
The best course of action is simply to be proactive and steer your child
clear of arsenic hazards from the start. Only if you suspect an exposure
(i.e., if you have an unsealed deck where your child loves to play) should you
look into testing.

Q *How do I know if I have pressure-treated wood in my yard?*

A As we said, if you have a wooden structure in your yard that was built before 2005, there is a good chance it contains arsenic. Naturally rot-resistant
wood like cedar and redwood have been on the market for many years, but
they're so expensive, pressure-treated wood came to dominante the market,
with the arsenical (CCA) formulation being the prevalent treatment chemical. Therefore, unless you know for sure your wood is cedar or redwood,
you should assume it's pressure-treated. You can test your wood by chipping off a piece and sending it to a lab for an arsenic analysis. Environmental testing labs certified with the state can be trusted to give you an accurate
arsenic result.

Q *Should I test my yard or well for arsenic contamination?*

A It's a proven fact that arsenic drips straight down from decks, treehouses,
and playscapes, so only the soil directly underneath those structures is at
risk of being contaminated. There is no need to test if you can remove the
top 6 inches of soil and replace it with clean fill—of course, after you seal
the wood above it. If you do test, be aware that arsenic naturally occurs in
soil, so you can expect 1-10 ppm as background level just about anywhere.
Also note that soil in the arid Southwest is naturally high in arsenic. For
the rest of the country, if you find soil in your yard with arsenic above
10 ppm, you likely have contamination that should be removed or made
inaccessible.

Your well is not at risk from arsenic leaching from wood. After it hits the
ground, most arsenic stays bound to soil in the top six inches. It won't make
it all the way down to the water table.

THE RISK INDEX FOR ARSENIC IN PRESSURE-TREATED WOOD

We give arsenic a high toxicity ranking, one befitting its historic reputa-
tion as a poison and the modern discovery that it's a human carcinogen.
Arsenic contamination of decks, playscapes, and other outdoor wooden
structures made from pressure-treated wood is an important exposure
source, the exact amount dependent upon many factors (e.g., age of the
deck, use of sealants, children's behaviors, climate, and season). These
exposures yield a moderately high risk for cancer. Bottom line, you need

to protect your family from arsenic-laden dust on your deck and contaminated soil underneath.

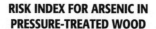

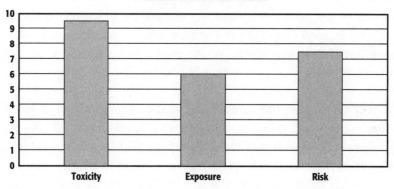

GARDEN BEDS AND COMPOST BINS

Because of their resistance to decay, pressure-treated boards are commonly used in backyard gardens for terracing and supporting raised beds, releasing arsenic into the soil. Gardeners can easily track arsenic-laced soil into the house. Like lead, arsenic can also be taken up into plants, the greatest concern being for contamination of carrots, potatoes, and other root crops (Cao and Ma, 2004). (And like lead, the highest concentration of arsenic will be in the peel of root crops, so if you do grow your own, make sure you wash and peel them well.) It's best to avoid the issue altogether by replacing any old pressure-treated boards in your garden beds with newer, safer boards. It's usually not necessary to remove the rich soil you've been building for years, even if it contains arsenic; mixing in a healthy amount of fresh soil and compost will sufficiently dilute the arsenic concentration.

At one time, pressure-treated wood was used to construct compost bins. This practice ended when it was discovered that arsenic could leach into the fermenting compost. If you've inherited an old composter made of treated wood, dismantle it, and don't use the compost.

Protecting Your Family from Arsenic in Pressure-Treated Wood

The solution Amanda came up with was to remove her old deck entirely. While removal is a valid option, most health officials don't think it's necessary. You can coat your deck with sealants that do a pretty good job of keeping the arsenic in the wood. However, the sealants need to be applied often, approximately once a year, to guarantee success. If you follow our advice below, you should be safe from arsenic contamination.

- Seal all existing pressure-treated structures in your yard, including picnic tables, benches, stairways, decks, or playscapes. Do not do any abrasive power washing or sanding. To prepare the surface, clean it with deck wash, then apply an oil-based stain to coat the wood. (This type has been shown to hold up longest in the elements.) Stain the deck every year in the spring.

- Remove contaminated soil from under the deck or playscape. Alternatively, create a barrier so that children and pets can't get to the contaminated soil.

- Replace wood liners for garden beds with newer pressure-treated products that don't contain arsenic. Dilute the existing soil with a large amount of clean soil and compost.

- Do not test your children for arsenic. Instead, keep them arsenic safe by sealing old pressure-treated structures.

- If you choose to remove an old deck or playscape, there are several replacement options that hold up well outside and do not contain arsenic:
  - pressure-treated wood that uses a quaternary ammonium compound (ACQ) instead of arsenic
  - naturally rot-resistant woods (cedar, redwood)
  - recycled plastic/wood composites

- When you dispose of pressure-treated wood, bring it to your town's transfer station; never burn it.

- If you must cut pressure-treated boards, put down tarp in the work area and collect all shavings to prevent soil contamination. Don't use the resulting wood chips or sawdust as compost or mulch.

Persistent Pesticides

CHLORDANE CONTAMINATION

If your house is one of the millions that has struggled with termite infestation, it may well have a related problem, chlordane. This pesticide was the treatment of choice for termites and ants during the 1970s and 1980s, until it was banned in 1988. Why are we talking about it today? Because chlordane breaks down so slowly, it's still easy to find it in yards across the country. This section addresses the residues left behind from the proper applicaton of chlordane. We are not going to cover the isolated cases where chlordane was injected into the interior wood beams of homes. Such houses had to be condemned, because it was impossible to remove chlordane once it was in the interior structure.

When properly used, chlordane was spread on or injected into the soil right at the house foundation, creating a chemical shield that could kill any crawling bug looking for an entry point. However, chlordane also caused high levels of contamination where it was applied (CAES, 1999). Over time, the soil around the foundation could have been mixed and dispersed by excavations for utility pipes or for shrub, garden, or tree planting, possibly spreading the chlordane contamination several feet out from its original limits.

Chlordane is a persistent chemical that can build up to high levels in the environment and within our bodies. Animal studies have shown it to be a carcinogen in the liver. It also has hormonal effects, and is capable of affecting reproduction—in-utero exposure to chlordane caused offspring to have a lifetime of hormonal and endocrine imbalance (Cranmer et al., 1984). In its heyday of the 1980s, annual chlordane use in the United States approached four million pounds; this included agriculture as well as residential use. Chlordane was a very popular termite treatment because of its long-term persistence—you wouldn't have to re-apply the pesticide for twenty years after a thorough initial foundation treatment.

Some of the pesticide found its way down to groundwater, where it still presents an occasional problem. However, most of the chlordane remained in the soil, where today, nearly twenty years later, it can be a source of exposure for those doing yardwork or gardening, and by young children. Pets can also become contaminated by digging in chlordane-contaminated soil, and then bring that contamination indoors.

The other pathway of exposure is through home vegetable gardens. Chlordane is taken up by plants, especially zucchini, lettuce, spinach, carrots, and potatoes (CAES, 1999; Mattina et al., 2004). We strongly advise against gardening or digging of any type in chlordane-contaminated soils, not only because of the pesticide in the vegetables themselves, but also because of risk of contamination on skin and clothing, and of accidental ingestion.

AVOIDING EXPOSURE TO CHLORDANE

Chlordane should not be a problem in the majority of your yard, or in houses built after 1988. Therefore, you can focus your attention on the soil within a few feet of the foundation of your pre-1988 home. The following are the keys to avoiding chlordane exposure from your yard:

- Avoid soil right next to the house foundation. Do not dig in this soil or use it for gardening. Keep pets from digging there as well. It is best left covered in grass, mulch, or crushed stone.

- If this is an area you want to dig or garden in, then test the soil for chlordane. Make sure you send some soil from deeper layers off to the lab. That's where chlordane is likely to be greatest.

- If you find chlordane contamination, contact an environmental consulting firm to have it removed and replaced with clean topsoil.

PERSISTENT PESTICIDES FROM THE FARM

The land your house sits on may have looked a lot different twenty-five or fifty years ago. Woods and farmland have been gobbled up in recent years to meet the housing needs of a growing population. The redevelopment of farmland has raised contamination issues because pesticides formerly used on the farm are highly persistent; residues of dieldrin, chlordane, DDT, and arsenic, all banned from agriculture at least fifteen years ago, can still be high. That is, high enough to cause a concern for cancer and endocrine effects in families that move onto affected properties, and garden and play in the soil.

There are no warning signs to alert the new homeowner that his land is contaminated. You should find out if the land you are living on, or are considering buying, was ever used for farming. If so, test the soil for persistent pesticides. If they are detected, contact your local and state health authorities to find out what the levels mean, and what actions you can take to avoid exposure. In general, make sure to use clean topsoil for gardening and children's play areas, and keep other areas that retain pesticides well covered with grass or some other barrier crop.

LAWN AND GARDEN PESTICIDES

Many people spend their summers keeping their lawns as green and as thick as their neighbors'. Others may have a vegetable garden, entrenched in warfare with a variety of fungi, weeds, worms, and bugs trying to live off their hard work. For decades, homeowners have used pesticides to win these backyard battles. However, they may have been paying a hidden price: increased chemical exposure and health risk, and not just to the applicator. When you spray a pesticide outside, everyone in your household gets exposed.

The research on how bad pesticide exposure is for you and your kids is far from decisive. If it were decisively bad, there would be fewer chemical ingredients to puzzle over in the hardware store. Lawn company trucks would pay fewer house calls. And if it were decisively good news, we wouldn't need little pesticide warning signs on our lawns after an application, and there wouldn't be so many notices and restrictions about pesticide use around schools.

This section will focus on the health issues associated with using herbicides, fungicides, and insecticides, whether sprayed by you or a lawn company. We're not going to focus on fertilizers, because they don't present a public health risk. However, we should mention that they carry an environmental consequence: they are often overused, with the excess leaching through soil to contaminate groundwater. When this groundwater reaches lakes and larger bodies of water such as Long Island Sound, the fertilizer stimulates the growth of algae that chokes out fish. So, keep in mind the "act locally, think globally" motto when considering how many fertilizer applications your lawn needs this season.

The major pesticides used in the yard and garden are insecticides and herbicides; fungicides are less commonly applied. The most prevalent pesticides within each category are listed in the following table, along with their toxic effects. While there are a myriad of organisms that attack grass, leaves, or fruiting produce, there are only three major types of insecticide; one of these types, organophosphates, has fallen out of favor due to toxicity concerns. In fact, formerly popular organophosphates diazinon and chlorpyrifos (Dursban) have been phased out because of risks to children. Pyrethroids have risen to the top of the market in their place. The third type, carbamates (carbaryl), have a similar action to organophosphates, but are somewhat safer and are still on the market.

Herbicides are even more commonly used than insecticides. Our desire to keep weeds out of our lawns and gardens has led to a heavy reliance on several different phenoxy acids and glyphosate (see table). Fungicides are occasionally used on lawns and gardens in warm, wet climates to control mildew and rust (a type of fungus). They are more heavily used in orchards to protect fruits from fungal diseases.

OVERVIEW OF YARD AND GARDEN PESTICIDES

The following table provides an index of the extent to which these chemicals are able to produce acute toxicity/poisoning, as well as more chronic effects. Typically, we are most concerned about acute toxic effects, because they're what could land someone in the emergency room after a misapplication or accident. However, some pesticides aren't immediately toxic (low acute toxicity), but could pose a cumulative risk from long-term exposure.

PESTICIDES IN YARD AND GARDEN PRODUCTS

PESTICIDE TYPE	PESTICIDE CLASS	COMMON AGENTS	TOXIC EFFECTS[1]	TOXIC POTENCY
Insecticide	Pyrethroid	Permethrin Cyfluthrin Resmethrin	Nervous system Irritation	Low
Insecticide	Organophosphate	Malathion Disulfoton	Nervous system Development[2]	Moderate to high
Insecticide	Carbamate	Carbaryl	Nervous system Development	Moderate
Insecticide	–	Rotenone	Nervous system Development Irritation	Moderate
Herbicide	Phenoxy acids	2,4-D MCPP Dicamba	Possible cancer risk Nervous system Development	Low acute toxicity; moderate for other effects
Herbicide	–	Glyphosate	No major effects	Very low
Fungicide	–	Chlorothalonil	Cancer Skin sensitization	Low acute toxicity; moderate for other effects
Fungicide	Carbamate	Thiophanate	Nervous system Thyroid	Low
Fungicide	Phthalimide	Captan	Development Reproduction Irritation Possible cancer risk	Low acute toxicity; moderate for other effects

[1] Toxic effects seen in animal studies at high dose. There is typically a low risk for these effects in the general population at normal usage rates.

[2] Development refers to toxic effects on the fetus.

SPRAYING PESTICIDES OUTSIDE LEADS TO EXPOSURE INSIDE.

TOXIC FACT

Studies of the general public find that most people have a mixture of pesticides in their body, although it can't all be blamed on lawn and garden sprays (CDC, 2005). While the greatest exposure comes from pesticide use indoors (Chapter 7), and some from pesticide residues in our diet (Chapter 5), an important source is also what we apply in the yard.

All else being equal, families that use backyard pesticides will have higher exposure than those that do not. This not only goes for the person doing the spraying, but also for the entire household. The applicator himself receives direct inhalation and skin exposure, although the latter can be minimized by wearing protective clothing; the rest of the household gets exposed because outdoor pesticides find their way indoors through different entry points, probably the most important being dogs and people tracking contamination into the house. Spray drift can also occur if the pesticide hangs in the air a few minutes after application and some goes into the house. Studies with several commonly used backyard pesticides demonstrate that indoor levels in house dust and air go up ten times after an outdoor application (Nishioka et al., 2001). The fact that pesticides move indoors guarantees that young children will become exposed, even if you keep them off a treated lawn. Furthermore, exposures can continue after application for a week or more.

MYTH: Any exposure to a pesticide is toxic, because these chemicals are designed to kill unwanted insects and plants.

REALITY: Yes, pesticides are designed to kill "pests," but the levels people are normally exposed to are far below that which causes serious illness or death. Just because you or your child mistakenly walk across a recently treated lawn does not mean you are going to get sick. The newer pesticides are less toxic, and some herbicides (e.g., glyphosate) inhibit plant growth in a way that makes them virtually nontoxic to people. While we can understand why people would be deathly afraid of pesticides, the reality is that most exposures will not lead to noticeable symptoms. However, when pesticides are not handled properly, there can be immediate and severe effects. And there are questions about the cumulative effects of even low-level pesticide exposures.

TOXIC EFFECTS FROM LAWN AND GARDEN PESTICIDES

Toxic effects from acute overexposure to pesticides have been well documented. The USEPA estimates that there are 10,000 to 20,000 pesticide poisonings in the United States per year in agricultural workers, and another 20,000 per year in the general public (CDC, 2004). Most of them probably stem from accidents or pesticide misuse. However, even if you handle the pesticide carefully, according to label directions, there's still a chance that your exposure could cause health risks.

One way to fathom the possible risks of pesticide use is to consider the effects in people who work with the chemicals day in and day out, the pesticide applicators. They range from crop dusters to the guys in the green suits working for lawn companies; they can be exposed to ten to one hundred times more pesticide than the general public. Farmers and workers in pesticide manufacturing are also at elevated exposure levels. Epidemiology studies of these workers have focused on three types of effects: developmental (effects on babies from fetal exposure), neurological (brain and nerves), and cancer, generally evaluating the link between disease and pesticide exposure, rather than studying the effects of individual pesticides.

Cancer

Cancer epidemiology studies provide a mixed bag of results, in part because the amount of pesticide exposure in these studies is not well defined. Several cancers seem to be associated more often than not with pesticide exposure: non-Hodgkin's lymphoma, muliple myeloma, and prostate cancer. Cancer epidemiology studies in children also find associations between household use of pesticides and leukemia or non-Hodgkin's lymphoma. However, it is unclear which pesticides may cause cancer. The most studied is the phenoxy herbicide, 2,4-D. While some studies suggest a link to non-Hodgkin's lymphoma, the associations are not strong (Toronto Public Health, 2002). In fact, the most commonly used pesticides around the home are generally not proven carcinogens in animals or people. Overall, the data are too inconsistent to draw conclusions for adult or child cancer risk from lawn and garden pesticides. But we still recommend minimizing your exposure on the basis of possible risk.

Effects on the Brain and Nervous System

Many pesticides, particularly insecticides, are designed to be toxic to the nervous system of insects. Although we have a much more complex nervous system than an insect, insecticides can be toxic for us as well. Acute overexposure to carbamates, organophosphates, and pyrethroid insecticides can overstimulate our nervous system, leading to potentially life-threatening symptoms. (The pyrethroids are less toxic in this regard, so it's a good thing they are replacing the organophosphates.) Long-term worker exposure to these pesticides has been linked to brain and nerve function deficits, although the effects have not been huge. Of potentially greater concern is the body of evidence linking pesticide exposure to Parkinson's disease among farmers (Toronto Public Health, 2002). Which pesticides might be behind this association is not clear, and the implications for the general population, which is exposed to much lower levels, is unknown.

Children may be more sensitive to the neurotoxic effects of pesticides, as suggested in a number of laboratory studies in which young animals were more severely affected by pesticide exposure compared to adult animals (Vidair, 2004). As with other toxins, children receive greater exposures per unit of body weight. Overall, we don't really know how our current use of lawn and garden chemicals is affecting brain and nervous system development in young children. It's prudent to assume that it might, and minimize pesticide use around kids as much as possible.

Developmental Effects
There is also a body of evidence that suggests that pregnant women working with pesticides have a somewhat greater risk of losing the pregnancy or having a child with a birth defect (Nurimen, 2001). The increase in risk in these studies was generally small, and the causative pesticides have not been identified. Additionally, the implications for pregnant women exposed to lower levels of pesticides around the home is unclear. However, recent epidemiology studies suggest that household exposure to organophosphate pesticides during pregnancy impairs fetal growth (Whyatt et al., 2004). As we said, these organophosphates have been phased out of the home market, but it's smart to be extra careful during pregnancy and avoid any possible risk factors. Minimizing pesticide use around the home should be part of your healthy pregnancy plan.

FORGOTTEN PESTICIDES CAN BE THE MOST DANGEROUS

TOXIC FILE

Fred finally agreed to clean out the garage after several years of accumulating clutter and his wife Jodie's constant coaxing. "Heck, there might be tag sale material buried in all that junk," she said, knowing he would get more interested if there was some money involved. Jodie was thrilled at Fred's garage pronouncement and decided to bake him his favorite pie. The garage was not well organized, so Fred spent most of that morning sorting through bric-a-brac of all shapes and sizes. He reached up to a top shelf to get down a long piece of two-by-four, and saw too late that he was inadvertently pushing a bottle on the shelf over the edge. In another instant, the bottle tumbled down, hit the cement floor with a thud, and broke, freeing the oily liquid. The liquid smelled pretty bad, but it was out of Fred's way. He decided to make more progress before lunch and deal with the cleanup later. After about a half hour, he couldn't put up with the odor anymore; he went over and picked up the broken bottle. In the dark corner of the garage, Fred couldn't read the label very well—something about mixing instructions for killing beetles and other garden insects. He didn't even remember buying the stuff. Maybe it was left here by the previous owners.

After putting the bottle back down, Fred noticed the oily, odorous liquid on his hands. He made a mental note to wash his hands thoroughly before touching things in the house. Finding some old rags, he sopped up the liquid, but as he straightened up, a wave of nausea and dizziness passed through him, and he felt a cold sweat break out on his forehead. His vision was no longer clear and a tremor was taking hold of his limbs. Alarmed, Fred looked down at the blurry rags emitting a heavy odor a few feet from his face. He dropped the cloth and staggered back, knocking over a bike and falling on top of it. Gasping for air, he summoned the strength to free himself from the bike and crawl toward the open garage door. When he reached the driveway, he lay still, moaning for help.

Jodie was horrified at the sight of Fred's prone body and feeble cries. A heart attack? Stroke? She raced outside as she dialed 911 on her cell phone. Fred was green and shaking, tears streaming from his eyes; his breathing was shallow and weak, and he reeked of some awful chemical odor. When the ambulance arrived, the EMTs examined Fred's desperate condition and heard Jodie's account. Smelling him and the garage, they realized he must have spilled a highly toxic chemical, his symptoms being consistent with insecticide poisoning. They knew that if they handled Fred in this state, they and their ambulance would be contaminated. But they had to act quickly: Fred was in serious condition, and his exposure was continuing due to the contamination of his clothes and skin. Organophosphates easily pass through the skin and attack the nervous system.

Fortunately, they had an antidote in the ambulance: atropine. They called the poison control center to be sure of how to proceed. Following instructions, the EMTs donned protective suits, then dosed Fred with the antidote. They stripped off his clothes and scrubbed him with copious amounts of soap and water. Finally, they wrapped him in a medical gown and whisked him off to the hospital.

Fred survived the severe pesticide poisoning, returning to health within a few weeks. The medical toxicologist said that the bottle he broke contained *a potent organophosphate insecticide that wasn't used much anymore. Cleaning up spills of such pesticides required protective clothing and a mask to prevent inhaling the chemical. The toxicologist said Fred was lucky the garage door was open. If not, Fred may not have survived.*

Organophosphates are highly toxic, and have been one of the leading causes of accidental poisoning and deaths in years past (which have decreased, now that they've been phased out of the homeowner market). However, as Fred found out, having an old pesticide bottle in the garage is a toxic accident waiting to happen. Search your garages, sheds, attics, and basements for stored pesticides. Keep them in a safe place until you can discard them properly.

THE RISK INDEX FOR LAWN AND GARDEN PESTICIDES

It's important to remember that all pesticides are toxic to some degree. They are more likely to have effects on vulnerable groups such as pregnant women, young children, or the chemically sensitive. The risk index chart below shows that pesticides merit a moderate toxicity ranking because the most potent kind (organophosphate insecticides) have been replaced in recent years by less toxic alternatives. However, pesticides can still cause serious effects, and even be fatal if there is a large accidental exposure. Even when you use them according to label directions, you risk the possibility of widespread household exposure and some health risk. Exposure should be minimized, especially for pregnant women and young children.

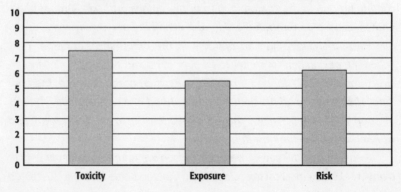

RISK INDEX FOR LAWN AND GARDEN PESTICIDES

AVOIDING EXPOSURE TO YARD AND GARDEN PESTICIDES

The most obvious way to decrease your exposure to outdoor pesticides is to simply use less, a move that's good not only for your family's health but also for your yard's environment. Some pesticides can go beyond the intended target and kill worms and other beneficial organisms. Furthermore, many people use more pesticide than is needed to control bugs or weeds; there are many instances where a pesticide isn't needed at all. The term given to describe commonsense pesticide practices is Integrated Pest Management (IPM). This approach heads the list of recommendations for decreasing your pesticide exposure and includes several techniques:

- Keep your lawn and garden healthy with good soil, proper pH, fertilizer, and watering. A healthy lawn and plants can outgrow weeds and resist insects, reducing the need for pesticides.

- Monitor the degree of pest infestation. A small amount may not do much damage and may be self-limiting. Do not use a pesticide until it is necessary.

- Optimize growing methods to decrease the likelihood of large pest infestations. This can include rotating crops and planting disease-resistant varieties.

- Use alternative control methods before resorting to a pesticide, including simple things like hand-picking bugs or using environmentally friendly pesticides such as dormant oils, soaps, and strains of bacteria that kill insects (e.g., *Bacillus thoringensis*—Bt).

- Check with the USEPA and other resources for more specific IPM techniques that address your particular situation (http://www.epa .gov/ pesticides/food/ipm.htm).

- Watch out for hidden pesticides. Many commercial fertilizers have a product line that is fertilizer "plus." The plus is often some granular form of pesticide that you may not want to have in your yard.

If you must resort to a chemical pesticide, decrease your exposure as follows:

- Follow label directions; use the minimal amount that will get the job done.

- Keep children and pets out of the area where pesticide is being applied.

- Wear protective clothing to avoid contact with your skin. Take this clothing off when entering the house and put it directly in the laundry.

- Wash hands and face thoroughly after handling pesticides.

- Do not spray on a windy day to hold down spray drift.

- Keep windows and doors closed during pesticide application and for several hours afterward.

- Do not walk on the treated lawn or soil for as long as possible.

- Keep children and pets off the treated parts of your yard for at least one day and preferably longer.

- Take off your shoes every time you come in the house after spraying and for several days thereafter. Keep a mat by the door for wiping in the event your guests don't adhere to your custom.

- The unused portion of all pesticide bottles should be stored in a safe place away from children.

- Discard any unnecessary pesticides at your town's next hazardous chemical collection day, which are usually held several times a year. Call town hall to find out the schedule.

Buried Heating Oil Tanks

It used to be fairly common for home heating oil to be stored in an underground tank in the side yard. The fill pipe would stick up out of the ground, and the tank would supply the furnace through a hole in the basement wall. These systems became an environmental problem when it was discovered that the tank, or the lines into and out of the tank, could leak heating oil into the ground, which could then migrate down to groundwater and affect drinking water quality in the area. Alternatively, the heating oil vapors can be swept into nearby basements and create indoor air problems.

You may be completely unaware that such a tank exists in your yard. Previous owners of the house may have switched to an aboveground or in-basement tank, or switched over to natural gas. If so, chances are good they left the tank in the ground. Oil-polluted soil and groundwater have become more than an environmental hazard—they've become a legal liability for homeowners. If you buy property that contains a buried tank, you may be buying into thousands of dollars in tank removal and cleanup costs.

Before you buy a house, find out what kind of fuel runs the furnace, both now and in the past. Town fire marshal records may show whether a buried tank was ever on-site. If your questions and a records search leave you unsatisfied, you can hire an environmental consultant to scan the yard with a large metal detector. If you find a buried tank, check with state officials about their requirements for removal, soil testing, and cleanup. Get a cost estimate and put it into the purchase agreement for the house.

CHECKLIST FOR YARD AND GARDEN CHEMICALS

❑ Focus on the foundation: If your home was built before 1988, test the soil around the foundation for lead and chlordane. If contaminated, limit access to the contaminated soil by covering with mulch, stones, or an intact grass layer. Do not garden or allow children or pets to play in the affected soil.

❑ Prevent more lead from contaminating the soil by encapsulating lead paint that is on the exterior of the house.

❑ Seal your deck and other wooden outdoor structures built before 2005. Use an oil-based stain every year in the spring. The stain will cut down on the amount of arsenic that can leach, and will also keep the wood in good shape, preventing splinters.

❑ Do not let children or pets play under decks where arsenic may have leached from pressure-treated wood.

❑ Minimize the use of pesticides for lawn and garden care by using IPM techniques.

❑ Avoid pesticide use around pregnant women, young children, and those who are chemically sensitive.

❑ Keep pesticides, lead, and arsenic out of the house by taking shoes off at the door and wiping mud off of the dog's paws.

❑ Carefully store unused pesticide bottles in a safe place. Discard any that's not needed at the town hazardous waste collection day.

❑ Find out if your land was farmland in the past. If so, consider testing the yard for persistent pesticides.

❑ Find out if your yard has a buried tank. If so, have it sealed shut or removed and conduct soil testing and cleanup as needed.

CHAPTER 13

Power Lines and EMF

They're an eyesore, and they're scary. In wet weather they crackle as if possessed by an eerie force you'd find in a horror movie. If you drive under them, they destroy the radio reception in your car. And of course they are associated with fires and electrocution. What are they? High-voltage power lines. Are they safe? Well, they're not as dangerous as they look, but they do raise health concerns.

This chapter is not going to talk about downed wires—those are an obvious danger. Instead, we're going to explore what is known about electric and magnetic fields (EMF) that come from power lines when they're up and running. EMF is a form of radiation (also given off by common household appliances) that has been studied intensively over the last twenty years. One very important question still remains: can EMF cause childhood leukemia? The short answer is, we don't really know. But you should read the whole story because it may help you decide which house to live in.

EMF is a form of radiation unlike any other in the radiation spectrum. That spectrum ranges from damaging forms like X-rays to innocuous forms, such as radio waves. But EMF wave energy is very low, much lower than radio waves (CalDHS, 2000). Rather than being bombarded by waves and rays, when you're exposed to EMF, your body is placed in a magnetic field. The theory is that this field has a subtle influence on the alignment and flow of chemicals in your body. We know for sure that metal objects are strongly influenced by magnetic fields; if we were made completely of metal, EMF might influence how we move and function. But we are not the Tin Man from the *Wizard of Oz*. It's possible that the metallic and charged ions in our body can be influenced by EMF, but the magnetic field strength we are routinely exposed to is very weak. And even if we could prove there was such an influence, it's unclear why it might lead to cancer. Therefore, many scientists have dismissed the risk of EMF on theoretical grounds. However, there are still some questions about what EMF might be able to do.

One unresolved issue has to do with the type of magnetic field produced by electricity. We already live in a large magnetic field created by the earth's crust—that's why our compasses always point north, to the magnetic north pole. Until electricity was invented, the Earth's field was our main magnetic influence. That all changed with the advent of electricity. Whenever electricity travels through a wire, a magnetic field is created around the wire. The more current in the wire, the stronger the field. Since our form of electricity is alternating current (AC), changing direction sixty times per second, that magnetic field oscillates rapidly, alternating polarity sixty times per second in step with the changing direction of the line current. By contrast, the earth's magnetic field always has the same direction, north one way and south the opposite; they never reverse. The argument has been made that EMF from power lines and appliances—reversing fields—are very different from the constant magnetic fields we've evolved with over millions of years. Of course, the influence of these oscillating fields is speculative, given how weak they are relative to the natural magnetic fields around us.

There has been much speculation on how magnetic fields affect the human body. Some people think they have a positive effect. In fact, there is a whole line of magnet-based healing products to treat everything from depression to arthritis (NCCAM, 2004). The efficacy of these products is the subject of a different book. Let's just say that the magnetic fields from power lines are far weaker than the magnets used in such products. The biomedical research is also uncertain. As described in this chapter, the epidemiology research raises enough red flags for us to cast a cautious eye on EMF, but we are far from having any proof of definitive health effects.

EMF IS ASSOCIATED WITH CHILDHOOD LEUKEMIA IN SOME EPIDEMIOLOGY STUDIES, BUT NOT OTHERS.

What do we really know about power lines and cancer? That is this multi-million dollar question, with at least that much spent trying to get the answer. After fifteen years of intensive study, we can still only say that the connection between power lines and cancer is possible, a big maybe. That's not very reassuring, especially since one reason the effects of EMF are so difficult to study is that we are all exposed to them, even if we don't live near a power line. If EMF *does* cause cancer, everyone will have some risk. That's precisely why it's so difficult to test.

Why? Because, when you're doing a cancer study, you need a group that is clearly exposed, and a group that is clearly not exposed, or at least exposed much less. But everyone has some level of exposure to EMF, whether it's around the house, at the supermarket, or at work. The levels of exposure are highly variable: high when you're standing in front of a whirring washing machine or walking past the bank of refrigeration units in the supermarket, low when you're relaxing on the couch or in bed, as long as you don't have the electric blanket turned on. Everyone gets a different dose, depending upon their daily habits. There's no zero exposure group.

Given all the obstacles, it's remarkable that several studies have shown a common thread: a link between living near power lines and one type of cancer in particular, childhood leukemia (NIEHS, 2002). And since the incidence of this disease has increased over the past several decades, it's tempting to speculate that our increased use of electricity has caused an increased exposure to EMF and an increase in childhood leukemia. While theoretically plausible, this connection is far from proven. In fact, there are a number of recent epidemiology studies that have failed to show any link between EMF and cancer (Linet et al., 1997; UK Childhood Cancer Study, 1999).

So, how are we supposed to draw any conclusions? All we seem to be doing is contradicting ourselves. Part of the reason why studies have conflicting results is that some may be more powerful at detecting a small increase in the odds of a human disease. In general, the more subjects enrolled in the study, the better chance the study has of finding an effect, if one truly exists. That's where pooling data across studies (meta-analysis) comes in. Many EMF scientists place their confidence in large-scale meta-analyses, since they have the greatest statistical power to find an effect. And in fact, they've given more veracity to the possible link to childhood leukemia (Ahlbom et al., 2000; Greenland et al., 2000; Wartenberg, 2001).

The best meta-analytical estimate is that a child's risk of leukemia doubles when EMF levels climb above the background range to readings of 5–10 mG or higher. The individual studies have had trouble showing that effect, because there were few children in any one study in the high range. But when the data are pooled, that's the trend that emerges.

Q *Have tests in animals shown a cancer risk?*

A The short answer is no. We know that epidemiology studies and meta-analyses are full of uncertainties. Animal testing is usually a good way to prove whether a suspect agent can produce cancer. The result? When animals are exposed to EMF for long periods of time, they do not get leukemia or other kinds of cancer. There have been a few high-dose studies suggesting that EMF can damage DNA, but overall, the evidence is that EMF is not an animal carcinogen (NIEHS, 2002; Lai et al., 1997; Lai and Singh, 2004). Does this mean we can stop worrying about this issue?

Unfortunately, no. One concern is that EMF may be like arsenic, chromium, or cigarette smoke—all examples where humans are more sensitive than the animals we test. Another problem is that the way EMF is generated and tested in a lab may not fully reproduce the human experience—the animals are not under a power line or caged in front of a washing machine 24/7. It's difficult to replicate the pulsating field generated by electric current in our wires and machines in a simplified lab test. So, the animal studies neither support nor fully negate the human epidemiology meta-analyses.

🅣 OUR HOUSE WON'T SELL

Judy and Bob lived in a great house for twenty-five years, raised three sons, and were all set with their retirement plans: sell the house and move to a warm-weather climate. They knew it would be hard to say good-bye to the neighborhood, old friends, and especially to the house where they had so many fond memories. But what they didn't realize was how hard it would be to sell the house. You see, Judy and Bob lived on a street that was bordered by high-voltage power lines—lines that brought electricity into the neighborhood. In fact, the lines ran right through the back end of their yard. They knew the lines didn't look appealing when they bought the house, but they figured they'd just plant trees to block the view. They had no idea the lines would affect their property value.

After two months on the market and an open house, Judy and Bob confronted their Realtor. "Why haven't we gotten a single bid? We priced the house to sell, it's springtime, so where are the buyers? What do we have to do to sell?"

Their Realtor told them they have a great house, but the word was that buyers were worried about the power lines. Some thought the lines could cause cancer or birth defects; others just seemed to be worried about the property value. The term EMF kept coming up. It was all very unsettling. Suddenly, Judy and Bob started wondering if they had been risking their own health over the past twenty-five years.

On the advice of their Realtor, Judy called the electric company and asked for customer service. After being transferred several times, she finally got to talk to someone who knew what EMFs are, and what they had to do with power lines. The power company official told her there was no health risk and that EMFs were really a non-issue, way overblown by people who saw gremlins everywhere. That made sense to Judy—they raised three healthy, strapping boys right next to those lines.

"But," she said to the utility official, "even if the lines are safe, nobody wants to buy our house. What can we do at this point?"

"You can test the yard for EMF," he replied. "In fact, we can come out and test for you, at no charge. There's a chance the wires don't produce that much EMF to start with."

Judy was hopeful as the company truck pulled up. She greeted the driver and followed him around as he used a small meter to take measurements around the yard, talking in terms of milligauss. The numbers on his meter bounced around a lot. They were definitely greatest under the power lines— she saw a number as high as in the nineties. Fortunately, it dropped quite a bit by the time they got back to her deck. The reading there was fifteen.

"Well, it's pretty much what you'd expect, being so close to the lines," the man said. "There's some extra EMF just about everywhere in the yard, including right here on the back deck and probably also inside the house. EMF is not stopped by walls and windows. But, you can get just as much EMF from standing in front of the refrigerator or washer when it's running. Let me show you." And sure enough, he proved that common appliances around the home, including the hair dryer that she used every day, created EMF.

Judy and Bob were really confused. They knew they had elevated levels of EMF in their yard compared to other people's yards. But what did it mean that they could get just as much exposure from household appliances? The *electric company said there was no health risk, but that's what you'd expect them to say. When they looked up EMF on the Internet, they found a ton of information, but still couldn't find the answers to their questions. Most of the websites said EMF was dangerous—an unnatural type of energy, stress to the body's cells, cancer, maybe other health effects. Some companies were even selling products that would rebalance your energy field to shield you from EMF. But, Judy also stumbled on her state health department website; it came up because the health department had posted a fact sheet on EMF. It sounded balanced, saying some of the things the electric company was saying, but also acknowledging some of the health questions. It left her with the impression that power lines might cause a small increased risk of child-hood leukemia, but no one could be sure.*

Seeing that they weren't going to get definitive answers to what their backyard readings meant, they had a heart-to-heart talk with their Realtor. They agreed that no one knows whether there is a real risk from power line EMF, but in any case, the elevated levels around their house were going to be an issue for potential buyers. They felt the issue was on a par with living near a landfill or a factory that raised pollution concerns. They decided to drop the price twenty-five percent, which brought it into the range of more industrialized parts of town. But they were worried that they might be set-ting up a young family for a tragedy by making the house affordable, but giving children some extra cancer risk. So they instructed their Realtor to steer older couples, or couples perhaps with grown children, to the house. The Realtor became more educated about EMF in the process. After many months, the right couple came along, one that wanted a quiet neighbor-hood and were not going to have children. They were happy to benefit from the reduced price and from all the upfront information on the EMF is-sue. Finally, Judy and Bob could move to their dream retirement home, and do it with a clear conscience.

Q *Should I test my house for EMF?*

A Yes, if you live within 300 feet of a high-voltage power line, roughly the length of a football field. Farther than 300 feet, the strength of the field will be very low. EMF levels will also depend on the height of the wires, the amount of current that runs through them, and how they are arranged rela-tive to one another.

Your EMF reading will be measured with a gaussmeter, and described in units called milligauss or mG. Electric companies have this equipment, and will measure when asked. We have always trusted their measurements as accurate. However, you should be wary of the company's likely "of course it's safe" interpretation. You can probably arrange for your own test by hiring an environmental consultant that has a gaussmeter. We've known some individuals who've rented a meter to take their own measurements. The devices are simple to use.

Note that background EMF levels in homes range from 0.5 to 3 mG. However, certain locations within the home can be much higher, such as right in front of major appliances (washer, dryer, refrigerator, TV set). The levels drop off quickly as you move a few feet away; in general, background levels away from major appliances are below 3 mG. Sleeping under an operating electric blanket can be a substantial exposure to EMF; it's prudent to warm up the bed first with the blanket and then turn it off to sleep. EMF levels will be considerably higher near high-voltage power lines.

There are no public health safety standards for mG levels. The best way to describe your EMF risk is that we are less sure of your safety the higher your EMF level gets above background.

MYTH: People can be sensitive to the energy fields from EMF and get immediate health effects.

REALITY: We have heard reports of a small number of individuals who claim to be so sensitive to EMF, they get splitting headaches, weakness, dizziness, and nausea. They claim this only occurs when they are close to major EMF sources; some even have their own gaussmeter to test levels in certain areas before deciding if they're safe. However, we know of no scientific data to support these health effects. Although they are possible, the cause is unknown. It could be fear or worry, or some other type of exposure. If these people are sensitive individuals, they would appear to constitute a very small group.

THE RISK INDEX FOR EMF

Given that there has been extensive study of EMF in both humans and animals, it's unlikely there will be much new research. Overall, we're left with more uncertainty than fact, a situation reflected in the risk index chart. The toxicity ranking for EMF is moderate, but with a question mark. It would be higher if we knew there was a concrete cancer hazard, and lower if we could prove there is no risk. The exposure rating is also moderate, reflecting the fact that very few people live close to power lines, but for those who do, exposures well above background are possible. As a result, we can only give EMF a middle-of-the-road, highly tentative risk ranking.

All the uncertainty surrounding EMF dictates prudent avoidance—in other words, minimizing exposure to the extent that is practical, especially when pregnant women and young children are involved. That's because childhood leukemia is the major question mark regarding EMF risk. However, since we can't be certain of whether there actually is a risk, we can't recommend that people go to great lengths (e.g., moving to a different house) to avoid exposure.

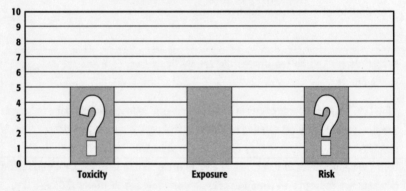

RISK INDEX FOR POWER LINES AND EMF

EMF CHECKLIST

IF YOU LIVE NEAR (WITHIN 300 FEET) HIGH-VOLTAGE POWER LINES:
❏ Arrange for EMF measurements.
  ❏ Test both indoors and out, since buildings do not block magnetic fields.
  ❏ To the extent practical and feasible, minimize the time pregnant women and young children spend in areas that are above 10 mG. Having them sleep in the opposite side of the house from the power line can make a difference.

❏ Ask the utility to help lower EMF.

THIS MAY BE AMBITIOUS AND MAY INVOLVE YOUR NEIGHBORS, BUT IT CAN DO SOME GOOD:
❏ Raise awareness among neighbors who are at a similar distance to the power line.

❏ Organize a meeting between concerned neighbors and the power company.
  ❏ Describe your EMF levels and health and property-value concerns.

❏ Ask the utility to alter the lines so they don't send as much EMF to your neighborhood.
  ❏ Possible options are split phasing of the wires (where the EMF from one wire cancels out the field from the adjacent wire), making the towers taller (and thus farther from you), or putting the wires underground.
  ❏ The goal is to get EMF levels everywhere on residential property down to 10 mG, and ideally, below 3 mG.

IF YOU ARE CONSIDERING MOVING INTO A HOUSE THAT IS NEAR HIGH-VOLTAGE POWER LINES:
❏ Find out if the house is within 300 feet of the power line.

❏ If within 300 feet, ask for EMF measurements at the time of home inspection.

❏ If levels of 10 mG or higher are found near the house, consider the uncertainties surrounding EMF risks along with all the other factors involved in your decision about which house to live in.
  ❏ Consider whether you will have young children or will be pregnant while living in the house; the possible health concern is less if this is not the case.
  ❏ Consider how the uncertainties about EMF may affect property values in the future.

THINGS TO DO TO MINIMIZE EXPOSURE TO EMF IN ANY HOME FROM HOUSEHOLD APPLIANCES:

❑ Keep your child at least two feet from TV sets and computer screens.

❑ Keep a two-foot distance from major appliances when they are running (e.g., washer, dryer, refrigerator, electric range) except as needed to use the machine.

❑ Use an electric blanket to warm up the bed, but turn it off when getting into bed.

CHAPTER 14

Hazardous Waste Sites

Time capsules are pretty neat. You put pictures, bumper stickers, newspaper clippings, and key artifacts into a container and store it away for a long time. Someday, when your grandkids find the capsule in the attic, they'll be puzzled and amazed at the story of a different era told by the relics inside.

Toxic waste sites are a time capsule of a different sort, a glimpse into an era when industry was unbridled in its ability to pollute. Amazing and unconscionable as it may seem, the evidence at abandoned factories, warehouses, landfills, and chemical dump sites does not lie. These sites document how chemical wastes were cast off into toxic lagoons or via effluent pipes into streams and ponds. It's not unusual to find an industrial burial ground where chemical drums, incinerator wastes, and debris were mounded into a landfill. Heavy metals, polycyclic aromatic hydrocarbons, asbestos, chlorinated solvents, PCBs, pesticides, and a host of other chemicals could have been left behind at any given site. Thankfully, as environmental regulation took hold in the 1970s and 1980s, chemical waste disposal was brought under control. What was once a common corporate practice became a serious crime.

Many sites—we hope the worst ones—have been cleaned up. Federal and state programs like CERCLIS and Superfund (described later in this chapter) have done a good job of identifying the major waste sites and getting them resolved. However, there are still hazardous waste sites lurking in communities yet to be investigated or remediated, possibly having sat for many years as orphans of industries that went bankrupt or moved overseas. Today, the impetus for cleaning up these time capsules is as much economic development as anything else. Developers and bankers want to know about the environmental liabilities that come with these undervalued tracts of land. In many states, developers are required to test the soil and groundwater and report results to state agencies that oversee site cleanup. But there may be no developers willing to buy an abandoned industrial eyesore (generally termed a "Brownfield Site") and turn it into new homes or businesses ("Greenfield development"). The cleanup costs may not be worth the risks. So, the land may go undeveloped and remain contaminated. There may be fences with warning signs, but at many sites, even those minimal precautions are missing.

For the people who live near a known toxic site, there are the issues of depressed property values and heightened environmental and health concerns. However, even people who live a quarter or a half mile away may still have something to worry about. Chapter 15, "Pollution from Below," describes how pollutants from toxic sites can travel via groundwater directly into your home. And then there's the aboveground transport mechanism covered later in this chapter: trespassing. While you may think there would be no reason to enter such a site, your children may think otherwise.

The dawning of the age of awareness about hazardous waste came in the late 1970s with revelations about the Love Canal, a project in Niagara Falls, New York, conceived by William T. Love. The canal was never completed—it was abandoned in the early 1900s, with the land falling into the hands of a local industry that turned it into a chemical dump site. The industry sold the property to the city for one dollar in the 1950s, and by 1960 a neighborhood of approximately one hundred homes and a school were built on the site (USEPA Journal, 1979). Over time, the elements went to work on buried drums of toxic chemicals lying in wait under the neighborhood. By the late 1970s, chemicals were oozing out of rusted barrels, across backyards, and into basements. Chemical odors permeated the neighborhood; residents reported skin rashes after contacting the soil, polluted rain puddles, and even mini-explosions when rocks hit the ground. When a newspaper sampled a resident's sump pit and reported that it was toxic waste, the authorities finally moved in. Subsequent findings of contamination of staggering proportions was the wake-up call America needed for congress to pass the Superfund law in 1980.

The Superfund refers to the set of laws and monies created by congress for the USEPA, together with the Justice Department, to go after polluters and make them clean up sites. A big part of the program was discovering the locations of these sites and ranking them in terms of health threat. All the waste sites discovered by the USEPA were put on a master list (CERCLIS list), which today totals approximately 40,000 sites. The highest-priority sites are put on the National Priority List (NPL). Superfund monies can only be spent on NPL sites, of which there are only 1,000. Thus, the vast majority of sites are left to the states, towns, or developers to address— sites in various stages of cleanup, from completely fixed to sitting dormant waiting for their day in the sun. And then there are sites that have slipped through the cracks and have never been discovered.

The 40,000 officially recognized hazardous waste sites are spread widely across the country. Most cities and towns have at least one site; some have ten or more. In addition to the ones on the federal list, many states keep a list of sites where a chemical spill or hazardous waste was reported. In Connecticut alone, the list has over 12,000 addresses. And Connecticut is not the only state that has so many contaminated sites, which can range from abandoned properties to active businesses sitting on top of historic pollution. While many of them have been brought under control, some are still releasing chemicals into the community.

TOXIC FACT

TRESPASSING IS OFTEN THE MOST IMPORTANT SOURCE OF EXPOSURE TO HAZARDOUS WASTE SITES.

Surprisingly, many people are tempted to walk on a waste site, especially children who are old enough to get out of the house on their own. To kids, an old abandoned factory with vestiges of fencing and warning signs might look like the perfect place to hang out after school, or play imaginary games. Sometimes, toxic sites don't look like waste sites at all—the buildings may have been knocked down or burned a long time ago, and brush and trees may have overgrown the asphalt. In many cases, old factory sites are near rivers, as water was the main power source in the early days of industry. Which means that the waste site may be the only semi-public access to the river for fishing, wading, stone skipping, etc. It's common to find footprints of all sizes at hazardous waste sites.

Obviously, it's incredibly dangerous to wander around on such sites because of the toxic chemicals you may be exposed to. But there are also a number of physical hazards in abandoned buildings, like broken glass or missing floorboards, and in debris that could be dug up by the young and curious. And then there's the trouble kids can get into on their bicycles.

DIRT BIKING MADE EXTRA DANGEROUS

TOXIC FILE

Eddie and his friends roamed the neighborhood with more swagger and confidence than the local police. This bicycle brigade of five buddies would head out after school to seek adventure until dark or suppertime, whichever came first. Being nine years old and curious, they were drawn to the old abandoned R&R Metals Reclamation site on Hilltop Drive. The rusted-out fence topped with barbed wire and "No Trespassing" signs didn't do much to dissuade them—in fact, they egged them on to find a way in. Bushwhacking around the perimeter of the ten-acre site, they found what they were looking for: an out-of-the-way section of fence was on a slope, and the ground underneath had eroded to the point that a dog could easily fit underneath. With some prying up of the fence, the boys were able to squeeze under and drag their bikes behind them. Once inside, the boys explored the site by bicycle and came across a peculiar sight: large, tan-colored piles of dirt, mounded up thirty feet high. The most curious part was that these mounds were housed in a large shed, evidently to keep the weather off. They looked as though they had not been disturbed in years.

A knowing glance went through Eddie and his gang, and they immediately headed off for the adventure of the day. Biking up the dirt piles was a chore, with loose dirt impeding their progress. However, coming down the other side was a complete blast and their momentum took them halfway up the next mound. They dirt-biked over the mounds for the better part of an hour, vowing not to tell anyone about their secret place. Biking had kicked up dust that hung in the shed like a fine cloud. It was Eddie who commented: "My eyes burn a little, maybe from the dust. I think I'll borrow my brother's ski goggles for next time."

The boys, outfitted in goggles, went back to their dirt-biking piles every day after school that week. After more of the same the next week, Eddie told the guys: "Hey, this place is great, but let's find some other cool places tomorrow; we don't want to get tired of coming here." In reality, Eddie needed a day off from the piles, as he had developed a sore throat and felt like the dust was making it worse. He even thought he wheezed a bit when he dashed up the stairs after dinner.

Several days later, the boys headed back to the R&R site and hit the dirt piles once again. After about ten minutes, Eddie knew something was wrong. He had difficulty getting up one of the piles, wheezing badly from the exertion. When he got to the top, he got off his bike to catch his breath, but his breathing only became more difficult. In fact, he felt like he was choking and began to cry. His friends came over to see what was wrong and were alarmed at his reddened face and loud wheezing. Eddie was panicking. One of the boys had a brother with asthma and recognized what Eddie was going through. He knew how serious a breathing attack could be. "Let's get Eddie home; he needs help." Eddie was in no shape to bike and could barely walk, spending most of his energy trying to breathe. When they got out of the shed, Eddie felt too weak to go on. He sat on a rock, doubled over. "Call for help," he groaned. The boys knew a call to a parent, or worse the police, would have them all in a pile of trouble. Breaking through a fence and trespassing would certainly get them grounded. But it was clear Eddie's situation was more serious than the discipline they would face later on. One friend whipped out his cell phone and dialed for help.

The call went to Eddie's home, where his mother picked up. Alarmed, she called 911. Police and an ambulance were on the scene in minutes and provided Eddie with oxygen to help his breathing. They took him to the hospital, where they gave him some drugs to open up his lungs; he stayed overnight. Meanwhile, the police lingered on the scene. They had never been on the R&R property and wished the town would do something useful with the abandoned site. Evidently, no one would touch it with a ten-foot pole. They noted the bicycle tire tracks running up and down the mounds of dirt; there was still a dust cloud hovering in the air. "Well, we know what the boys were doing here. Those dirt piles were made for nine-year-olds with bikes." The police officer then mused, "I wonder what's in those dirt piles; it's strange that they would be in this shed. A nine-year-old who never had asthma before suddenly comes down with a serious attack while dirt-biking on an industrial dirt pile. Maybe we should call in the environmental and toxics people."

It didn't take state officials long to figure out what had happened to Eddie. R&R had run a metal reclamation business up until 1991, when they went out of business. The covered dirt piles were loaded with cadmium, chromium, nickel, cobalt, and other heavy metals. When inhaled as a dust, these metals could accumulate in the lungs and cause damage, or even more worrisome, an allergic reaction that looked like asthma, but could be severe, even life-threatening. The metal allergy hit Eddie, which was bad for him, but good for the other boys: it got them out of the metal waste piles before they experienced long-term lung damage.

The state found a pot of money to remove the waste piles and the old factory building, and clean up other contamination that was found around the property. A developer then bought the land and decided to build luxury homes on the spacious site. The townspeople who knew the story of how the site was discovered and cleaned up would always call the development "Eddie's Estates." That's because without Eddie's toxic mishap, the site might never have been cleaned up and developed.

Dirt-biking over toxic waste piles is only one of the hazardous activities an adventurous child may find attractive at an abandoned factory. You should teach your children that trespassing is illegal and potentially dangerous. Explore the neighborhood with them and point out any sites that may harbor physical hazards or hazardous waste. Contact town officials to encourage them to get these sites cleaned up and moving in the "Brownfields" to "Greenfields" direction. In the meantime, get the town to secure toxic sites with fencing and patrols to keep kids out.

MYTH: You can choose which town to live in based upon how many hazardous waste sites it contains.

REALITY: If you are worried about toxics, the natural temptation is to choose a town where there are no waste dumps, thinking you're ensuring clean water, air, and a healthy environment for you and your family. Many people call state environmental offices or search websites looking to avoid "toxic town." But the reality is that you can't go by townwide statistics in thinking about contaminated sites—it's really a localized issue, and you need to look at every neighborhood or street individually for potential pollutant sources. A town may have a number of polluted sites in an industrial area, but may feature another area that's suburban or rural of high environmental quality. Alternatively, a neighborhood may look great and have no industry, but be too close to highways (Chapter 11), high-voltage power lines (Chapter 13), or be located on reconverted farmland that still contains pesticide residues (Chapter 12). So, don't look at statistics, but rather at each neighborhood or street on its own merit.

Q *How risky is living near a toxic waste site?*

A In spite of appearances, living next to a hazardous waste site is not as big a worry as you might think, assuming you're not physically entering the site. Contamination such as asbestos, lead, or arsenic remains concentrated in the soil, and that soil isn't going anywhere. Neighbors worry about it turning into dust that on windy days might blow contamination into their yard. Except in extreme cases like Libby, Montana (see Chapter 4), that's not an important factor. In some cases, soil contaminated with polycyclic hydrocarbons or VOCs can release toxic gases into the air, gases that have the potential to produce health symptoms (Ozonoff et al., 1987). However, the amount put into the air is usually too small to be a health risk to downwind residents. The more serious concern is that these chemicals can migrate underground into the neighborhood and get into basements the way radon also moves indoors (see Chapters 2 and 15). Finally, there is the potential for certain chemicals to leach through soil and get to groundwater, which then gets into your home via drinking water (see Chapter 6).

All in all, the amount of exposure associated with living near a hazardous waste site depends on many factors: which chemicals are present, how mobile/toxic they are, how close people live, whether or not you have children. Be careful when looking at studies conducted on neighborhoods near waste sites because fear and outrage may exaggerate people's reports. Remember, some symptoms can be stress induced. For example, it's a given that sites that emit odors will cause increased headache and respiratory symptoms in the surrounding community, but that may have as much to do with the odor as with an actual toxic effect (Shusterman, 1992). Larger studies of multiple waste sites have provided suggestive evidence of more serious health effects, including heart disease and birth defects (Sergeev and Carpenter, 2005; Dolk et al., 1998; Geschwind et al., 1992), but other studies have not found adverse effects (UK Committee on Toxicology, 2001). The studies done on waste sites are not definitive, because they've not actually measured chemical exposure, just proximity to the waste site. This makes it impossible to show that chemicals from a site caused a problem. Therefore, with the exception of extreme cases like the Love Canal or Eddie's biking incident, the risk for serious health effects from simply *living* near hazardous waste sites represents an area of uncertainty.

IN THE PAST, TOXIC WASTE WAS PASSED OFF AS "CLEAN" FILL.

TOXIC FACT

The hazardous waste time capsule we've presented so far is probably pretty difficult for you to fathom, regardless of your views about the environment. However, there's another element that goes even farther into the unbelievable. Not only were hazardous waste sites created by industrial abuses and government neglect, and not only were some neighborhoods built on top of such sites, but waste materials were actually sold or given away as "clean" fill. If you were a builder and needed to backfill around a foundation or level a field, you may have used some cheap fill material that came from a local industry. Thirty years ago, no one tested fill or thought about its source— if it wasn't obviously contaminated (odorous, stained, containing lumps of debris), you could pass it off as clean material and spread it around an entire neighborhood. Whether this was the work of scoundrels or just very naive people, we don't know. What we do know is that this unnecessary and unfortunate distribution of toxics led to the creation of some of the largest hazardous waste sites in the country.

One classic example is the town of Grand Junction, Colorado. Radioactive material was spread throughout the town in the 1950s and '60s when uranium mining wastes were used as "clean" fill and sand for yards and construction sites. It was also used as an ingredient in concrete for the construction of schools and other buildings. The uranium it contained formed radon gas that was released into the buildings at hazardous levels. A total of 4,200 buildings and lots were affected, and required cleanup or demolition at a total cost of $450 million.

Just as unfortunate was the fate of Times Beach, Missouri. The entire town was condemned due to soil contamination stemming from the use of dioxin-containing waste oil as a dust suppressant in the 1970s. After farm animals died and test results showed widespread dioxin contamination, the town was bought out by the federal government. Residents were moved out and the area cleaned up, all to the tune of $80 million. An example on the east coast is Stratford, Connecticut, where lead- and asbestos-containing waste materials were passed off as "clean" fill, turning an entire neighborhood into a Superfund site. All of these misuses of industrial waste led to elevated human exposure and health risk, not to mention mass community disruption and multi-million dollar cleanups, even outright condemnations.

What does all this mean to you? Fortunately, such hazardous waste horror stories are rare. From time to time, a new one surfaces when, for one reason or another, soil is tested and shows the tip of a toxic iceberg.

Therefore, it's important to be aware of toxic issues in the neighborhood and have a thorough soil test done at least once in your yard, just to make sure you are not the victim of toxic "recycling."

THE RISK INDEX FOR HAZARDOUS WASTE SITES

Each hazardous waste site is unique in terms of what has been dumped there, whether chemicals will move off-site, and how close the nearest neighbors live. Therefore, it's difficult to formulate an overall level of risk. The following chart reflects the fact that the toxicity level of wastes left behind at old industrial sites can be quite high. It presents the rankings for three different scenarios: living near a waste site, trespassing on a waste site, and living in a house in which toxic wastes were used in the past as "clean" fill to landscape your yard. The exposure potential and overall risks go up across these three scenarios, ranging from moderate to high. It's definitely prudent to look into the waste sites in your neighborhood, and avoid exposure by following our advice in the checklist.

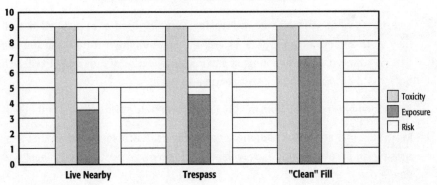

RISK INDEX FOR HAZARDOUS WASTE SITES

KEEPING YOURSELF SAFE FROM HAZARDOUS WASTE SITES

FIND OUT WHAT SITES HARBOR HAZARDOUS WASTE IN YOUR AREA:

❑ Ask your local health department or state environmental agency if they know of any sites that are or were contaminated in your area. Ask them if there is a statewide listing of such sites. A number of states do make this list available on the Web and at town halls across the state.

❑ Find out if there are any federal Superfund sites in your town by going to http://www.epa.gov/superfund/ and http://www.cleanuplevel.com/. These websites will give you the street address for any hazardous waste site listed by the federal Superfund program, whether it's on the NPL or not. These websites will also give you status information and contact names for USEPA staffers involved with the site.

❑ Remember, you are the first line of defense. Always be on the alert for possible toxic sites. If you see something suspicious, don't be afraid to report it to local officials.

SAFEGUARD YOUR FAMILY BY DOING THE FOLLOWING:

❑ Test your soil to find out if any contaminants from the site may have been used as "clean" fill at your property.

❑ Investigate what types of chemical wastes were disposed of at polluted sites. If they were volatile organics (VOCs), ask the state whether it has data proving that pollutants are not migrating off-site in your direction. If they don't have such data, ask them to begin an investigation and get it.

❑ Report any odors coming from the site to local and state environmental authorities.

❑ Make sure you and your children stay off the sites. Teach your children that trespassing on an abandoned factory, landfill, or chemical waste site is illegal and dangerous.

❑ Call for an external investigation. If you are unsatisfied with the local response, either because it is underfunded or less than responsive, you can contact the federal Agency for Toxic Substances and Disease Registry (ATSDR: http://www .atsdr.cdc.gov/2p-hazardous-waste-sites.html). They have regional offices around the country and can provide an independent investigation of the site in your neighborhood.

CHAPTER 15

Pollution from Below

This book describes many environmental concerns around the home, from consumer products to pesticide use to living near a toxic waste site. However, the least obvious and thus easiest to overlook is "pollution from below." This phrase refers to pollutants that have spilled into the ground and seeped down to deep layers of soil and groundwater. Over time, some of these pollutants are capable of rising from the depths and invading homes that are one-quarter mile or more from the initial spill, contaminating indoor air and becoming a health risk.

The industrial and commercial culprits are scattered across the landscape of our country. As described in Chapter 14, there may be thousands of locations in your county alone where the past practices of business and industry have caused pollution, ranging from old abandoned factories to businesses such as dry cleaners and gas stations. Contamination from a spill that occurred twenty years ago may just now be reaching your property. Without asking the right questions, you would have no clue about pollution that could end up affecting your property value, or worse, your family's health.

People looking to buy a house know that the first three rules of real estate are "location, location, location." The environmental version of this real estate axiom is "transport, transport, transport." If pollution has an easy means of transport to your home, then you have a "location, location, location" problem.

Chemicals spilled onto the ground either bind to the soil or are washed downward by rainwater, eventually reaching groundwater. Since groundwater is always flowing from one direction to another, the chemicals move—possibly into your neighborhood. Neighbors who are downhill of a spill are most likely to receive the pollution. When pollution flows onto a property, it may contaminate the drinking water well, if there is one (Chapter 6). And even if your water supply is from a reservoir, and you have no plumbing connection to groundwater, you may still get exposed—that's because chemicals can not only move in groundwater, but also, under certain circumstances, leave it.

Many chemicals that reach groundwater are volatile, meaning they readily vaporize to form a gas. Think of the way water evaporates off the street on a hot summer's day after a rain—if the ground is hot enough, you can see steam rising off the surface as the water turns into vapor and dissipates into the air. Volatile organic chemicals (VOCs), like those in gasoline, can also easily evaporate. That's why if you spill a drop of gasoline on the ground when you're at the gas station, the spot dries up quickly but still smells strong—the chemical changed from a liquid to a gas and rose up to your nose. Similarly, volatile chemicals that escape groundwater are then free to move back up through the soil, where they can be drawn into your house.

Monitoring studies have found VOCs to be common in groundwater, with results generally greater in urban/suburban zones than in rural areas (Moran et al., 2004). Those data correspond with the locations of most gas stations and industries, the two main sources of VOCs in groundwater. The levels found were generally low, but the study purposely stayed away from known contamination areas in order to characterize background levels. In fact, it's not unusual to find VOC hot spots in communities adjacent to polluting industries or businesses. If you are unlucky enough to live in such a zone, you may be breathing VOCs coming up through the soil under your house.

> **MYTH:** Those who live closest to a contaminated waste site will have the greatest health risks.
>
> **REALITY:** Pollution can travel considerable distances, and those living closest may not be right in its path. Those living farther away may have greater health risks but be totally unaware.

UNDERGROUND VOCs ARE DRAWN TOWARD OVERLYING BUILDINGS.

It sounds like some kind of environmental conspiracy theory. Why should a chemical spill that started across town head directly toward your basement? As unlikely (and unfortunate) as it may seem, it's true (Little et al., 1992), and it's happened in houses across the country. In its most severe form, this phenomenon has resulted in buildings actually *blowing up* because they were located too close to landfills, as illustrated by cases in Pennsylvania, Ohio, and North Carolina (ATSDR, *Fact Sheet*). Methane is a flammable gas that builds up inside landfills and can travel underground toward a nearby house; if enough methane accumulates in the basement, any spark can set off a chemical explosion. Fortunately, most people do not live or work that close to a landfill. However, these examples show that VOCs really can move underground and get into buildings, where they can become a hazard.

The reason that methane gas or any VOC would head toward a house is because the house naturally exhales or breathes out air, especially in the wintertime. As the air in the house is heated, it rises toward the rafters to find cracks where it can exit. This "exhale" requires replacement air, with drafty windows and doors often providing the source for your house to "inhale" fresh air. However, if your house is airtight and energy efficient, there's probably very little draftiness, which may be good in terms of your heating bills but not so good in terms of your exposure to chemicals. That's because your airtight house will draw air from the soil, bringing soil gas into your home through cracks, drains, and sump pits in the foundation. In fact, studies in the Pacific Northwest have estimated that up to one-third of the makeup air for a weather-tight house in the winter comes from the soil gas (Turk et al., 1990). In most cases, this is not a health concern, because soil gas is not normally contaminated with high levels of VOCs, and hopefully you've done a radon test (see Chapter 2) to make sure the radioactive gas isn't lurking under your house, either. However, as we've said, certain homes may be in a hotspot area where the soil gas does have high levels of VOCs.

RIVER BEND ESTATES

John and Fran were immediately sold—one look at River Bend Estates was enough. Lovely homes on half-acre plots with river views and plenty of privacy. They could afford the high price tag; it was worth it for the peaceful surroundings, quality of life, and solid long-term investment. The house would have the conveniences of town water and sewer. John and Fran bought in, watched their new house get built, and lived happily there for six years. Then one day they read in the local newspaper that chemical contamination was discovered in an old industrial park nearby. It wasn't in an area where they ever drove or walked. Interesting, but of no concern to them, they thought. That all changed when they received a letter from town officials two months later, saying the town wanted to take "soil gas" samples near their home. The reason? Because there were signs that the pollution may have spread out toward River Bend Estates. After months of testing and worry, their fears were realized when their entire development was found to have enough soil gas contamination to cause increased health risks; contamination was found in groundwater and soil gas, and was also very likely indoors. The town recommended that residents take immediate steps to stop toxic gases from entering their home from the soil. At a town meeting there was a lot of emotion, finger-pointing, and media attention, the latter ingredient leading to the story being broadcast across the state. Property values fell within the week.

Several years later, the contamination problem was fixed, the furor died down, and John and Fran were finally able to sell and get their investment back. However, they still worried about how much health risk they accumulated by living in a contaminated house for six years.

A WIDE VARIETY OF BUSINESSES AND INDUSTRIES HAVE CREATED INDOOR AIR VOC PROBLEMS FOR THEIR NEIGHBORS.

The following table provides a short list of the industries that are most often involved in VOC pollution of groundwater. The table is organized by the types of sources and chemicals that may be released. Note that if you're also drinking the water, you have to take into account a larger number of businesses and chemicals, since here we are only dealing with volatile chemicals. See Chapter 6 for a listing of groundwater contaminants that could pose a risk to those drinking from a private well.

SOURCES FOR POLLUTION FROM BELOW
- **Industries that perform metal plating, metal refinishing, or the manufacture of machinery or parts**
- **Dry cleaners**

POLLUTANTS THAT MAY HAVE BEEN RELEASED:	WAYS POLLUTANTS MAY HAVE BEEN RELEASED:	POSSIBLE HEALTH EFFECTS	SAFE DISTANCE FROM SOURCE
Degreasing solvents such as trichloroethylene (TCE), trichloroethane (TCA), perchloroethylene (PCE)	Leaking drums, spills/sloppy handling, deliberate disposal into soil **Note:** Most of these types of releases happened years ago, when there was less awareness of pollutant transport and fewer (if any) fines. We'd like to think that, in this environmentally enlightened age, industries large and small are much more careful in the way they handle chemicals and wastes.	**TCE:** cancer; damage to nervous system, liver, and kidney; may cause reproductive harm and birth defects if exposed during pregnancy **PCE:** similar to TCE but generally milder form of toxicity **TCA:** less potent still; mostly high-dose liver and nervous system effects	One-half mile for metals working shops. One-quarter mile for dry cleaners, because they would have only released PCE, which is less toxic than TCE

SOURCES FOR POLLUTION FROM BELOW
- **Gas stations and auto repair shops**

POLLUTANTS THAT MAY HAVE BEEN RELEASED:	WAYS POLLUTANTS MAY HAVE BEEN RELEASED:	POSSIBLE HEALTH EFFECTS	SAFE DISTANCE FROM SOURCE
Gasoline, whose major toxic ingredients are benzene, ethylbenzene, xylene, toluene, and oxygenates such as MTBE	Leaking underground storage tanks beneath the gas pumps; spills **Note:** Gasoline leaks from underground tanks should now be under control, as many states have required the installation of tanks that are much less likely to rust even with many years of service. However, gasoline already in groundwater can be a health risk today and for years to come.	**Benzene:** damage to blood cells, leukemia **Toluene, Ethylbenzene, Xylene:** much less toxic than benzene but can cause effects on nervous system at high doses **MTBE:** possible carcinogen and kidney toxicant at high doses **Gasoline overall:** kidney toxicant, possible carcinogen, odors	Approximately one-tenth of a mile (500 feet)

SOURCES FOR POLLUTION FROM BELOW
■ Landfill (municipal or industrial) or Superfund or hazardous waste site

POLLUTANTS THAT MAY HAVE BEEN RELEASED:	WAYS POLLUTANTS MAY HAVE BEEN RELEASED:	POSSIBLE HEALTH EFFECTS	SAFE DISTANCE FROM SOURCE
Many different chemicals possible, including hydrogen sulfide, ammonia, methane, chloroform, chlorinated solvents, industrial chemicals	Disposal of chemical wastes into landfill; chemical reactions in the landfill that generate toxic gases; rainwater percolating through landfill bringing chemicals to groundwater. At Superfund sites, chemical discharges to ground via floor drains, lagoons, leaking drums, industrial landfills. **Note:** Town chemical waste collection days and tougher environmental laws have cut down on how much toxic waste is discarded at landfills. However, numerous old landfills exist that can still be a source of underground pollution that can travel in soil gas or groundwater.	**Hydrogen Sulfide:** strong odorant (rotten egg smell) and irritating to nose, throat, and eyes **Ammonia:** strong odorant and irritant **Methane:** flammable and explosive **Chloroform/Chlorinated Solvents:** toxic to kidney and liver; some are carcinogenic	Approximately one-half mile. That's the distance that landfill gases can travel aboveground and get into neighborhoods to affect air quality outdoors and in. Hydrogen sulfide is a very strong odorant, and if the wind is blowing toward your house from the landfill, you can likely detect the landfill from a half mile or more away. If the landfill is capped with liners, so that no gases can escape to the outside air, the safe distance can be decreased to roughly one-fifth mile (1,000 feet), which is the distance landfill gases have been found to travel underground. Superfund sites are generally zones of high-level chemical contamination, such that contaminated groundwater may extend out one-half mile.

Notes About Keeping a Safe Distance:

The table should give you a rough estimate of how large a buffer zone you need to feel safe if there is a polluting industry in the vicinity. The estimates are based upon how toxic the contaminants from these industries tend to be and how far they can travel. However, there are other factors to keep in mind:

Contamination may reach farther locations:

■ If the amount of contaminant spilled was large, leaving behind very high levels in the spill area. Starting from such a high concentration, you run the risk of exceeding cleanup criteria farther out from the spill site.

- If you are in a downhill direction from the source area, groundwater usually flows from higher to lower areas, often toward a stream or lake. Even gently sloping land can be a sign of which way the groundwater will flow. Look at the slope of the land for blocks around your new house. Walking is better than driving through a neighborhood to evaluate the terrain.

Contamination may not get as far:

- If the soil type beneath your house is clay. Clay soils are tightly packed and very dense, leaving little room for air. They form a fairly good barrier to the upward movement of VOCs coming from groundwater, leaving you with less potential for exposure. Sandy soils provide very little barrier.

- If there is an intervening stream or river between you and the pollution source, it is unlikely the pollution will reach you. As we said, groundwater generally flows downhill toward open water and drains into a creek, stream, or river; the water and the VOC contaminants would then be carried downstream rather than toward your house.

RAINFALL AND SEASON CAN AFFECT VOC ENTRY INTO YOUR HOME.

We've seen time and again that the weather can affect how much soil gas pollution gets into someone's house. A case in point was a lovely and rather pricey condominium complex that was built at the bottom of a hill—not just any hill, but a landfill. In general, landfills are not good neighbors, a fact that became obvious in certain units where the residents began smelling objectionable odors. At first they were baffled: the odors were inconsistent, there one day, gone the next. But soon, the residents' health began to suffer; people experienced insomnia, body aches, headaches, and cold/flulike symptoms. Finally, one resident noticed that the odors were worse after a heavy rain; another noticed they were worse just after the lawns had been watered. The evidence led to the conclusion that rainfall had flushed landfill chemicals into the groundwater, where they flowed downhill to the condominium foundation.

Another factor was probably at work: when rainwater fills up the soil, it drives soil gas out of the ground and up toward the surface. Think of worms rising up after a heavy rainstorm—they're chasing the oxygen that has been driven out of the soil. The fact that just watering the lawn also brought on the odor suggested that landfill chemicals had already moved onto the condominium grounds and were poised to move into the units.

This example should teach you how the weather can affect the levels of pollutants in soil gas and indoor air. Remember, a single test is only a snapshot—pollution levels could change if testing were done in another season or weather condition. Therefore, if polluted groundwater is a strong possibility, it's wise to test several times (e.g., once in each season for a year) before concluding you don't have a problem.

Q *Can pollution from below be stopped?*

A Yes. A current homeowner or prospective home buyer doesn't need to give up on a house because of this pollution problem. There are two primary ways to make the residence safe and save the property value.

1) Groundwater Cleanup Ordered by Governmental Agencies

The government fix is ultimately the best because it removes pollution at its source and takes care of the problem for the whole neighborhood. However, it's also the most time-consuming and complex. It requires town and state authorities to test soil and groundwater until they can identify where the pollution is centered, and how it is moving through the neighborhood. The cleanup technology can be complex, and paying for everything involves getting the cooperation of the offending industry, which of course could mean bringing them to court. There may be spill funds in your state, which would allow the environmental agency to take on the cleanup job proactively and worry about reimbursement later. Government cleanups are important long-term solutions that you, as the current or prospective resident, should make sure are being pursued by the authorities.

2) Individual Action You Can Take

Property owners can take a different, more direct approach to solving their groundwater problem, one that's simpler, quicker, and highly effective. It involves installing a sub-slab ventilation system, similar to what was described in Chapter 2 for radon. The venting system will prevent soil gas from coming into your basement; no matter what type of pollutant you may be facing, it won't be able to enter. That is, so long as your basement stays dry and doesn't get flooded by a rising water table. Which brings us to another important point: if you have a sump pit, you may have groundwater sitting for long periods of time during the wetter parts of the year. If the groundwater is contaminated, the VOCs may move into your basement right from the sump pit. This can be solved by installing a secure, airtight cover over the pit, in addition to the sub-slab venting system.

If the problem is radon, you as the homeowner will have to pay for the venting system. However, with VOC pollution, the state may require the polluting industry to pay for the system at your house. Be sure to ask state officials if you can receive assistance with venting system installation.

MYTH: Testing my home's indoor air is the best way to discover pollution from below.

REALITY: While this is how you test for radon, it doesn't work well for VOCs that come up from below. In fact, it should be the last option you consider.

Unlike radon, VOC testing is rather expensive. Furthermore, there are background sources of VOCs in most homes (e.g., glues, paints, solvents, petroleum products—see Chapter 7), so that it's not always easy to tell where a chemical is coming from. Therefore, you should only pursue indoor air testing after you've taken the initial steps of finding out whether VOC pollution is likely to be under your house, and even then it may not be necessary.

How to Investigate Whether There Is Pollution from Below

Step 1: Walk and drive the neighborhood to find out if there are any industries or landfills within one-half mile, or gas stations within one-tenth mile of your home. Ask neighbors about any unusual odors or environmental concerns.

Step 2: Evaluate the slope of the yard and surrounding neighborhood. Are there potential sources uphill of your house? Write a list of these addresses.

Step 3: Contact the local health department and state environmental agency. You may find out quickly with a phone call whether pollution has been documented at a particular address. You may want to follow up with a visit to the state's environmental agency to look at its records. Look for the following types of information:

- Reports of improper handling or disposal of wastes at any of the addresses you noted in your neighborhood walk-around.

- Environmental investigations, violations, fines, or cleanup orders.

- Listed hazardous waste sites, such as those within the Superfund, RCRA (Resource Conservation and Recovery Act), Brownfields, or LUST (leaking underground storage tank) programs.

- Reports of illegal dumping of garbage or wastes in the area. Roadside dumping of chemical wastes was an unfortunate way for garbage haulers to not pay landfill fees and make illegal profits.

- Statewide listing of addresses that have some evidence of environmental pollution. A number of states maintain a "contaminated sites list" organized by town and made available on the state environmental agency web page. The list can be a very useful starting point.

Getting this type of information may not always be straightforward, depending upon the way the state environmental and health agencies keep (or do not keep) records. The information you seek may be present in different bureaucratic silos, in which case it won't be one-stop shopping. Our state recently developed a comprehensive listing of "contaminated sites," so if you're buying a house in Connecticut, you'll have a big head start. It is certainly worth inquiring at both the local and state level to find out what is readily available, and to ask town and state officials to do their job and provide you, the public, with assistance. After all, what you are seeking is public information.

Hopefully, the first three steps will lead you to the conclusion that there really isn't much to worry about in the neighborhood. And we do think that this will be the outcome in most cases. However, if your observations and inquiries lead you to the opposite (high-risk) conclusion, then you should consider the next steps in the process.

Step 4: Environmental testing: This involves hiring (or requiring the seller in a house sale to hire) an environmental consultant to look into underground contamination in the area, which could involve a thorough search of town records, and if necessary, testing the groundwater and soil gas on the property you want to purchase. The testing should include a wide range of volatile chemicals to cover all possible types of underground pollution. Groundwater testing is the most reliable, followed by soil gas. Indoor air testing inside the basement is also possible, but probably the least reliable because it is the most variable over time due to seasonal/weather effects. Hiring a consultant and testing the groundwater and soil gas can be expensive and time consuming. Fortunately, as we described, there is a solution that can be more cost and time efficient. Therefore, you may opt to spend minimal effort on Step 4 and jump right into Step 5.

Step 5: Install a radon-style sub-slab venting system that ensures contaminated soil gas will not enter your basement. A basic system is not terribly expensive (approximately $1,000), although there may be cases in which adequate protection of the house may require a more sophisticated system. Many states maintain a listing of companies that are approved to do this type of work. Sub-slab systems work well, but you need to make sure that the fan that drives the system is always left on and is replaced promptly when it wears out.

THE RISK INDEX FOR POLLUTION FROM BELOW

The risk index chart indicates that the VOCs that may intrude upon your house can be highly toxic. However, this exposure pathway does not prove to be a significant health concern very often, so the exposure rating is only low to moderate. The combination yields a moderate overall risk ranking, although the risks can potentially be high for those right in the path of groundwater carrying pollution. Use the checklist in the next section to make sure pollution from below is not an important risk at your house.

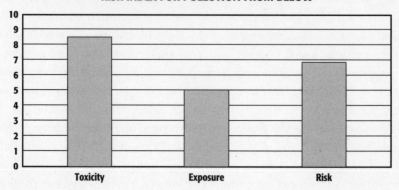

RISK INDEX FOR POLLUTION FROM BELOW

CHECKLIST FOR AVOIDING VOC POLLUTION FROM BELOW

❑ Walk, then drive through the neighborhood, looking for possible toxic sites, as well as noting the slope of the neighborhood. Talk to your neighbors to see if there were pollution issues in the past.

❑ Note the names and addresses of industries, landfills, or suspicious sites (e.g., abandoned industrial properties) within one-half mile of your home, or the house you are interested in.

❑ Note the names and addresses of any gas stations within one-tenth mile of the house.

❑ Pay particular attention to those sites that are closest, and also uphill of the house.

❑ Ask town and state environmental and health officials about the addresses you are most concerned about. Also ask about any other Superfund, RCRA, LUST, or Brownfields sites in town that could potentially affect your house.

❑ Report any unusual odors in your basement to town officials and ask to have them evaluated.

❑ If there are outstanding contamination issues involving VOCs, ask state officials to test the groundwater and soil gas; consider hiring an environmental consulting firm if the state cannot do the testing.

❑ If testing turns up groundwater pollution underneath your house, check with state officials about what it might mean for indoor air and health risks. Consider installing a sub-slab venting system if risks are high.

CHAPTER 16

Cancer Clusters

You have every reason to worry about air pollution, toxic waste dumps, tainted groundwater, and power lines in your neighborhood: But the most frightening concern is that your neighborhood is a hotbed of environmental cancer. This fear usually spikes when someone does an informal survey, and discovers that people up and down a particular street are getting cancer. There may be no obvious source of pollution in the area, but when everyone seems to be coming down with this dread disease, people start looking around for answers.

Imagine your worst nightmare: your wife is diagnosed with breast cancer. She's led a healthy lifestyle; consumed a diet of vitamin-rich, high-fiber foods; drank in moderation; exercised daily; and never smoked. How could she, of all people, get sick? There must be a reason, something beyond her control. Then you find out that a neighbor had breast cancer last year. You start asking, and find out about cases of skin, colon, and lung cancer, all in your immediate vicinity. This can't be a coincidence! You call the state health department and your education on "cancer clusters" begins.

Nationwide, government agencies receive an estimated 1,000 cancer cluster calls each year (Thun and Sink, 2004). And that's probably a low estimate, since many states and most local health departments don't track such calls. A big reason behind the volume of calls is that cancer is so common. You may be shocked to learn that one out of two men will develop some form of cancer in their lifetime. For women, the statistics are only slightly more in their favor, at one out of three (SEER, 2004). Such high rates can make it seem like every neighborhood is a cancer cluster. The most common cancers in men are prostate, lung, colon, skin, and bladder, while in women they are breast, lung, colon, and uterine. As described below, there can be many different and highly individual reasons for cancers. The percentage caused by the environment has been a decades-long debate, difficult to resolve because so many factors combine to determine total cancer risk.

Popular movies like *A Civil Action* and *Erin Brockovich* put cancer clusters on the map, and squarely placed the blame on industries illegally dumping hazardous waste. Unfortunately, although those movies are based on true stories, simple answers to what causes a cancer cluster are usually hard to come by. Most reported cancer clusters are not related to environmental contamination. In fact, most reported cancer clusters are not even clusters at all!

A cancer cluster can be defined as an excess number of cancers of one particular type in a specific neighborhood, occurring within several years of one another. The cancers don't have to be connected by where the victims live, as there can be clusters at work or based upon some common exposure or experience.

Cluster investigations have led to the discovery of workplace and environmental hazards, but the main application has been in the area of infectious disease. Outbreaks of food poisoning, hepatitis, meningitis, and emerging conditions like Legionnaire's disease (in the 1970s) and SARS (severe acute respiratory disease from a virus imported from China in 2003) have been solved by cluster investigations. This kind of detective work has taught us how serious infectious outbreaks can be, even from everyday sources like bacterial pollution of a well or having turkey casserole sit out during a summer picnic.

There are far fewer examples of cluster investigations leading to discovery of a specific pollution source causing cancer. Most examples have occurred in the workplace:

- Lung cancer and mesothelioma—asbestos exposure—in shipbuilders

- Bone cancer: radiation from radium in clock dial painters

- Scrotal cancer: PAHs from soot in chimney sweepers

- Liver cancer: vinyl chloride in chemical workers

However, cancer cluster studies in communities are far less likely to turn up associations with chemical contamination. Among the thousands of cancer clusters reported to health officials over the past thirty years, only a handful have produced clear associations with an environmental chemical. That's because, in many cases, the reported cluster is not real, and even in cases where it is real, the limitations of epidemiology make proving cause and effect very difficult. For example, if ten people all came down with the same cancer on the same street and it was due to a common drinking water supply, the odds would be against finding the link. The latency period to develop most cancers is twenty years or longer; by the time a cancer diagnosis could be made, a number of these people will have moved away and been lost from the study. Furthermore, exposure estimates for people you could still locate would be difficult to reconstruct from so long ago. Another problem is that if the cancer is fairly common, the incidence in those you track down might not seem very different from the background rate. The best chance of finding a cluster and a cause is to study a collection of tumors that are rare in the general public.

Breast cancer is a prime example of the difficulty in linking cancer to environmental factors. Breast cancer rates have increased over the past several decades, with one in nine U.S. women now likely to develop the disease in their lifetime. While these statistics might suggest an environmental cause, there are a variety of risk factors that have changed over the same time frame. For example, the trend has been for women to start a career after college and have children later in life. Having children affects a woman's hormone balance, decreasing estrogen levels for prolonged periods of time. Since high estrogen is a risk factor for breast cancer, having children earlier in life and having numerous children can be protective. So the current trend of delaying childbearing can increase cancer risk. Just to clarify, we are not saying women should have more children and at younger ages. We are just pointing out that subtle factors can affect breast cancer risk and rates. Other factors that have varied over the decades include dietary patterns (higher fat), level of obesity (increasing), and age at onset of puberty (earlier), all potential risk factors for breast cancer. Add genetics to the mix of personal risk factors, and you can see why it can be difficult to pluck out the environment as a cause.

WHILE IT'S DIFFICULT TO PROVE THAT CANCER COMES FROM OUR ENVIRONMENT, THERE ARE TWO CLUSTER INVESTIGATIONS THAT SHOW US HOW CLOSE WE CAN COME.

The two clusters that have been most strongly associated with an environmental cause occurred in Woburn, Massachusetts, and Dover Township, New Jersey. In both cases, associations were found between VOCs in drinking water and childhood leukemia. Childhood leukemia is somewhat easier to study because it has a short latency period (generally from 1 to 10 years), which means people are more likely to still be in the neighborhood when they come down with the disease. That doesn't mean that every leukemia cluster will have an environmental cause, but these two did.

1) **Woburn, MA:** If you saw the movie *A Civil Action* (starring John Travolta) or read the book, then you learned about the infamous cluster in Woburn. In 1979, six cases of childhood leukemia were found in a small area that was served by public wells contaminated with trichloroethylene (TCE), perchloroethylene, and chloroform. As the cluster was investigated, additional cases were identified, increasing the rate to more than three times that expected for childhood leukemia (Mass DPH, 1997). The increase was large enough to stand up to various statistical tests. The studies suggested that the greatest risk occurred if mothers drank the contaminated water during pregnancy. Which means that childhood leukemia may start, at least in some cases, with fetal exposure to toxic chemicals.

The strong associations coming out of the Woburn cluster were made possible by the high levels of TCE in the water, much more than are typical in contaminated areas today. Additionally, as mentioned above, childhood leukemia is easier to study because of its short latency period. These findings put TCE and related solvents on the map as possible human carcinogens, which is consistent with findings in animals (ATSDR, 1997). The contaminated wells were closed in 1979, and health officials did not find any new cases between 1986 and 1994, so it appears the cluster ended when the water was cleaned up.

2) **Dover Township, NJ:** Similar cancer results have been found in the Dover Township portion of New Jersey, also referred to as Toms River: childhood leukemia patterns emerged there between 1974 and 1995. The cancers were shown to be associated with maternal consumption of contaminated drinking water during pregnancy and with air pollution from a nearby chemical plant (New Jersey DHSS, 2003). A number of contaminants were identified, most notably TCE and a contaminant unique to the

site called styrene-acrylonitrile trimer (SAN). While the NJ cluster has not gained the notoriety of Woburn, it suggests that even low levels of TCE and other solvents in groundwater can be a risk for childhood leukemia.

The investigations at Woburn and Dover Township provide the best cancer-environment associations to date in the United States. Note that we use the term "association". Even these particularly successful studies do not actually prove cause and effect. However, they were sufficient to send a warning to cities and towns across the country about drinking water contaminants (also see Chapter 6), and about not taking cancer cluster calls lightly. You never know where the next Woburn will be.

Q *What is a real cluster, and what should be done about it?*

A Most calls are not based upon actual cancer clusters. People often report different kinds of cancer in a given neighborhood: for example, two breast cancers, five prostate, one colon, and one brain cancer. What many don't realize is that cancer is not a single disease. Each cancer type has its own set of risk factors and causes. Only cancers of the same type can be counted toward a cluster and compared against background rates. Cancers that are very common, such as prostate, breast, colon, skin, and lung, are usually not worthy of investigation. Health departments will become more animated over a reported cluster of brain, kidney, or liver cancer, certain leukemias or mesothelioma. When such rare tumors appear as a cluster, there may well be environmental links to explore.

But even when rare cancers occur as a cluster, there may not be an environmental cause. Called "perceived clusters," they occur by random chance. There are over one million cases of cancer diagnosed in the United States each year, and these cases are not evenly distributed across the country. It's inevitable that some will occur close to each other, just by chance, and appear to be a cluster. Separating such perceived clusters from true environmental clusters usually requires finding a pollution source that could logically be at fault. But again, you might never end up with absolute proof of cause and effect.

For a cluster investigation to take off, the following conditions usually have to be met:

- Numerous cases of a single type of cancer in a small geographic area.

- The cancer type occurs infrequently in the rest of the population.

- There is a particular source of environmental chemical(s) in the community that might logically connect to the cancer.

If a cluster jumps all of these hurdles, the state health department may come on the scene and collect more detailed information on the cases and the exposures. They will try to locate additional people with the disease, both locally and those who have moved away, and map their addresses in comparison to pollution sources.

CHILDHOOD LEUKEMIA CLUSTER IN FALLON, NEVADA

Fallon, Nevada, is a town with 7,500 residents, located near the center of the state. It was like so many anonymous small towns, until the summer of 2000, when citizens reported to state health officials that five children had developed Acute Lymphocytic Leukemia (ALL). During the ensuing investigation, ten more ALL cases were found around town.

On face value, this rate of childhood leukemia in such a small population stuck out as unusual. The state health department calculated that only one leukemia case should have been expected, and not just for Fallon, but for the whole county. Thus, the fifteen Fallon cases was a major finding. The next piece of detective work was to find the cause. Since there was a Navy Air Station not far from town, local suspicion turned in that direction. Most of the jet fuel that went to the air station was piped under Fallon, so some thought there may have been underground fuel leaks and contamination of groundwater. However, the town water was tested regularly and no jet fuel compounds were found.

Numerous other possible explanations were pursued—agricultural pesticides, arsenic in the drinking water, and radiation from atomic bomb tests run in the 1950s. All were ruled out, either because Fallon was never exposed to the suspect agents, or the chemicals were not known to cause ALL. The CDC even went so far as testing the blood and urine of residents in the county where Fallon was located. Since they did not really know what they were looking for, they tested for a wide variety of chemicals, including metals, pesticides, PCBs, and volatile organic compounds.

Despite the extensive testing, no obvious cause was found. One surprising result was elevated levels of a particular metal, tungsten, in the blood of residents. Further testing showed tungsten was present in the town water supply. While tungsten is not known to be a carcinogen, the Fallon data have spurred renewed toxicologic study of tungsten in animals.

The lack of an environmental association to the leukemia was particularly frustrating because the odds of a cluster of that magnitude occurring strictly by chance was one in 232 million (Steinmaus et al., 2004). Not giving up, investigators turned toward viruses. Viruses are known to cause a few types of cancer, but not ALL. Theories were developed explaining how a virus may have been involved anyway, but they remain speculative. The bottom line is that after extensive testing of the environment and the people of Fallon, no explanation for the dramatic cancer cluster was found.

What does this Toxic File tell us about cancer clusters in general? That even when you have a well-defined cluster, linking it to an environmental source can be difficult. But in spite of the difficulties, this kind of investigative work needs to go on, because you never know when it will lead to associations and interventions that protect public health.

MYTH: Most cancers are caused by exposure to chemicals in the environment.

REALITY: About eighty percent of all cancers are related to lifestyle factors such as tobacco and alcohol use, high fat intake and other dietary patterns, obesity, exposure to sunlight, and lack of exercise, all of which are controllable.

The following listing provides estimates of how much cancer is caused by different factors (updated from Doll and Peto, 1981):

Tobacco 35%
Diet 30%
Infections 10%
Reproductive and sexual behavior 7%
Occupation 4%
Alcohol 3%
Geophysical factors* 3%
Pollution 2–5%
Medicine 1%
Food additives . . . . less than 1%
*Sunlight causes a much greater percentage of nonfatal cancers

Most people are surprised when epidemiology studies suggest that "pollution" accounts for less than five percent of all cancer. Keep in mind, these kinds of estimations are rather crude. But no matter how you cut the cancer pie, environmental pollution from such sources as drinking water or a nearby waste dump is a relatively small piece. What the listing does show is why there has been so much emphasis on lifestyle factors such as smoking cessation, weight loss, lower-fat diets, and using sunblock. Of course, we can't entirely ignore environmental carcinogens. But it's also important to keep these statistics in mind when you hear someone claim that a neighbor's cancer, or an apparent clustering of cancers, is caused by the environment, because our best science suggests that environmental chemicals are not the major cause of most cancers.

Should My Neighborhood Be Studied?

A concerned community often wants a "cancer study" to be done to see if they have elevated disease rates, and if so, what the cause might be. However, you can't just rush in—there needs to be evidence of a clustering of cancer and plausible environmental links to justify a major investigation. In fact, cluster investigations are warranted in only a small number of situations. When conducted, they are almost always negative and usually do not lead to answers or interventions that will protect public health. This being said, it is still important to identify carcinogens in the environment and reduce exposure whenever possible.

As a resident of a "suspect" neighborhood, you should evaluate the need for a cancer cluster study by going through the following checklist. Feel free to contact your local and state health officials to help you answer the questions on this checklist.

CANCER CLUSTER CHECKLIST

Do the cancers in your area add up to a real cluster? The following steps will help you evaluate this possibility:

☐ Keep in mind that most "clusters" are not real and are not worth investigating.

☐ Consider whether cancers are of the same type and occur in a small geographic area; only cancers that fit both criteria should be counted toward a cluster.

☐ Consider whether the cancer that seems to be appearing is common or rare; rare cancers are much easier to study than common cancers.

☐ Consider whether there is a plausible environmental exposure that might explain why the cancers occurred; i.e., if there are sources of carcinogens that are not typically found in other neighborhoods.

☐ Consider whether enough time has passed (a latency period) between exposure to the chemical and cancer onset; remember, the latency period for most cancers is twenty years or more.

☐ Consider whether there are other likely causes for the cancers, such as smoking or diet.

☐ Call your local or state health department to discuss your concerns.

SECTION 5

Tying It All Together

CHAPTER 17

Home-Buyer's Guide

We've given you lots of safety tips regarding toxics in the home, yard, and neighborhood, on how to recognize a toxic concern and how to address it. We expect that these tips will help you size up chemical risks in your current dwelling. But beyond that, we hope that they can be useful to those looking to buy a house. It's obviously much better to find out about risks before you move in, as you don't want to inherit someone else's toxic problems. You can prevent that situation if you know what to look for.

Fortunately, toxics in homes can often be removed; they are not the deal-breaker that a "bad neighborhood" or flood zone may be. However, fixing toxic hazards can take time, effort, and money. If you know about them up front, you may be able to make the remediation costs part of the purchase agreement, just as you would a new roof. Or in some cases, you may decide against a house because of toxics concerns and uncertainty over whether they can be fixed.

We've written this chapter not only for home buyers, but also for inspectors and Realtors, who are usually aware of some, but not all, of the toxics issues in a home. As the buyer, seek out a Realtor and home inspector who are interested and knowledgeable and have your safety in mind. The last thing you need is an inspector who misses an important issue, or an agent who thinks you are silly to be worried over an imaginary toxic risk.

Many home purchase agreements already cover four toxics issues: lead, radon, asbestos, and UFFI (urea-formaldehyde foam insulation). We start our checklist with these four basic issues, and then go on to concerns that can be just as risky, depending upon the house and its environment. If you follow all the steps, you should feel confident that you're buying a toxic-safe home. Good luck!

LEAD IN PAINT
Risk: Toxic lead levels can build up in children from flaking paint (Chapter 1).

❏ Assume any house built before 1978 still contains lead paint unless the seller can document that it was de-leaded.

❏ Ask whether the lead paint has been sealed with encapsulants. If so, when?

❏ Inspect the condition of painted surfaces. Are they in good condition or dilapidated? Check window wells; are they loaded with dirt and paint chips?

❏ If these lead hazards exist, plan on having the house professionally cleaned and painted surfaces encapsulated before moving in. This is especially important if you are moving in with young children.
    ❏ Estimate the cost of the procedures and consider making it part of the purchase agreement.
    ❏ Encapsulating or completely removing lead paint within reach of young children is a good idea, even if the paint is in good condition.

❏ If the house was built before 1978, assume that the soil right next to the house is lead contaminated. Do not grow a garden in this soil until it is tested and remediated.

RADON
Risk: A radioactive, carcinogenic gas that comes in through the basement (Chapter 2).

❏ Arrange for your home inspector to do a radon test of the basement. The test should be done with the house sealed up to maximize the chance of detecting radon.
    ❏ If the test is done in warm weather, recognize that it could be higher in the winter. Borderline results merit a retest the following winter.
    ❏ If the results are above 4 pCi/l, get an estimate for installing a radon-mitigation system. Consider making this part of the purchase agreement.

ASBESTOS
Risk: Fireproofing insulation that has caused cancer in workers (Chapter 4).

❑ Assume insulation around pipes and hot water tank is asbestos if the house was built before 1975.

❑ Inspect the condition of this insulation; if poor, it will need to be removed by a professional contractor. If good, it can be left in place.

❑ Other asbestos-containing materials that may be in the house (e.g., drop ceiling tiles, floor tiles) can be left in place unless damaged.

CARBON MONOXIDE (CO)
Risk: A toxic gas that can build up to lethal conditions if the furnace is not operating properly (Chapter 8).

❑ Find out if there is at least one CO detector in the house. If not, make sure you install one after you move in.

❑ Find out when the furnace was last tuned up, and make sure it is tuned up before the next heating season.

UREA-FORMALDEHYDE FOAM INSULATION (UFFI)
Risk: Blown-in insulation that contained a toxic, carcinogenic gas (Chapter 8).

❑ Do not worry about it. UFFI was discontinued in the early 1980s. There has been plenty of time for the formaldehyde to have vaporized and left the house.

MOLD
Risk: Damp conditions can cause chronic mold problems and health effects (Chapter 3).

❑ Inspect the house from top to bottom looking for evidence of mold, water intrusion, or excess condensation/moisture. Don't bother testing the air.

❑ Require that any water problems be addressed and mold be removed as a condition of purchase; this may involve:
　❑ Fixing plumbing or roof leaks;
　❑ Discarding water-damaged structural materials and furnishings;
　❑ A thorough mold cleanup.

DRINKING WATER
Risk: Pesticides, metals, and VOCs may contaminate private wells (Chapter 6).

❑ Find out what type of water supply the house is on.

❑ If it's a private well, ask to see water test results.

❑ If no testing has been done within the past year, consider getting a test done before moving in.
  ❑ You may be able to make the purchase agreement contingent on the test results.

❑ This testing is more important if the house is within one-half mile of any potential contamination sources: gas stations, dry cleaners, factories (current or abandoned), farms, garden shops, or landfills.

❑ Ask if the current occupants now or in the past have used a water filter and why.

❑ If on public water, ask to see the latest consumer confidence report from the water company with recent testing results.

THE NEIGHBORHOOD
Risk: Various sources of pollution may increase your environmental risks.

❑ Local sources of outdoor air pollution (Chapter 11):
  ❑ Try to stay away from major sources, the most important being busy roads, landfills, sewage treatment plants, and factories;
    ❑ homes more than 500 feet away from such sources are less likely to have a concern.

❑ Watch out for sources of volatile chemicals (VOCs) that can enter the house from groundwater (Chapter 15):
  ❑ Tour the neighborhood looking for landfills, gas stations, dry cleaners, factories (current or abandoned), or hazardous waste sites that are within one-half mile of your candidate house; make special note of those closest and uphill of the house.
  ❑ Check with local and state officials to find out if there have been contamination issues at these addresses; some states may already have a statewide "contaminated sites" listing.
  ❑ If the house is on a private well, find out if it has ever been tested for VOCs (see above).
  ❑ Make note of any unusual odors when inspecting the basement.

❑ If these inquiries lead to concerns about neighborhood sources of groundwater pollution, more testing may be needed; environmental consultants can test for VOCs in shallow groundwater and soil gas under the house.

LOOK FOR LOCAL SOURCES OF HAZARDOUS WASTE (CHAPTER 14).

❑ Ask town and state officials whether toxic waste is present on any sites in the neighborhood (e.g., abandoned factories, landfills, areas of chemical dumping).

❑ Ask whether soil or other material from the sites were ever used in the neighborhood as "clean" fill.

❑ Ask whether VOCs are present at the sites, and whether they may be leaching toward your candidate house.

❑ Inspect to make sure the sites are well secured so that your children will not be able to gain access.

❑ Find out what future cleanup plans there are for the sites.

❑ Power lines and EMF (Chapter 13):

❑ Consider proximity to high-voltage power lines.

❑ Have the yard tested for EMF if the house is within 300 feet of the lines.

❑ Levels above 10 mG are well above background and present greater uncertainty that the home is safe for young children.

THE BACKYARD

Risk: Previous residents may be leaving you with toxic chemicals in wood decks, in soil, or in the garage (Chapter 12).

❑ Ask when any decks or wooden play structures were built and what type of wood was used. Chances are good that it was arsenic-containing pressure-treated wood.

❑ Consider that such structures will need to be sealed every 1 to 2 years to prevent arsenic leaching.

❑ Consider that soil directly beneath the structure is likely contaminated with arsenic, and will need to be removed or kept off-limits.

❑ Find out if the land had ever been used for farming; if so, consider testing soil for persistent pesticides (chlordane, dieldrin, DDT, lead arsenate).

❑ If these pesticides are found in soil, contact state health department to find out if the levels are above cleanup standards.

❑ If so, get a cost estimate for their removal and make this part of the contract agreement.

❑ Old chemicals left around house:
  ❑ Inspect the garage, basement, and attic to make sure old paint, pesticides, and solvents have not been left behind.
    ❑ Bring any residual chemicals to your town's hazardous waste collection day.

❑ Buried heating oil tank:
  ❑ Find out if the the property contains a buried fuel oil tank.
  ❑ If there is one, ask for soil sampling to demonstrate that it has not leaked in the past.
    ❑ Find out what local laws require for buried tanks.
    ❑ Find out the costs for removal or sealing of the tank and for testing the soil for spilled oil.
    ❑ Consider applying these costs to the purchase agreement.

CHAPTER 18

Consumer's Guide

Whether you are headed for the hardware, art supply, carpet, furniture, or even grocery store, the choices you make will determine how many toxic chemicals you bring home. Government regulations and corporate efforts to reduce toxics in the marketplace have not gone far enough to ensure risk-free products and foods. Armed with a little information, you can become a smarter shopper and avoid much of the risk.

We hope this book provides that information. The chapters on food (Chapter 5) and consumer products (Chapter 7) are the most obvious places to look, but other chapters also touch on consumer products. This Consumer's Guide gathers our most important recommendations in one place for quick reference. For more details on any of these topics, go to the relevant chapter. Happy shopping!

GUIDING PRINCIPLES:

❑ Do not assume that all products are safe. Consumer products are not tightly regulated and can contain toxic and carcinogenic ingredients.

❑ Buy Green! A variety of manufacturers have developed alternative product lines that boast low- or nontoxic ingredients. Look for these healthier products and read the label to make sure that they really do deserve the green designation. Volatile organic chemicals such as benzene, toluene, ethylbenzene, xylene, trichloroethylene, and perchloroethylene are some of the chemicals to watch out for.

❑   Consider whether you need the product at all. Reduce your use of products with toxic chemicals, especially pesticides.

❑   Follow product use instructions, especially when using them indoors. Adequate ventilation and protective clothing recommendations are usually important precautions.

❑   Keep toxic products away from children and stored safely.

❑   Stop using any product that irritates your eyes, nose, or throat.

CLEANING PRODUCTS (CHAPTER 7)

❑   Avoid harsh cleaners such as ammonia or bleach.

❑   Never mix products that contain ammonia and bleach.

❑   Stop using any product that causes irritation to your eyes, nose, or throat.

❑   Air out your dry-cleaned clothes in a ventilated area, since most dry cleaners use perchloroethylene (PERC). Better yet, go to a dry cleaner that does not use PERC.

PAINTS, COATINGS, AND GLUES (CHAPTER 7)

❑   Use water-based paints and wood finishes wherever possible. Remember that even products labeled as water-based have some VOCs, so always use them in well-ventilated areas.

❑   Keep family members away from the work area until the odors have dissipated, usually a few days to be safe.

❑   Conduct small glueing and painting projects outside; only bring the object in after it has fully cured.

ART SUPPLIES (CHAPTER 10)

❑   Do not let children use solvent-based glues (e.g., rubber cement) or spray fixatives. These should only be applied by adults and with adequate fresh air.

❑   Take care when handling a variety of other art supplies, including powdered paints, pottery glazes, and photography supplies. These should not be used by children.

CARPETS AND FURNISHINGS (CHAPTER 8)

❏   Look for green-labeled carpets that are low in VOCs.

❏   Let a new carpet air out prior to installation.

❏   Minimize the amount of particleboard or veneer furniture that you buy; ventilate the room they are placed in for days to weeks to decrease formaldehyde exposure.

INDOOR AND OUTDOOR PESTICIDES (CHAPTERS 7 AND 12)

❏   Only use pesticides when absolutely necessary. Choose integrated pest management (IPM) and other natural control methods before resorting to more toxic measures.

❏   If you must use a pesticide, only purchase the minimum quantity needed. Apply only enough to treat the specific area or problem rather than widespread spraying.

❏   If whole-house application is needed, plan to evacuate the house for a few days and cover household items, particularly food and things that children handle (toys).

❏   If you're applying pesticides yourself, carefully follow the manufacturer instructions.

❏   Local county and college extension offices often have websites and pamphlets with tips on safe application of pesticides.

AIR PURIFIERS, WATER FILTERS, AND CARBON MONOXIDE / RADON DETECTORS (CHAPTERS 2, 6, 8)

❏   Purchase a carbon monoxide detector and install it in your basement outside the furnace room.

❏   Purchase a radon test kit and determine the level of radon in your home, if you didn't when you bought the house.

❏   Do not rely on air purifiers to fix an indoor problem. Most purifiers are not effective in cleaning large areas, and no filter is capable of removing all types of contaminants; in fact, some may add contaminants such as ozone.

❏   Use a water filter to remove harmful contaminants detected in your drinking water.

❏   Choose a filter designed for the problem you have: carbon filters for most VOC contaminants, reverse osmosis for metals. Proper maintenance is critical to keep the filter working properly.

COMBUSTION APPLIANCES (CHAPTERS 8 AND 9)

❏   Do not purchase a backyard furnace, as these are more polluting than other heating appliances.

❏   Do not buy unvented gas logs or other unvented combustion appliances; only use kerosene heaters and electric generators with adequate ventilation.

COSMETICS AND PERSONAL CARE PRODUCTS (CHAPTER 7)

❏   Use less cosmetics before and during pregnancy to reduce exposure to various chemicals, including reproductive toxins (phthalates) and a carcinogen (1,4-dioxane).

❏   Use green or homemade products. Look out for bubble baths that contain 1,4-dioxane and formaldehyde.

FOOD (CHAPTER 5)

❏   Eat fish as part of a healthy diet, but be careful. Find out about consumption advisories for the fish you eat, both those you catch locally and those you buy at the supermarket. It is most important for women of childbearing age and children to follow the U.S. Food and Drug Administration's advice not to eat shark, swordfish, and king mackerel, which tend to be highly contaminated.

❏   Canned tuna is okay in moderation (one to two meals per week) for women and children, but choose light rather than white meat tuna for safer mercury levels.

❏   Eat less high-fat animal products; instead choose leaner meat, vegetarian options, and low-fat dairy.

❏   Pesticide levels on fresh fruits and vegetables are generally low, so don't be overly concerned. However, washing and peeling vegetables and buying organic produce are still good precautions.

LEAD (CHAPTER 1)

❑   Do not drink out of leaded crystal glassware or eat or drink out of handmade glazed pottery; remember, lead risk seems to be greatest for pottery made in Mexico and other foreign countries.

❑   Handle hair dyes with caution, as many contain lead.

Resources

CHAPTER 1

Lead in Drinking Water:
USEPA Fact Sheet: (http://www.epa.gov/safewater/lead/index.html).

Lead in Mexican Pottery:
For more information, visit http://www.co.yakima.wa.US/Health/documents/
    press/05-080-Lead-pottery-candy.pdf.

Lead Poisoning:
Washington DOH, Fact Sheet: (http://www.doh.wa.gov/topics/lead.htm).

Lead-Safe Painting and Renovations:
CTDPH Fact Sheet: (http://www.dph.state.ct.us/BRS/Lead/Lead-
    Safe/lswp_brochure.pdf).

USEPA Requirements: (http://www.epa.gov/lead/pubs/renovation.htm).

Use of Lead Encapsulants—NYS Fact Sheet: (http://www.nyc.gov/html/
    hpd/downloads/pdf/nys-doh-tech-fact-sheet-encapsulants.pdf).

CHAPTER 2

State Radon Contacts: To find contact information for your state radon office, use
    the link www.epa.gov/iaq/whereyoulive.html, or call the Indoor Air Quality
    Information Clearinghouse (IAQ INFO) at 800-438-4318. The USEPA's
    radon home page (www.epa.gov/radon) also includes links to publications,
    hotlines, consultant certification programs, and more.

CHAPTER 3

Centers for Disease Control, "Protect Yourself from Mold.":
    (http://www.bt.cdc.gov/disasters/mold/protect.asp).

New York City, "Guidelines on Assessment and Remediation of Fungi in Indoor Environments.": (http://www.nyc.gov/html/doh/html/epi/moldrpt1.shtml).

USEPA, "A Brief Guide to Mold Moisture and Your Home.": (http://www.epa.gov/iaq/molds/moldguide.html).

USEPA Mold Resource web page: (http://www.epa.gov/mold/moldresources.html).

CHAPTER 4

Asbestos in drinking water: USEPA Safe Drinking Water Hotline: 800-426-4791.

For general information on asbestos, go to the USEPA website: (www.epa.gov/asbestos); USEPA asbestos line: 800-471-7127; USEPA ombudsman: 800-368-5888.

For information on asbestos in consumer products, contact the U.S. Consumer Product Safety Commission (CPSC) or 800-638-CPSC.

For information on state certification programs for professionals, call the USEPA at 202-554-1404.

Health effects of asbestos: Centers for Disease Control/Agency for Toxic Substances and Disease Registry (ATSDR): (www.atsdr.cdc.gov/asbestos).

CHAPTER 5

ATSDR (Agency for Toxic Substances and Disease Registry) Toxicological Profile for Chlorinated Dibenzo-p-dioxins (1998).

Center for Science in the Public Interest (CSPI): (www.cspinet.org).

USEPA Fish Advisory website (www.epa.gov/waterscience/fish).

USFDA, Center for Food Safety and Applied Nutrition: (www.cfsan.fda.gov).

CHAPTER 6

American Water Works Association Fact Sheets: (http://www.awwa.org/advocacy/learn/).

Clean Water Action: (http://www.cleanwateraction.org/).

NSF Drinking Water Information and Certification of Filters: (http://www.nsf.org/consumer/drinking_water).

Purdue University Fact Sheet—Understanding Consumer Confidence Reports: (http://www.ecn.purdue.edu/SafeWater/drinkinfo/WQ-33.htm).

USEPA Safe Drinking Water Hotline (800-426-4791) and website: (http://www.epa.gov/safewater).

CHAPTER 7

FDA Consumer Home Page: (http://www.fda.gov/opacom/morecons.html).

Listing of green product alternatives: (www.thegreenguide.com).

National Institute of Health's Household Products Database: (http://household products.nlm.nih.gov/).

CHAPTER 8

AERIAS—IAQ Resource Center. In-depth information on IAQ topics online: (www.aerias.org).

California Indoor Air Quality Program: (www.cal-iaq.org). Information, research, and guidelines for numerous IAQ issues.

Green Seal: (www.greenseal.org). Information on environmentally friendly consumer products and low-VOC-emitting products.

USEPA Indoor Air Pollution Hotline: 800-438-4318.

USEPA Indoor Air Quality website: (www.epa.gov/iaq/). Links to USEPA websites and fact sheets and IAQ topics.

USEPA, *The Inside Story: A Guide to Indoor Air Quality*, 1995. General background on a wide variety of indoor air topics.

CHAPTER 9

Association of Occupational and Environmental Clinics (AOEC): (www.aoec.org).

For office and other commercial buildings, the USEPA has an IAQ management tool called I-BEAM. Find out more at 800-438-4318: (www.epa.gov/iaq/largebldgs/I-BEAM_html).

National Institute of Occupational Safety and Health (NIOSH). International chemical safety cards: (www.cdc.gov/niosh/ipcs/icstart.html).

National Institute of Occupational Safety and Health (NIOSH). NIOSH pocket guide to chemical hazards: (www.dcd.gov/niosh/npg/default.html).

U. S. Occupational Safety and Health Administration (OSHA): (www.osha.gov).

CHAPTER 10

Avoiding Hazardous Art Materials in the Classroom, California USEPA: (http://www.oehha.ca.gov/education/art/artguide.html).

USEPA Indoor Air Quality Education and Assessment Guidelines (I-BEAM): 800-438-4318: (www.epa.gov/iaq/largebuildings/I-BEAM_html).

USEPA Indoor Air Quality Hotline: 800-438-4318.

USEPA Tools for Schools: (www.epa.gov/iaq/schools/toolkit.html).

U.S. Green Building Council, Leadership in Energy and Environmental Design (LEED): (www.usgbc.org).

CHAPTER 11

American Lung Association: (www.lungusa.org).

AIRNOW—Air Quality Index (AQI): (www.airnow.gov).

California Air Resources Board: (www.arb.ca.gov).

EDF Toxics Scorecard: (http://www.scorecard.org/).

USEPA NATA website, Air Toxics information: (http://www.epa.gov/ttn/atw/nata/).

USEPA—(particles, ozone, toxics): (www.epa.gov.air).

Toxic Release Inventory (TRI) database maintained by USEPA: (http://www.epa.gov/tri/).

CHAPTER 12

CDC Pesticides Fact Sheet, 2004: (http://www.cdc.gov/nceh/hsb/pesticides/activities.pdf).

CDC Pesticides website: (http://www.cdc.gov/health/pesticides.htm).

USEPA Fact Sheet on Chlordane: (http://www.epa.gov/safewater/contaminants/dw_contamfs/chlordan.html).

CHAPTER 13

Electric Power Research Institute (electric company trade group): (http://www.epriweb.com).

National Institute of Environmental Health Science (NIEHS), *EMF RAPID Research and Brochure*: (http://www.niehs.nih.gov/emfrapid/booklet/youremf.htm#field).

Updates on EMF research from *Microwave News*: (http://www.microwavenews.com/).

See also links listed in the references for this chapter.

CHAPTER 14

Site contamination and cleanup information for over 10,000 CERCLIS (Comprehensive Environmental Response, Compensation and Liability Information System) sites: (http://www.cleanuplevel.com/).

USEPA Superfund website: (http://www.epa.gov/superfund/).

CHAPTER 15

State of Wisconsin Fact Sheet on Vapor Intrusion for Homeowners: (http://www.dhfs.state.wi.us/eh/Air/pdf/VI.pdf).

USEPA Guidance for Evaluating the Vapor Intrusion Pathway: (http://www.epa.gov/correctiveaction/eis/vapor.htm).

USEPA Indoor Air Publications: (http://www.epa.gov/iaq/pubs/targetng.html).

CHAPTER 16

National Cancer Institute (NCI), Fact Sheets on Cancer Clusters: (www.cancer.gov).

Surveillance, Epidemiology, and End Results (SEER), National Cancer Institute, *U.S. Cancer Statistics*.

U.S. Center for Disease Control, Cancer Clusters: (www.cdc.gov/nceh/clusters/).

Contact your state health department to get the cancer incidence statistics for your town.

References

CHAPTER 1

Azcona-Cruz, M.I., et al. "Lead-Glazed Ceramic Ware and Blood Lead Levels of Children in the City of Oaxaca, Mexico." *Archives of Environmental Health* 55 (2000): 217–222.

Bellinger, D., et al. "Low-Level Lead Exposure and Children's Cognitive Function in the Preschool Years." *Pediatrics* 87 (1991): 219–227.

Blumenthal, D. "An Unwanted Souvenir: Lead in Ceramic Ware." *FDA Consumer* (1989): (http://www.fda.gov/bbs/topics/CONSUMER/CON00081.html).

CDC (Centers for Disease Control). *National Report on Human Exposure to Environmental Chemicals* (2005). Available at: (http://www.cdc.gov/exposure report/3rd/pdf/thirdreport.pdf).

CPSC (Consumer Product Safety Commission). *News Bulletin* 96–150 (1996).

Farley, D. *FDA Consumer*, January to February 1998.

Landrigan, P.J. "Pediatric Lead Poisoning: Is There a Threshold?" *Public Health Reports*, November 2000.

Lewis, Jack. "Lead Poisoning: A Historical Perspective." *USEPA Journal*, May 1985.

Meyer, P.A., et al. "Surveillance for Elevated Blood Lead Levels in Children—United States, 1997–2001." *Morbidity and Mortality Weekly Report* 52 (2003): 1–21.

CHAPTER 2

Field, R.W. "A Review of Residential Radon Case-Control Epidemiologic Studies Performed in the United States." *Reviews on Environmental Health* 16 (2001): 151–167.

Gregory, B., and P.P. Jalbert. *National Radon Results: 1985 to 2003*. (October 2004).

NRC (National Research Council). *Health Effects of Exposure to Radon: BEIR VI*. (Washington, D.C.: National Academies Press, 1999).

USEPA Fact Sheet: Radon: (http://www.epa.gov/radiation/radionuclides/radon.htm).

CHAPTER 3

IOM (Institute of Medicine of the National Academies). *Damp Indoor Spaces and Health* (2004).

Kowalski, W.J. "Indoor Mold Growth: Health Hazards and Evaluation." *HPAC Engineering* (September 2000).

New York City Department of Health, Bureau of Environmental and Occupational Disease Epidemiology. *Guidelines on Assessment of Fungi in Indoor Environments* (2000).

Occupational Disease Epidemiology. *Guidelines on Assessment of Fungi in Indoor Environments* (2000).

Ponikau, J.U., D.A. Sherris, E.G. Kern, et al. "The Diagnosis and Incidence of Allergic Fungal Sinusitis." *Mayo Clinic Proceedings* 74 (1999): 877–884.

USEPA. *Mold Remediation in Schools and Commercial Buildings* (2001).

CHAPTER 4

ATSDR (Agency for Toxic Substances and Disease Registry). *Toxicology Profile for Asbestos* (1999).

HEI (Health Effects Institutes). *Asbestos in Public Buildings* (1991).

CHAPTER 5

ATSDR (Agency for Toxic Substances and Disease Registry). *Toxicological Profile for Chlorinated Dibenzo-p-Dioxins.* (1998): PB/99/121998.

"Baby Alert." *Consumer Reports*, May 1999.

Becker, et al. "German Environmental Survey 1998 (GerES III): Environmental Pollutants in Blood of the German Population." *International Journal of Hygiene and Environmental Health* 205(2002): 297–308.

Consumer Reports. "Bottled Water Test Results." August 2000.

Dohoo, I.R., L. DesCôteaux, K. Leslie, A. Fredeen, W. Shewfelt, et al. "A Meta-analysis Review of the Effects of Recombinant Bovine Somatotropin 2. Effects on Animal Health, Reproductive Performance, and Culling." *Canadian Journal of Veterinary Disease* 67 (2003): 252–264.

"EU Scientists Confirm Health Risks of Growth Hormones in Meat." Associated Press, April 23, 2002: (http://www.organicconsumers.org/toxic/hormone 042302.cfm).

EWG (Environmental Working Group). *Report Card: Pesticides in Produce* (2003): (http://www.foodnews.org/reportcard.php).

FDA. *Total Diet Study* (2005): (http://www.cfsan.fda.gov/~comm/tds-res.html).

Foran, J.A., D.O. Carpenter, M.C. Hamilton, B.A. Knuth, S.J. Schwager. "Risk-based Consumption Advice for Farmed Atlantic and Wild Pacific Salmon Contaminated with Dioxins and Dioxin-like Compounds." *Environmental Health Perspectives* 113 (2005): 552–556.

Grandjean P., P. Weihe, R.F. White, F. Debes, S. Araki, K. Yokoyama, K. Murata, N. Sorensen, R. Dahl, R.J. Jorgensen. "Cognitive Deficit in Seven-Year-Old

Children with Prenatal Exposure to Methylmercury." *Neurotoxicology and Teratology* 19 (1997): 417–428.

Herman-Giddens, M.E., E.J. Slora, R.C. Wasserman, C.J. Bourdony, M.V. Bhapkar, G.G. Koch, and C.M. Hasemeir. "Secondary Sexual Characteristics and Menses in Young Girls Seen in Office Practice: A Study from the Pediatric Research in Office Settings Network." *Pediatrics* 99(4)(1997): 505–512.

Hites, R.A., J.A. Foran, D.O. Carpenter, M.C. Hamilton, B.A. Knuth, and S.J. Schwager. "Global Assessment of Organic Contaminants in Farmed Salmon." *Science* 303 (2004): 226–229.

IFIC (International Food Information Council). *Food Ingredients and Colors* brochure (2005): (http://www.ific.org/about/results.cfm).

Jensen, E., and P.M. Bolger. "Exposure Assessment of Dioxins/Furans Consumed in Dairy Foods and Fish." *Food Additives and Contaminants* 18 (2001): 395–403.

MMWR (Morbidity and Mortality Weekly Report). "Aldicarb Food Poisoning from Contaminated Melons." *MMWR* 35 (1986): 254–258. (http://iier.isciii.es/mmwr/preview/mmwrhtml/00000721.htm).

Mutter, J., J. Naumann, R. Schneider, H. Walach, and B. Haley. "Mercury and Autism: Accelerating Evidence?" *Neuroendocrinology Letters* 26 (2005): 439–446.

NAS (National Academy of Science). *Dioxins and Dioxin-like Compounds in the Food Supply: Strategies to Decrease Exposure*. (Washington, D.C.: National Academies Press, 2003).

———. *Toxicological Effects of Methylmercury*. (Washington, D.C.: National Academies Press, 2000).

Oken, E., R.O. Wright, K.P. Kleinman, D. Bellinger, et al. "Maternal Fish Consumption, Hair Mercury, and Infant Cognition in a U.S. Cohort." *Environmental Health Perspectives* 113 (2005): 1376–1380.

SCVPH (Scientific Committee on Veterinary Measures Relating to Public Health). *Hormones in Bovine Meat* (2001): (http://europa.eu.int/comm/dgs/health_consumer/library/press/press57_en.pdf).

Semenza, J.C., P.E. Tolbert, C.H. Rubin, L.J. Guillette, and R.J. Jackson. "Reproductive Toxins and Alligator Abnormalities at Lake Apopka, Florida." *Environmental Health Perspectives* 105 (1997): 1030–1032.

Silva, M.J., D.B. Barr, J.A. Reidy, et al. "Urinary Levels of Seven Phthalate Metabolites in the U.S. Population from the National Health and Nutrition Examination Survey (NHANES) 1999–2000." *Environmental Health Perspectives* 112 (2004): 331–338.

Swann, S.H., K.M. Main, F. Liu, S.L. Stewart, et al. "Decrease in Anogenital Distance among Male Infants with Prenatal Phthalate Exposure." *Environmental Health Perspectives* 113 (2005): 1056–1061.

Toth, B., L. Wallcave, K. Patil, I. Schmeltz, and D. Hoffman. "Induction of Tumors in Mice with the Herbicide Succinic Acid 2,2-Dimethylhydrazide." *Cancer Research* 37 (1977): 3497–3500.

Tsuda, S., M. Murakami, N. Matsusaka, K. Kano, et al. "DNA Damage Induced by Red Food Dyes Orally Administered to Pregnant and Male Mice." *Toxicological Sciences* 61 (2001): 92–99.

USEPA. *Draft Risk Assessment on the Potential Human Health Effects Associated with Exposure to Perfluorooctanoic Acid and Its Salts* (2005).

CHAPTER 6

ATSDR (Agency for Toxic Substances and Disease Registry). *Toxicological Profile for Fluorides, Hydrogen Fluoride, and Fluorine* (2003).

AWWA (American Water Works Association). *Fact Sheet: Trihalomethanes* (2006): (http://www.awwa.org/advocacy/pressroom/thms.cfm).

Betts, K.S. "Showering Data May Help Expose Miscarriage Link." *Environmental Science and Technology (ES&T) Science*, March 13, 2002.

Bove, F., Y. Shim, and P. Zeitz. "Drinking Water Contaminants and Adverse Pregnancy Outcomes: A Review." *Environmental Health Perspectives* 110, Supplement 1 (2002): 61–74.

Cochrane, J.A., C.E. Ketley, I.B. Arnadottir, et al. "A Comparison of the Prevalence of Fluorosis in Eight-Year-Old Children from Seven European Study Sites Using a Standardized Methodology." *Community Dentistry and Oral Epidemiology* 32, Supplement 1 (2004): 28–33.

Corso, P.H., M.H. Kramer, K.A. Blair, D.G. Addiss, et al. "Cost of Illness in the 1993 Waterborne Cryptosporidium Outbreak, Milwaukee, Wisconsin." *Emerging Infectious Disease* 9 (2003): 426–431.

Hileman, B. "New Studies Cast Doubt on Flouridation Benefits." *Chemical and Engineering News*, May 8, 1989.

King, W.D., and L.D. Marrett. "Case-Control Study of Bladder Cancer and Chlorination By-products in Treated Water." *Cancer Causes Control* 7 (1996): 596–604.

NAS (National Academy of Sciences). *Fluoride in Drinking Water: A Scientific Review of EPA's Standards* (2006): (http://fermat.nap.edu/catalog/11571.html).

NRDC (Natural Resources Defense Council). "Bottled Water, Pure Drink or Pure Hype?" (1999): (http://www.nrdc.org/water/drinking/bw/bwinx.asp).

OK DEQ (Oklahoma Department of Environmental Quality). *Trihalomethane Fact Sheet* (2005).

Villanueva, C.M., K.P. Cantor, S. Codier, et al. "Disinfection By-products and Bladder Cancer: A Pooled Analysis." *Epidemiology* 15 (2004): 357–367.

Whelton, H.P., C.E. Ketley, F. McSweeney, and D.M. O'Mullane. "A Review of Fluorosis in the European Union: Prevalence, Risk Factors and Aesthetic Issues." *Community Dentistry and Oral Epidemiology* 32, Supplement 1 (2004): 9–18.

Woffinden, B. "Fluoride Water Causes Cancer." *The Observer*, June 12, 2005.

CHAPTER 7

ATSDR (Agency for Toxic Substances and Disease Registry). *Toxicological Profile for Trichloroethylene* (1997).

Campaign for Safe Cosmetics / Environmental Working Group. *Skin Deep: A Safety Assessment of Ingredients in Personal Care Products* (2004): (http://www.ewg.org/reports/skindeep/findings/index.php).

CDC. *Third National Report on Human Exposure to Environmental Chemicals* (2005): (www.cdc.gov/exposurereport).

"Dry Cleaning Alternatives." *Consumer Reports,* February 2003.

Duty, S.M., R.M. Ackerman, A.M. Calafat, and R. Hauser. "Personal Care Product Use Predicts Urinary Concentrations of Some Phthalate Monoesters." *Environmental Health Perspectives* 113 (2005): 1530–1535.

Hore, P., M. Robson, N. Freeman, J. Zhang, et al. "Chlorpyrifos Accumulation Patterns for Child-Accessible Surfaces and Objects and Urinary Metabolite Excretion by Children for Two Weeks after Crack-and-Crevice Application." *Environmental Health Perspectives* 113 (2005): 211–219.

Houlihan, J., C. Brody, and B. Schwann. "Not Too Pretty, Phthalates, Beauty Products and the FDA." (2002): (http://www.nottoopretty.org/images/NotToo Pretty_final.pdf).

Lindberg, N., and E. Lindberg. "Painter's Syndrome." *American Journal of Independent Medicine* 13 (1988): 519–520.

RAIS (Risk Assessment Information System). *Toxicity Summary for Naphthalene* (1993): (http://risk.lsd.ornl.gov/tox/profiles/naphthalene_f_V1.shtml#t3).

SCCNFP (Scientific Committee on Cosmetic and Non-Food Products). *Draft Pre-opinion Regarding Fragrance Allergy in Consumers* (1999): (http://dr-baumann.com/dokumente/Study%20Europ%20Gem%20Parfum%20en%20Conserv%20Allergie.pdf).

Swann, S.H., K.M. Main, F. Liu, S.L. Stewart, et al. "Decrease in Anogenital Distance among Male Infants with Prenatal Phthalate Exposure." *Environmental Health Perspectives* 113 (2005): 1056–1061.

TESS (Toxic Exposure Surveillance System). *Annual Report of the American Association of Poison Control Centers* (2002): (http://www.aapcc.org/Annual%20Reports/02report/Annual%20Report%202002.pdf).

CHAPTER 8

ATSDR (Agency for Toxic Substance and Disease Registry). *Toxicology Profile for Formaldehyde,* 1999.

CARB (California Air Resources Board). *Air Cleaning Devices for the Home: Frequently Asked Questions,* March 15, 2001.

"Getting Through the Filter." *New York Times Sunday Magazine,* January 22, 2006, 28.

IARC (International Agency for Research on Cancer). *IARC Classifies Formaldehyde as Carcinogenic to Humans,* press release, June 15, 2004.

National Institute of Medicine. *Clearing the Air: Asthma and Indoor Air Exposures,* (Washington, D.C.: National Academies Press, 2000).

"New Concerns about Ionizing Air Cleaners." *Consumer Reports,* May 2005, 22–25.

USEPA. *Ozone Generators That Are Sold as Air Cleaners: An Assessment of Effectiveness and Health Consequences*, May 2002.

———. *Project Summary: The Total Exposure Assessment Methodology (TEAM) Study*, 1987b.

———. *Residential Air Cleaning Devices: A Summary of Available Information*, February 1990.

———. *Sources of Indoor Air Pollution: Nitrogen Dioxide*, 2006: (www.epa.gov/IAQ/NO2.html).

———. *Unfinished Business: A Comparative Assessment of Environmental Problems*, 1987a.

Weintrub, L.N., B.F. Toal, and D.R. Brown. "Reassessment of Formaldehyde Exposures in Homes Insulated with Urea-Formaldehyde Foam Insulation." *Applied Industrial Hygiene* 4(6) (1989): 146–152.

CHAPTER 9

Congress of the United States, Office of Technology Assessment. *Screening and Testing of Chemicals in Commerce* (1995), OTA-BP-ENV-166.

Nighswonger, T. "Where Do You Set the Standard?" *Occupational Hazards* 5(1) (2000).

U.S. Department of Labor, Bureau of Labor Statistics. *Survey of Occupational Injuries and Illnesses, 2003*.

USEPA. *Fact Sheet: Should You Have the Air Ducts in Your Home Cleaned?* October 1997.

———. "Indoor Air Quality and Work Environment Study: USEPA Headquarter Buildings." *Volume 4: Multivariate Statistical Analysis of Health, Comfort, and Odor Perceptions as Related to Personal and Workplace Characteristics.* USEPA Atmospheric Research and Exposure Assessment Laboratory (June 1991), 21M-3004.

———. *Notice Regarding Use of Disinfectants and Sanitizers in HVAC Systems*, March 14, 2002.

CHAPTER 10

California Department of Education. *Science Safety Handbook for California Public Schools*, 1999.

"Hysteria-Hysteria." *New York Times Magazine*, June 2, 2002.

U.S. Department of Education. *A Summary of Scientific Findings in Adverse Effects of Indoor Environments on Students' Health, Academic Performance, and Attendance*, 2004.

CHAPTER 11

Brown, W. "Deaths Linked to London Smog." *New Science* 1931 (1994): 12–13.

EWG (Environmental Working Group). "Smokestacks and Smoke Screens." 1997.

Hemminki, K., et al. "Cancer Risk of Air Pollution: Epidemiologic Evidence." *Environmental Health Perspectives* 102(4) (1994): 187–192.

Janssen, N.A.H., et al. "The Relationship between Air Pollution from Heavy Traffic and Allergic Sensitization, Bronchial Hyper-Responsiveness and Respiratory Symptoms in Dutch Schoolchildren." *Environmental Health Perspectives* 111(12) (September 2003): 1512–1518.

Lomat, L., et al. "Incidence of Childhood Disease in Belarus Associated with the Chernobyl Accident." *Environmental Health Perspectives* 105(6) (1997): 1529–1532.

NAS (National Academy of Sciences). *Rethinking the Ozone Problem in Urban and Regional Air Pollution.* (Washington, D.C.: National Academies Press, 1991).

NCI (National Cancer Institute). *Fact Sheet—No Excess Mortality Risk Found in Counties with Nuclear Power Plants* (1991).

New York State Office of the Attorney General. "Outdoor Wood Boilers in New York State" (2005).

Nuclear Regulatory Commission. *Fact Sheet—Backgrounder on Radiation Protection and the "Tooth Fairy Issue."* (http://www.nrc.gov/reading-rm/doc-collections/fact-sheets/tooth-fairy.html).

Samet, J.M., et al. "The National Morbidity, Mortality and Air Pollution Study Part II." *Health Effects Institute Report* 94, Part II (2000).

U.S. Department of Transportation. "Transportation Related Air Toxics." (http://www.fhwa. dot.gov/environment/airtoxic/casesty6.htm).

USEPA. "Smog—Who Does It Hurt? What You Need to Know about Ozone and Your Health" (1999).

———. *The Particle Pollution Report: Current Understanding of Air Quality Data and Emissions through 2003* (2004).

———. *Toxic Release Inventory Public Data Release Brochure* (2003): (http://www.epa.gov/tri/tridata/tri03/brochure.htm).

———. web page: Relative Emissions of Fine Particles (2006): (http://www.epa.gov/woodstoves/refp.html).

CHAPTER 12

ATSDR (Agency for Toxic Substances and Disease Registry). *Toxicological Profile for Arsenic* (2005).

CAES (Connecticut Agricultural Experiment Station). *Research on Chlordane* (1999): (http://www.caes.state.ct.us/FactSheetFiles/AnalyticalChemistry/FSA C002f.htm).

Cao, X., and L.Q. Ma. "Effects of Compost and Phosphate on Plant Arsenic Accumulation from Soils Near Pressure-Treated Wood." *Environmental Pollution* 132 (2004): 435–442.

CDC (Centers for Disease Control). *National Report on Human Exposure to Environmental Chemicals* (2005): (http://www.cdc.gov/exposurereport/).

———. *Pesticides Fact Sheet* (2004): (http://www. cdc.gov/nceh/hsb/pesticides/activities.pdf).

Cranmer, J.M., M.F. Cranmer, and P.T. Goad. "Prenatal Chlordane Exposure: Effects on Plasma Corticosterone Concentrations Over the Lifespan of Mice." *Environmental Research* 35 (1984): 204–210.

Jacobs, D.E., H. Mielke, and N. Pavur. "The High Cost of Improper Removal of Lead-Based Paint from Housing: A Case Report." *Environmental Health Perspectives* 111 (2003): 185–186.

Mattina, M.J.I., B.D. Eitzer, et al. "Plant Uptake and Translocation of Highly Weathered, Soil-Bound Chlordane Residues: Data from Field and Rhizotron Studies." *Environmental Toxicology and Chemistry* 23 (2004): 2756–2762.

Nishioka, M.G., R.G. Lewis, M.C. Brinkman, et al. "Distribution of 2,4-D in Air and on Surfaces Inside Residences after Lawn Applications: Comparing Exposure Estimates from Various Media for Young Children." *Environmental Health Perspectives* 109 (2001): 1185–1191.

Nurimnen, T. "The Epidemiological Study of Birth Defects and Pesticides." *Epidemiology* 12 (2001) 145–146.

Peryea, F.J. "Gardening on Lead- and Arsenic-Contaminated Soils." *Bulletin of Cooperation Extension at Washington State University*. (1999) (http://www.ecy. wa.gov/programs/tcp/area_wide/AW/AppK_gardening_guide.pdf).

Prenney, B. "Community Lead Exposure." *American Journal of Industrial Medicine* 23 (1993): 191–195.

Stillwell, D., and K. Gorny. "Contamination of Soils with Copper, Chromium and Arsenic under Decks Built from Pressure-Treated Wood." *Bulletin of Environmental Contamination and Toxicology* 58 (1997): 22–29.

Toronto Public Health. *Lawn and Garden Pesticides: A Review of Human Exposure and Health Effects* (2002): (http://www.toronto.ca/health/pesticides/health_effects.htm).

Vidair, C.A. "Age Dependence of Organophosphate and Carbamate Neurotoxicity in the Postnatal Rat: Extrapolation to the Human." *Toxicological and Applied Pharmacology 2004* 196 (2004): 287–302.

Whyatt, R.M., V.A. Rauh, D.B. Barr, et al. "Residential Pesticide Exposure, Fetal Growth and Neurocognitive Development among Urban Minorities." *Neurotoxicology* 25 (2004): 683.

CHAPTER 13

Ahlbom A., N. Day, M. Feychting, E. Roman, J. Skinner, J. Dockerty, M. Linet, M. McBride, J. Michaelis, J.H. Olsen, T. Tynes, and P.K. Verkasalo. "A Pooled Analysis of Magnetic Fields and Childhood Leukemia." *British Journal of Cancer* 83 (2000): 692–698.

CalDHS (California Department of Health Services). Fact Sheet: Electric and Magnetic Fields (2000): (http://www.dhs.ca.gov/ps/deodc/ehib/emf/longfactsheet. pdf).

Greenland, S., A.R. Sheppard, W.T. Kaune, C. Poole, and M.A. Kelsh. "A Pooled Analysis of Magnetic Fields, Wire Codes and Childhood Leukemia." EMF Study Group, *Epidemiology* 11 (2000): 624–634.

Lai, H., et al. "Acute Exposure to a 60 Hz Magnetic Field Increases DNA Strand Breaks in Rat Brain Cells." *Bioelectromagnetics* 18 (1997): 156–165.

Lai, H., and N.P. Singh. "Magnetic Field-Induced DNA Strand Breaks in Brain Cells of the Rat." *Environmental Health Perspectives* 112 (2004): 687–694.

Linet, M.S., E.E. Hatch, R.A. Kleinerman, L.L. Robison, W.T. Kaune, D.R. Friedman, R.K. Severson, C.M. Haines, C.T. Hartsock, S. Niwa, S. Wacholder, and R.E. Tarone. "Residential Exposure to Magnetic Fields and Acute Lymphoblastic Leukemia in Children." *New England Journal of Medicine* 337 (1997): 1–7.

NCCAM (National Center for Complementary and Alternative Medicine). "Research Report: Questions and Answers about Using Magnets to Treat Pain" (2004): (http://nccam.nih.gov/health/magnet/magnet.htm).

NIEHS (National Institute of Environmental Health Sciences). EMF Rapid Questions and Answers (2002): (http://www.niehs.nih.gov/em frapid/booklet/results.htm).

U.K. Childhood Cancer Study Investigators. "Exposure to Power Frequency Magnetic Fields and the Risk of Childhood Cancer: A Case/Control Study." *Lancet* 354 (1999): 1925–1931.

Wartenberg, D. "Residential EMF Exposure and Childhood Leukemia: Meta-analysis and Population Attributable Risk." *Bioelectromagnetics* 22, Supplement 5 (2001): S86–S104.

CHAPTER 14

Dolk, H., M. Vrijheid, B. Armstrong, L. Abramsky, F. Bianchi, E. Garne, V. Nelen, W. Robert, J.E.S. Scott, D. Stone, and R. Tenconi. "Risk of Congenital Anomalies Near Hazardous Waste Landfill Sites in Europe: The EUROHAZCON Study." *Lancet* 352 (1998): 423–427.

Geschwind, S.A., J.A. Stolwijk, M. Bracken, et al. "Risk of Congenital Malformations Associated with Proximity to Hazardous Waste Sites." *American Journal of Epidemiology* 135 (1992): 1197–1207.

Ozonoff, D., M.E. Colten, A. Cupples, et al. "Health Problems Reported by Residents of a Neighborhood Contaminated by a Hazardous Waste Facility." *American Journal of Industrial Medicine* 11 (1987): 581–597.

Sergeev, A.V., and D.O. Carpenter. "Hospitalization Rates for Coronary Heart Disease in Relation to Residence Near Areas Contaminated with Persistent Organic Pollutants and Other Pollutants." *Environmental Health Perspectives* 113 (2005): 756–761.

Shusterman, D. "Critical Review: The Health Significance of Environmental Odor Pollution." *Archives of Environmental Health* 47 (1992): 76–87.

U.K. Committtee on Toxicology. "Study by the Small Area Health Statistics Unit (SAHSU) on Health Outcomes in Populations Living around Landfill Sites" (2001): (http://www.advisorybodies.doh.gov.uk/landfill.htm).

USEPA Journal. *The Love Canal Tragedy* (1979): (http://www.epa.gov/history/topics/lovecanal/01.htm).

CHAPTER 15

ATSDR (Agency for Toxic Substances and Disease Registry). *Fact Sheet: Landfill Gas Primer*: (http://www.atsdr.cdc.gov/HAC/land fill/html/appe.html).

ATSDR/CDC. *Toxicological Profile for Trichloroethylene* (1997).

Little, J.C., J.M. Daisey, and W.W. Nazaroff. "Transport of Subsurface Contaminants into Buildings." *Environmental Science and Technology* 26 (1992): 2058–2066.

Moran, M.J., et al. *U.S. Geological Survey Water Resources Investigation Report No. 03-4200* (2004): (http://pubs.usgs.gov/wri/wri034200/wri034200.pdf.).

Turk, B.H., R.J. Prill, D.T. Grimsrud, et al. "Characterizing the Occurrence, Sources, and Variability of Radon in Pacific Northwest Homes." *Journal of the Air and Waste Management Association* 40 (1990): 498–506.

CHAPTER 16

ATSDR (Agency for Toxic Substances and Disease Registry). *Toxicological Profile for Trichloroethylene* (1997).

Doll, R., and R. Peto. "The Causes of Cancer: Quantitative Estimates of Avoidable Risk of Cancer in the United States Today." *Journal of the National Cancer Institute* 66 (1981): 1191–1308.

Massachusetts Department of Public Health. *Woburn Childhood Leukemia Follow-Up Study*, July 1997.

New Jersey Department of Health and Senior Services. *The Case-Control Study of Childhood Cancers in Dover Township (Ocean County) New Jersey*, 2003.

Steinmaus, C., M. Lu, R.L. Todd, and A.H. Smith. "Probability Estimates for the Unique Childhood Leukemia Clusters in Fallon, Nevada, and Risks Near Other U.S. Military Aviation Facilities." *Environmental Health Perspectives* 112 (2004): 766–771.

SEER (Surveillance, Epidemiology and End Results), National Cancer Institute. *U.S. Cancer Statistics*, 2004.

Thun, M. J., and J. Sinks. "Understanding Cancer Clusters." *Cancer Journal for Clinicians* 54 (2004): 273–280.

Index

(Page numbers in bold indicate charts or tables)